C000001113

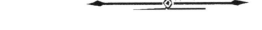

ISBN 978-0-484-61766-6
PIBN 10840504

This book is a reproduction of an important historical work. Forgotten Books uses
state-of-the-art technology to digitally reconstruct the work, preserving the original format
whilst repairing imperfections present in the aged copy. In rare cases, an imperfection in
the original, such as a blemish or missing page, may be replicated in our edition. We do,
however, repair the vast majority of imperfections successfully; any imperfections that
remain are intentionally left to preserve the state of such historical works.

THE JOURNAL OF

OPHTHALMOLOGY

OTOLOGY AND LARYNGOLOGY.

ISSUED QUARTERLY

CHARLES DEADY, M. D., Editor.

ASSOCIATE EDITOR :

A. W. PALMER, M. D.

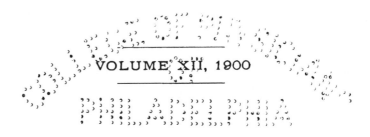

VOLUME XII, 1900

A. L. CHATTERTON & CO.,
156 Fifth Avenue, New York.
LAHIRI & CO., Calcutta.

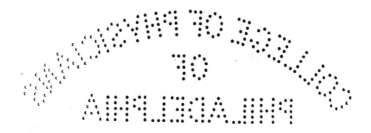

Vol. XII.   JANUARY, 1900.   Part I.

THE JOURNAL OF OPHTHALMOLOGY, OTOLOGY AND LARYNGOLOGY.

EDITOR.

CHARLES DEADY, M. D.

ASSOCIATE EDITOR,

A. W. PALMER, M. D.

THE DEVELOPMENT OF HEARING IN THE CONGENITALLY DEAF.

BY L. MOFFAT, BERKELEY, CAL.

"THE Development of Hearing" is a phrase that may often be found in the advertisements of "Teachers of the Deaf," yet it is one which seems to be decidedly misleading.   It has been gravely stated that "by means of a daily drill of from thirty to sixty minutes for the space of three months," a certain class "were able to recognize words and sentences spoken across the room; and frequently I [the teacher] stood in the hall, having the door slightly ajar, and spoke sentences which they heard and repeated."   Now, the class here spoken of were not simply hard-of-hearing pupils, but were children being educated in one of the largest deaf-and-dumb institutions in the United States.   The speaker goes on to say: "As to what takes place in a scientific point of view—whether the auditory nerve develops as a muscle develops by use, or whether there is simply an education of the partial hearing, or both, I do not now discuss.   This much I will say, however, that the sense of hearing which has lain dormant and useless up to this time is now sufficiently developed to be of great benefit to these children; and nobody is more conscious of it than they themselves.   They know that *heretofore they heard not and that now they do hear.*"

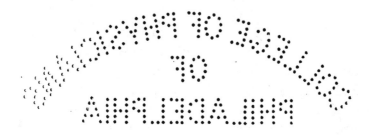

Vol. XII.   JANUARY, 1900.   PART I.

THE JOURNAL OF OPHTHALMOLOGY, OTOLOGY AND LARYNGOLOGY.

EDITOR.

CHARLES DEADY, M. D.

ASSOCIATE EDITOR,

A. W. PALMER, M. D.

THE DEVELOPMENT OF HEARING IN THE CONGENITALLY DEAF.

BY L. MOFFAT, BERKELEY, CAL.

"THE Development of Hearing" is a phrase that may often be found in the advertisements of "Teachers of the Deaf," yet it is one which seems to be decidedly misleading. It has been gravely stated that "by means of a daily drill of from thirty to sixty minutes for the space of three months," a certain class "were able to recognize words and sentences spoken across the room; and frequently I [the teacher] stood in the hall, having the door slightly ajar, and spoke sentences which they heard and repeated." Now, the class here spoken of were not simply hard-of-hearing pupils, but were children being educated in one of the largest deaf-and-dumb institutions in the United States. The speaker goes on to say: "As to what takes place in a scientific point of view—whether the auditory nerve develops as a muscle develops by use, or whether there is simply an education of the partial hearing, or both, I do not now discuss. This much I will say, however, that the sense of hearing which has lain dormant and useless up to this time is now sufficiently developed to be of great benefit to these children; and nobody is more conscious of it than they themselves. They know that *heretofore they heard not and that now they do hear*."

Parents reading such statements as these bring their children with gladness only to find, alas! too often that their own are not benefited, the simple reason being that the amount of hearing the child possesses is too small to be "developed." Like a singer's voice, the range is too limited. The promises made are, in some instances, seemingly fulfilled, yet to my mind scarcely any more actual hearing is possessed at the end of the term than at the beginning. More knowledge is there and a greater power of perception, but that is all. Let me illustrate. I enter a certain building; a peculiar sound meets my ear. I ask and am told what it is. Another noise of a differing kind is also explained, and that also my memory retains. The following day, hearing the same sounds, I recognize and can name them, yet my hearing is no greater than on the day previous. More knowledge I have, and a greater power of perception, for I can now separate these sounds which I know from other and unknown ones. The leader of an orchestra detects which one of the fifty instruments has caused the discord, while the novice though possessed of a sensitive ear may only note the discord. Herr Wolfschlag —a canary expert—can distinguish and judge a single bird's notes even when hundreds of others are trilling and warbling around it. Repeated visits to a factory will enable one to resolve into distinctive sounds that which was at first but a confusing whirr. A child enters a classroom of deaf-mute pupils. The teacher soon discovers that he has considerable hearing, yet for all its present availability he might as well be totally deaf. A spoken word presents somewhat the same difficulty to the ear of the partially deaf as a written word does to the eye of the uneducated hearing child. Neither child will connect it with the object of which it is the name, any more than we ourselves would a word in an unknown tongue.

The pupil is told to watch the mouth of the teacher, and see that when certain motions are made certain vibrations follow which produce a sound, and these sounds constitute a word. Presently when he has become familiar with the

fact that *b* and *oy* mean *boy*, the sound is made in his ear
—either with or without a hearing-tube—and his attention
is called to the fact that the noise he now hears is the word
he lately learned. We say "noise," as all vocal sounds
are as truly noises to the child with imperfect hearing as
any produced by inanimate objects and, at first, he makes
no distinction between them. Gradually one word after
another is added to his vocabulary, and one *noise* after
another withdrawn from the unknown "hum" to which he
has so long been listening. Visitors may remark, "But that
child has hearing; why is he in a school for the deaf?"
For the reason that the child has not yet advanced far
enough to analyze for himself the multitudinous sounds of
life. One of my pupils who gives readily, without a glance
at the face, words that are spoken in his ear with which he
has become familiar, fails completely to understand other
combinations though equally simple in construction and
spoken equally loud. Once while testing him I paused for
a moment to determine what new combination to give him,
and in the interval of silence on my part he gave the names
of three objects, thinking I had spoken, and failed utterly
on every unfamiliar word given. In some instances he
gave known words which approximated in sound the unknown ones desired ; *on* (*ah n*) being given for *awl* (*aw l*).
The degree of hearing seems to be equally good in either
case, but the perceptive faculty had not yet grasped the—
to him—new sound. It may be argued that his hearing
perhaps is dull to certain sounds and keen to others.
True ; but the same result follows if the known sounds are
placed in reverse order. (*K*)*nif*(*e*) he will give, but *fin*(*e*)
will not be spoken, or else *fan* may be substituted for it.
Again, when both words are known, a child will give in the
earlier stages of training—if the elements are the same as in
(k)n-*i*-f(e) and f-*i*-n(e)—either combination which suits his
fancy, more often perhaps giving the former for the latter,
as if wishing to seize the one nearest at hand (latest heard)
and then seeking the others. In "fine," the *n* being the
latest element caught by his ear he will pronounce that,

then take up the *i* and then the initial *f* making as said before a reversal of the elements. Leap in this way would be returned as peal and team become meat.

One child was taught the powers of s and sh by drawing the picture of a sky-rocket and pretending to light it, then making with the mouth the long ssssssss and broadening it into the *sh* as the explosion came. Rockets and their noises he was perfectly familiar with, yet when the same sound was produced by the mouth he would not repeat it until the picture was drawn and he was told the same sound was represented by the letters.

Dr. Alexander Bell tells of a congenitally deaf young man who was taught speech in adult life, and who, it was then found, could hear sentences spoken about a foot behind his head, and who said he had heard the people talking in the factory where he worked, but had not been able to understand what they said. Had he been a hearing child and then become deaf to the same extent as now, this could not have happened, as he would have associated the word-sounds with their meanings. A hard-of-hearing adult is classified simply as hard of hearing, but a-hard-of hearing infant is relegated to the ranks of the dumb and becomes to all intents and purposes a deaf-mute.

It is difficult to ascertain just how much hearing a deaf child possesses even when tested scientifically. He does not know what to expect nor what is expected of him. While witnessing the testing of individual members of a class, I found that in many instances an observer could discover in the eyes of the child when the first sensation was felt or heard. It seemed to be recorded there several seconds before the impulse came to lift the hand in signification of having heard. This I was led to observe from the fact that I myself had blundered as to the exact moment when my own very sensitive ears had perceived the vibrations; I was too busy watching the mechanism of the recording instrument, and it was only when the buzzing became painfully loud that I realized it, and said, " Please stop."

On the other hand, a child who is known to be totally deaf may, apparently, show signs of hearing. One little boy said that his dog said ou-ou-ou when it was hurt and that the cat said m-ou when he spoke to it, yet he had only reasoned it out from the movements of his own mouth in producing those sounds; still, it gave the impression that he heard. Again, a child may repeat the word papa after having it spoken in the ear, but only recognizes it by the two puffs of air—which he feels as the *p* is sounded. All these things mislead the unskilled investigator.

Partial deafness is of a varying kind, and a child who may be able to hear a deep tone may fail to hear a high shrill one. As there is color-blindness, so is there "element"-deafness. John Kitto of England—the deaf Biblical scholar—believed that total deafness was an impassable barrier to the writing of poetry, yet many deaf-mutes have written poems as rhythmical as those produced by the hearing. I fancy, though, if careful tests were made it would be found that the writers were sensitive to vibrations, and in that way found the path to the land of rhythm. I believe great good may be accomplished and the deaf much benefited by careful teaching along the lines of *perception*, but let it be done fairly and squarely and under no false titles or misrepresentations.

OCULAR MASSAGE.

BY H. WELLS WOODWARD, M. D., WASHINGTON, D. C.

ABOUT a year and a half ago my attention was called to a system of eye massage claiming to ameliorate and cure near-sightedness. The claim was made by Professor Dion of Paris, a gentleman who has some reputation as a scientist and inventor in this country as well as in France. I was much interested in his claim, particularly as he stated that he could reduce by pressure the anterior-posterior meridian measurement of the eyeball. An opportunity was afforded me this summer to visit his institute. Taking advantage of it, I observed him treat a number of patients; and upon returning home I brought an instrument with me, determined to give the method a good trial in Washington.

It is for the purpose of bringing this subject before the profession that this paper is written. Having searched the literature extensively on this subject, I have found but little, and that not satisfactory at all. Dr. Pagenstecher of Weisbaden has reported some cases treated successfully by massage with the fingers.

The Dion method is not practiced with the hand or fingers, but by a specially constructed scientific instrument designed to give a graded amount of pressure on the eye-ball, alternating with relaxation. This instrument resembles a large trial-frame with two sliding cylinders extending forward, between which is a dial registering the position of the cylinders, or, when adjusted, the amount of pressure upon the eyes. The pressure is regulated by a thumb-screw. The instrument is carefully adjusted so that the

14

pressure is made in the line of the visual axis upon the closed eyelids. When it is in perfect position the treatment is not painful, although generally attended by an appearance of lights before the eyes, varying in color, more often white; but sometimes red, yellow, green, or violet. At times there will be circles of light, stars, and checkerboard effects, but they all soon pass away, leaving no discomfort whatever. The treatment lasts about three minutes.

The first intention of the originator of this method was to treat myopia only; but he now uses it in all cases having defective vision. He was very sanguine when I saw him, showing me many remarkable records of cases and letters from people whose vision had been improved and restored.

As yet my experience has not extended over long enough time to make this a thoroughly scientific paper; but think I can demonstrate efficiency in the following cases, enough to demand an investigation by all oculists.

Before reporting these cases I must state by way of explanation that the system of measurements used is the French or decimal—employed because it is the easiest to compute in and the most accurate. The type are those devised by Snellen, excepting one which was often employed, and which so far as I know was originated, by Mr. Dion. It consists of two black circles 1.5 cm. in diameter arranged side by side, the two white centers giving the effect of the double light in the well-known sight-perception test. Its simplicity makes it easy for the oculist to determine at just what point the patient can see it.

CASE I. Rev. C. C. M., age thirty-seven. Near-sighted; wearing for twenty years R. E. —2.75 sph. L. E. —3.00 sph. Vision $\frac{3}{21}$. Could see circles at 160 centimeters. After the second treatment saw them at 170 cm. After the third treatment saw them at 180 cm. After the eighth treatment saw them at 200 cm. After the seventeenth treatment saw them at 385 cm. After the twentieth treatment saw them at 575 cm. After the twenty-fourth treatment the 15 m. type could be seen at five meters, making his vision $\frac{3}{12}$.

The patient is still under treatment, and I expect from the past record that vision will be $\frac{5}{5}$ soon. He wears glasses no longer and expresses himself enthusiastically to his friends that he has received over fifty per cent. benefit from the treatment.

CASE II. Miss A. S., age seventeen ; compound condition of myopia and astigmatism ; wearing for three years R. E. -4 sph. $\bigcirc$ -0.5. Cyl. ax. 180°, L. E. -7. sph. $\bigcirc$ -1.00. Cyl. ax. 180°. More unfortunate than the last case on account of the higher degree of myopia and her very poor vision, which was scarcely $\frac{5}{30}$. The circles were only seen at 75 cm. After the fifteenth treatment she was able to see them across the room 575 cm. After the twentieth treatment her vision was $\frac{5}{15}$. She is still under my care, and acknowledges that she sees nearly as well without her glasses as she did formerly when she wore them.

CASE III. Mrs. R. B., age about twenty-seven ; myopia for many years; wearing R. E. -6 sph., L. E. -7.50. Complains of much aching in eyes and great effort to see even with glasses. Her vision was scant $\frac{5}{60}$. After the fifth treatment her vision was $\frac{5}{21}$. Her glasses have been reduced one-half and she is getting about fairly well, and the indications are that she will improve as the treatment advances.

CASE IV. F. B., schoolboy ; hyperopic astigmatism of high degree left eye ; wearing for over a year L. E. $+1.50$.Cyl. ax. 135°. Vision $\frac{5}{18}$. Saw circles at 310 cm. After the thirteenth treatment saw them at 575 cm. and vision was $\frac{5}{15}$. After the twenty-fourth treatment it was $\frac{5}{12}$.

CASE V. Mrs. T. H. D. ; presents probably the most marked improvement of any case, the gains of vision being from $\frac{5}{36}$ to $\frac{5}{5}$ scant in seven treatments. The condition was hypermetropic astigmatism of the left eye, amblyopic in nature rather than spasmodic, as medicines did not improve the vision. There was a chalazion on both the upper and lower lids and much headache. The latter has almost disappeared.

CASE VI. Miss L. V. F., government clerk ; myopia of 0.50D. in right eye, 0.75D. in left. Vision but little improved, but frequent headaches, conjunctival congestion, and sticking together of the lids. She has received twelve treatments, and notwithstanding working hard all the time, her eyes have given her but little annoyance, and she has had but one headache during the past fifteen days.

I have had other cases suffering from headache who have been benefited, but will not take the time in reporting them in this paper.

To me the above results were very gratifying, and from my investigation of this method I am forced to conclude that if it will not bear out all that the originator claims, it is certainly a step in the right direction in the treatment of the eyes, and adds one more thing to the armamentarium of the oculist. Furthermore, it demonstrates the fact that many of our patients are not using one-half of their visual power; that they are often made more blind by a pair of strong glasses, which, taking from them the reliance in their own faculty of seeing, leaves them pitiably dependent. It gives promise also that spectacle-fitting will be diminished in the future; that it will be used as a temporary expediency rather than a life-long condemnation.

Why should an eye *not* be changed in form and function? It is not made of bone, but on the contrary of soft delicate tissue; and the same force which built it can, if assisted, readjust it toward the normal.

SHALL WE CUT THE OCULAR MUSCLES?

BY FRANK D. W. BATES, M. D., HAMILTON, ONTARIO.

I HAVE read with a great deal of pleasure Dr. Linnell's article on " Shall We Cut the Ocular Muscles? " in the October number of your journal, and, while I thoroughly agree with him in the main, would like to offer one suggestion in connection therewith. Some of your readers who heard my paper on " Eye-strain as a Cause of Disease " read at the meeting of O. & O. Society in June last, may look upon me as a tenotomy enthusiast, and imagine that I lose no opportunity to operate upon the eye-muscles. But they are mistaken ; I am very conservative and operate only as a last resort. I believe, with Dr. Linnell, that a very large percentage, if not the majority of cases of heterophoria, are due to errors of refraction (and in some cases very slight errors) and are corrected by correcting the trouble with refraction. Other cases (but a very small percentage, I believe) are reflex from troubles with organs remote from the eyes, and are corrected by curing the troubles of these organs. But a large percentage of the cases of heterophoria are independent of these causes, and lie in the muscles themselves ; and when we are certain that such is the case, and are thoroughly satisfied as to which muscle or muscles should be operated upon, I think we should have no hesitation about operating. But when to operate, how to operate, and how much to operate, are very important questions, and require some experience and good judgment. What has brought the operation of tenotomy for heterophoria into disrepute has been the want of good judgment on the part of many of those who have operated for the same. They have in many cases operated upon a muscle in a condition of tonic spasm instead of a short muscle,—thereby making matters worse instead of better, and in other instances they have operated too much upon the right muscle. The suggestion I was going to offer in connection with Dr. Linnell's paper is this: The doctor mentions two ways of treating a case of heterophoria, one by the systematic exercise of the weak muscle by means of prisms with the apex toward the weak muscle, the other by wearing prismatic glasses with the base toward the weak muscle. Some years ago I wrote a short article for your journal, condemning the use of prismatic glasses and advocating the systematic exercise of the weak muscles by means of prisms; and have many cases on my record books where I have developed the internal recti muscles up so that they could overcome easily a prism of 50, 60, and even 70°. I thought at the time that I was doing a good thing; and certainly I did have good results in one direction, for the persons could use their eyes with more comfort. But for the past three or four years I have discarded this method, believing it to be wrong; and if there is anything in the theory of the expenditure of nerve force through the eyes, it is decidedly wrong. The strain, in cases of heterophoria, does not come upon the short muscle, but upon the opposing muscle; and the more we strengthen that opposing muscle, the more work we put upon it and the more nerve force we use up. The wearing of prismatic glasses with the apex of the prism towards the short muscle is, I think, far preferable, and I have had many good results from same. Still, when we are certain of the condition present, a slight operation gives better results than either exercising with prisms or the wearing of prismatic glasses; for if the operation is rightly done we then have relief of all tension. Now, I think when we read an article in one of our journals, and there is any point in it with which we disagree, it is not only our privilege but our duty to let it be known. We may be wrong ourselves, but we will have given expression to our views, and some-one may take advantage of the opportunity to set us right. We are none of us infallible, and all have a great deal to learn, and will be more or less benefited by the inter-change of views. The subject of heterophoria I look upon as the most important subject that has ever come up in medicine, either in the department of ophthalmology or any other department, for there is no doubt that there is more nerve force used up through the eyes than in any other way—probably more than all other ways put together; and it is the using up of nerve force which undermines the system and renders it more susceptible to disease.

The using up of nerve force through the eyes includes, of course, that used in the endeavor of Nature to overcome troubles with the refraction as well as in her endeavor to keep the eyes in alignment with each other.

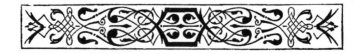

CLINICAL REPORT OF A CASE OF ETHMOID-ITIS NECROTICA.

BY J. W. DOWLING, M. D., NEW YORK.

IN presenting the history of this case it is not claimed that there is anything of special interest in the symptoms and pathology. It is the story of the patient, presented to me at his own instance, in grateful recognition of his relief under the homeopathic remedy and nothing else. It is encouraging to us who believe in the law of similia to encounter at odd times such an evidence of satisfaction at the results of its operations, particularly when compared with the incomplete methods of our brethren of the other school. And, furthermore, this little history will tend to encourage the practitioner who is not a specialist, in that, even though he lack the skill and manipulative dexterity of the expert, he may yet hope to cure his patient with the properly indicated remedy. This by no means is intended to belittle the results of those who, besides being homeopathic prescribers, are also experts in methods of local treatment.

Patient's statement of his cure, under date of May I, 1898:

Four months ago came under your treatment. Case had been diagnosed as a necrotic ethmoiditis from a trauma five years previously; and for three years terminating December 30 last had been treated by an expert of some standing in the old school. Treatment had been exclusively local, viz.:

Operative.—Removal of bony spur from septum, and occasional cutting away of tissue, bony or cartilaginous.

Aseptic.—Ortho-chloro-phenol spray.

Palliative.—Compound menthol ointment dressing.

Results.—Three years of above treatment effected in results nothing. Right up to December 30 last a muco-purulent discharge, to the extent of filling two handkerchiefs daily; had continued unabated for three years. The discharge was offensive and breath unpleasant. On December 30 homeopathic treatment was begun, and all other treatment ceased, and, reversing method of old school, was exclusively internal. A powder was taken twice a day for five weeks, without effect to the patient noticeable, when of a day, abruptly, the discharge diminished in quantity one-half, and so maintained itself till again, some seven weeks later, abruptly, it again diminished one-half, and so continued for three weeks, when it again dropped to the amount of three small blows of the nose in twenty-four hours, and has so continued until to-day, May 1.

P. S.—December 25, 1898. Ever since May 1, a period of eight months, discharge has been limited to this small and inconsiderable amount, except in short periods of passing colds. Patient notices, as characteristic, the abrupt and lasting diminution in the quantity of discharge; and in view of the very small amount for the past eight months, views himself to have been practically cured in three and a half months, after three years of no result from old-school treatment. His astonishment is only less than his gratitude.

The remedy was prescribed on the following indications:

1. Acuteness of smell extreme, even of smell of his own nostrils.

2. Better in open air.

3. Mental—Disgust for life; thinks he can succeed in nothing; morbidly depressed.

4. Head—Bruised feeling in bones of head.

5. Eyes—Constant lachrymation.

6. Nose—Sore feeling internally; putrid smell in nose when blowing it; purulent discharge.

7. Mouth—Taste putrid.

You will all recognize the one remedy having this peculiar combination, and that one is aurum metallicum. It was given in the third potency. Could anything more prettily illustrate the action of the single remedy, given with persistence, and unaided by any local treatment whatever?

Appreciating as I do the value of local treatment as a *help* to the remedy, I believe the two combined would have cured him much more quickly had they been together employed in the very beginning.

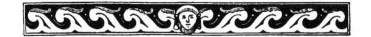

CANCER OF THE LARYNX.

BY A. WORRALL PALMER, M. D.

INSTEAD of prefacing the clinical histories of the following cases with original comment, I deem it will be more instructive to give the translation of the conclusions deduced by Dr. John Sendziak (Warsaw) in his book· " The Malignant Laryngeal Tumors (Carcinomata, Sarcomata), Their Diagnosis and Treatment."

These deductions are made from a study of the clinical records of four hundred and fifty-two cases of carcinoma and fifty of sarcoma :

NOTE.—The writer takes the liberty of making this lengthy quotation, because this book is the most thorough on its subject and that he is unable to find any English translation thereof.

1. The history of laryngeal cancer shows that they were known even in the earlier times, but, thanks to the discovery of the laryngoscope, commences the greatest development in the knowledge of laryngeal cancer, which have been extirpated only during the last ten years, thanks to the interest which was taken at the time of the illness and death of the German Emperor Frederick.

2. The ætiology of laryngeal cancer, as of cancers in general, is still dark. Long-lasting irritation seems to have a certain influence in the ætiology of this disorder. Endolaryngeal operations, however, are without influence in the development of laryngeal cancers from other tumors (papillomata, etc.) The parasitic origin which has been ascribed to the cancers is not yet proved.

3. There exist observations of Baratoux, Newmann,

Semon, which seem to speak in favor of the contagious-ness of laryngeal cancer, as well as of the possibility of the so-called auto-infection.

4. Heredity seems to have some signification in the ætiology of this disorder.

5. Advanced age, especially above fifty years, predisposes particularly to the disease. Women more rarely suffer from laryngeal cancer than men.

6. In general, cancers of the larynx are not frequent in comparison with the cancers of other organs, and with other laryngeal tumors (benign).

7. The laryngeal cancers are divided into intrinsic, which are more frequent; and extrinsic, more rare; and lastly, mixed forms.

8. Mostly they are localized on the true vocal cords, more seldom on the epiglottis and ventricular bands, rarest in sinus pyriformis.

9. According to the histological structure the laryngeal cancers are divided in epithelioma, carcinoma medullare, and scirrhus.

10. Laryngeal cancers are primary and secondary. The latter arise *per continuitatem* or by metastasis.

11. We offer the following initial forms of the primary laryngeal cancers: (*a*) Carcinoma polypoides et diffusum on the true vocal cords, as well as on the ventricular bands; (*b*) carcinoma ventriculare (B. Fraenkel); finally (*c*) the latent forms of laryngeal cancers (Schmidt.) Mostly we have to do with the advanced forms of this disorder.

12. Not one symptom is an absolutely certain diagnostic sign of this disease. Hoarseness, as well as pain, dys-phagia, fœtor ex ore, cough, secretion, salivation, bleeding, dyspnœa, and even affection of lymphatic glands, likewise cachexia, can exist or not in this disorder.

13. In the course of laryngeal cancer we discern three phases: formation of the tumor, ulceration, and destruction of the cancer. Mostly the development of the laryngeal cancer is fairly slow.

14. In the diagnosis of the cancer of the larynx, besides

the above symptoms, which have only a relative signification (just as also the trans-illumination of the larynx), above
all is important the laryngoscopic examination, which permits to state the appearance and localization of the tumor,
as well as the diminished or entirely deprived mobility of
the affected cord, or half of the larynx (Semon).

15. The most important method of deciding in most
cases of laryngeal cancers is the microscopical examination
of the extirpated fragments of the tumor, although also
here one may be mistaken, which appearances depend upon
the anatomo-pathology or are quite independent. The
latter is the case with too small or too superficially extirpated fragments given to be examined; further, in cases of
the existence of the so-called mixed tumors of the larynx
(carcinoma and papilloma, etc.).

16. The differential diagnosis of laryngeal cancer from
laryngitis, chorditis hypertrophica, from benign laryngeal
tumors (papilloma, polypus, cyst), finally, from the so-
called pachydermia and perichondritis of the larynx, is
pretty difficult. Most important, besides the diminished
mobility of the affected vocal cord, is the microscopical
investigation of fragments of the laryngeal tumor.

17. From syphilis of the larynx—namely, from its ulcerating forms. It is in most cases very difficult to distinguish
from the ulcerated laryngeal cancer, the more so as there
exist also mixed forms (Hunter Mackenzie).

A very important method is here the so-called *ex juvanti-
bus—i. e.*, application of specific mixed treatment (Kr.
and Hg.)

18. It is likewise hard to distinguish the laryngeal cancer
from the tuberculosis of the larynx, as here also the combination of both these affections is possible (case of Wolfen-
den); but not frequent, besides the laryngeal cancer, the
tuberculosis of the lungs can exist.

19. By far the easier is the diagnosis of layngeal cancer
from lupus, catarrhal ulcerations, sarcoma, finally from
secondary cancers.

20. The prognosis of laryngeal cancer is not so bad as it

was formerly supposed. Without doubt this disease, naturally in the early periods, is curable.

21. In the history of the treatment of laryngeal cancer I discern four phases: (1) The therapeutic nihilismus (ancient times); (2) birth of the rational therapy (from 1873, *i. e.*, since Bilroth first executed total laryngectomy); (3) the period of great oscillations in our opinions in regard to the therapy of laryngeal cancer (from 1881, *i. e.*, since the International Congress in London); (4) the phase of the sober critic (from 1888 to the present time).

22. The statistic ciphers have only relative signification in the appreciation of the operative results in regard to the cancer of the larynx. The collection of a good statistic is very difficult.

23. My statistics comprise four hundred and fifty-two cases of laryngeal cancers, and fifty of sarcoma, operated by means of difficult methods. (In the statistics, many inexact observations, as also the cases which have been operated after 1894, are excluded.)

24. The endolaryngeal method in laryngeal cancer (thirty-two cases in my statistics) gives twenty-five per cent. of favorable result, *i. e.*, such where after one year no relapse ensued, further 40.7 per cent. of relapses. It deserves to be applied in suitable cases (polypoid cancer).

25. Tracheotomy, as a therapeutic method, has no value in laryngeal cancer. It is, however, important to relieve the dyspnœa in case of suffocation, likewise as a preliminary method before greater operations.

26. Thyrectomy (ninety-two cases in my statistics) is a very valuable therapeutic method in the treatment of cancer of the larynx. It gives 21.7 per cent. of favorable results (of which 8.7 per cent. of definitive recoveries); further, 53.3 per cent. of recidives. It is almost harmless (9.8 per cent. of deaths after operation). Besides the therapeutic importance, this method has also a valuable diagnostical signification (before the extirpation of the larynx).

27. Subhyoid pharyngotomy (eight cases) can be success-

fully applied in cases of cancers of epiglottis, pharynx, and tongue, *i. e.*, above all in cases of external cancers.

28. Partial laryngectomy in laryngeal cancer (one hundred and ten cases in my statistics) gives 22.7 per cent. of favorable results, of which 11.8 per cent. of definitive recoveries. It is most decidedly the best therapeutic method in this disease, naturally in proper cases (only 28.2 per cent. of relapses and 26.3 per cent. of deaths).

29. Much worse results are given by total laryngectomy in laryngeal cancer (one hundred and eighty-eight cases). Favorable results have been obtained in 12.8 per cent., of which only 5.85 per cent. of absolute recoveries. At any rate, this method should be applied without hesitation in the suitable cases. It gives 32.45 per cent. of relapses, and 44.7 per cent. of deaths.

30. The most frequent cause of death after laryngectomy is the septic inflammation of the lungs (Schluck pneumonia), further collapse, etc.

31. As regards the technique of this operation, the tracheotomy (inferior) must be above all executed a couple of weeks before, then the windpipe tamponed, in order to avoid the trickling of blood into the respiratory ways, which can be attained best by means of Trendelenburg's tampon-cannula, or still better with Hahn's press sponge cannula. Then the larynx will be separated best in the direction from above down, without leaving behind the epiglottis.

32. There exist different modifications of extirpation of the larynx (laryngectomie sans trachéotomie préalable, Périer: méthode sous-perichondréale, Péan; modified laryngectomy of Solis-Cohen, etc.).

33. The post-operative treatment is in this disease of the greatest importance, and likewise the nutrition of the patients after operation.

34. The artificial larynx (of Czerny, Billroth, Gussenbauer, Hueter, Foulis, Von Bruns, Labbé, Cadier, Wolff, Périer, and finally E. Krauss, and prothetic apparatus of

Péan) can be applied, although they are not necessary, as is proved in the cases of Schmidt, Solis-Cohen, etc.

35. The indications and contra-indications to the operative treament of laryngeal cancer are of great importance. As a rule the patient must be operated on as soon as possible. One contra-indication, and only to a certain degree, is a very extended pathologic process (great affection of glands, pharynx, etc.) ; further, a very bad general state and complications on the part of other organs, especially of the lungs.

36. The symptomatic treatment must be employed only in cases where the operation cannot be performed. It is generally unsuccessful.

37. The laryngeal sarcomas happen much more seldom than the cancer of the larynx.

38. In regard to structure, they are mostly sarcoma fusi et globocellulare.

39. The course of the laryngeal sarcoma is quicker ; the symptoms similar to those with which we meet in cases of laryngeal cancer.

40. The diagnosis of sarcoma of the larynx is very difficult. The most important criterion here also is a microscopical examination of the extirpated fragments of the tumor.

41. The prognosis is much better than in laryngeal cancer.

42. The treatment can be : endolaryngeal extirpation of the tumor, pharyngotomia subhyoidea, thyrectomy, and finally, extirpation of the larynx (total or partial).

43. So, as in laryngeal cancer, the method of partial laryngectomy proved to be the most successful. The total extirpation of the larynx in sarcoma gave the best results (36.3 per cent., of which 27.3 per cent. were absolute recoveries).

44. The remaining operative methods (partial laryngectomy, laryngo-fissure, and endolaryngeal extirpation of the sarcomatous tumor of the larynx) can also give rela-

tively good results. In this manner, in suitable cases, they must be applied without hesitation.

45. In general, basing upon the ciphers obtained from my statistics of four hundred and fifty-two operated cases of laryngeal cancers and fifty of sarcoma, in which there were obtained good results in fifty cases of cancer and eighteen of sarcoma (of which thirty-seven and six were absolute recoveries), we must come to the conviction that there is only one rational—operative—treatment of malignant laryngeal tumors, and it should be the more often applied in suitable cases.

CASE I. H. B., male æt. fifty-one years, a healthy-appearing, strongly built man, slightly gray, presented himself at my clinic complaining of pain at the base of the tongue both on swallowing and articulating, which was aggravated by cold or sour fluids, but relieved by warm drinks ; cough with slimy expectoration ; duration of the above symptoms four weeks.

Laryngoscopic examination revealed a rough, lobulated grizzly-appearing tumor about one inch long by five-eighths inch in diameter, attached to the right arytenoid cartilage. The tumor apparently filled the right half of laryngeal space, overlying the anterior portions of the rima glottis, and the left true and false cord.

Although there were no constitutional symptoms, on account of the whitish-gray, shiny cartilaginous appearance we suspected it to be an epithelioma or malignant growth of some variety, on which account a specimen the size of a medium-sized pea was removed for microscopical examination. This confirmed the supposed diagnosis.

The subjective symptoms were so much relieved by either the removal of the small portion of the tumor or the bell. 2x that he did not return to hospital until February 27, (two months and a half), although he was informed by post that his throat needed immediate attention.

February 27, 1896.—Family history : Good. Father alive, seventy-nine years of age. Mother died at thirty-seven years of puerperal fever. Three sisters and a brother, all healthy. Weight 165 pounds ; apparently well nourished. Married twenty-nine years ; no children. Denies having syphilis, but had gonorrhea thirty years ago, followed by enlarged lymphatics in groins. Hemorrhoids of eight years' duration cured ten years ago. Until two years ago occupation in open air for eighteen years.

Status Presens. Since last September attacks of prosopalgia dextra. Immediately after excising microscopical specimen he had a little soreness which soon disappeared. Recently there is a sticking pain extending from top of naso-pharynx to larynx ; throat feels sore and obstructed on swallowing, but no choking.

Examination showed that about half of the tumor formerly present had ulcerated away, the whole right side of the larynx much tumefied and partly covered with ulceration from the epiglottis and ary-epiglottic fold to the upper part of the trachea ; entire laryngeal mucosa hyperæmic ; right cervical lymphatics and a few under head of right clavicle tumefied ; discharge is yellow, putrid, non-viscid and purulent in character ; on palpation all the diseased tissue was very hard and resistant.

On account of the implication of the extrinsic lymphatics and the extended area of ulceration, it was not considered advisable to operate. ℞, con. mac. 30.

March 13. Laryngeal congestion less..

March 30. ℞, pot. iod. sat. sol., gtt. x., t. i. d.; increasing one drop a dose each day.

April 20. Ulceration on ary-epiglottic fold healing ; when took 30 drops per dose the pain ceased, now taking 120 drops a day. ℞, ditto diminish gradually to 60 drops per diem.

May 18. The tumefaction in larynx increased and lymphatics on posterior wall of pharynx inflamed.

May 22. Occasional slight hemorrhage for a week.

June 10. Patient stopped medicine of own volition, and says he feels better without it.

July 20. From this time till decease occasional hemorrhages.

August 10. The tumor is noticeably ulcerating away, while the submaxillary and sublingual glands, as well as the cellular tissue within the thyroid cartilage, and in the base of the tongue, around the hyoid bone and in left tonsilar region, are being rapidly infiltrated.

The latter part of August the ulceration interfered far more with deglutition, the patient was not nourished as well, and from this and the progress of the disease he now commenced to weaken, which gradually increased until death on October 22. For two weeks before decease the characteristic pains were especially severe.

Necropsy.—A partial autopsy was consented to. The cancerous ulceration had spread above to the lower part of the tonsil, the lateral pyriform sinus, destroyed the epiglottis and ary-epiglottic fold, encroached slightly upon the left side of base of tongue, the whole left and posterior surface of the laryngeal box, extending down the trachea as far as the inner surface of the third tracheal cartilage, also over the upper margin of the laryngo-esophageal partition about a quarter of an inch onto the anterior wall of the esophagus.

Beside the glandular infiltration and cellular tissue inflammation given under date of August 10, there were found infiltrated lymphatics on both sides of the posterior wall of the pharynx and naso-pharynx, those under both clavicles and in the anterior mediastinum.

CASE II.—Mrs. S. A. T., æt. fifty-six years.—April 9, 1898. The patient's father died of cholera, and mother of phthisis, no history of malignant disease could be found in any of her relations. Two years previous she says she had la grippe while at the seashore, which was followed, the patient claims, with an attack of aphonia similar to the present, continuing four months.

Status Presens.—She complains of a continuous hoarseness of seven months' duration ; it was preceded by an acute otitis media suppurativa. Collection of tenacious phlegm in lower throat. Throat dry, great thirst, desire for acidulated drinks, tongue feels swollen, slight dyspnœa, frequent attacks of epistaxis for a year.

Objective Symptoms.—On right cheek opposite molars patch of mycosis aspergillis.

Larynx.—A dry, gray, tough, leathery membrane, like ozena scurfs, over the left false and true cords extending down left side of trachea. After the removal of this membrane by persistent use of peroxide spray the left false and true cords were congested, roughened, and thickened, and the excurtions of the latter were somewhat restricted.

Upon the first examination I thought it a case of that infrequent disease, laryngeal ozena. But the keeping of the larynx clear of membranea by peroxide spray and steam vapor of tinct.

benzoin comp., and the internal use of potash iod. for the anchylosed arytenoid joint for a month, was of no avail.

Then, on account of the above symptoms, coupled with a slight loss of strength, cancer was suspected two weeks before the following symptoms began to gradually appear : Soreness in region of the left cervical glands and the upper outer portion of the left breast, and glands between it and the clavicle, "nipping pains" in the throat and breast, which later became burning, both breasts sensitive to pressure ; strange it was there was no induration of any glandular tissue until very near the end.

On account of the disease having encroached upon the upper part of trachea as well as larynx, and the subjective symptoms showing it to have infected the cervicle and mammary glands it was deemed too widespread to be advisable to operate.

Early part of June the characteristic appearance of the skin showed itself, and she commenced to rapidly lose her strength, while the last of June the dyspnœa became much more severe, so that tracheotomy was considered a probable necessity in the near future.

About this time the diagnosis and prognosis was confirmed at a consultation with Dr. Robt. C. Myles of New York City.

The larynx was kept as clear as possible by cleansing and detergent spray ; tonic remedies internally and very nutritious diet were administered, but the patient rapidly weakened and died of exhaustion about August 1.

Of the internal medication will only mention the drugs from which the greatest relief was obtained, the dyspnœa was ameliorated most by the action of kali bich. 2x or 6x upon the copious viscid cancerous discharge ; the pains by phyto. 6x ; while the tincture of cinch. gave best result as a tonic.

It was impossible on account of the patient's aversion to the use of instruments to obtain a specimen for microscopical examination, therefore the exact diagnosis is impossible ; but from appearance I should judge it to be an ulcerating epithelioma. Furthermore, any cutting except thorough extirpation I believe only hastens the progress of the disease.

In closing would say that I only present these cases hoping they will impress upon the readers, as they have upon the writer, the great importance of both early diagnosis and early and thorough extirpation.

If the first case had returned to hospital and had a partial laryngectomy performed as we desired, his life would have been lengthened a few years. Or if the last case had come under observation of a specialist sooner operative procedure would probably have benefited her.

The early and thorough extirpation of any even suspicious tumor of the larynx is impressed upon one's mind by the perusal of Mackenzie's account of the case of Emperor Frederick, although it was written to explain the reasons of his temporizing treatment.

LOCALIZING FOREIGN BODIES IN THE EYE BY THE X-RAY.

BY GEO. H. TALBOT, M. D., NEWTONVILLE, MASS.

WITH the proper apparatus it is not only possible to determine the presence or absence of foreign bodies in the eye or orbit, but further to accurately locate them and calculate their size, even if they be so small as one or two mm. square. The difficulty is in correctly interpreting the result that is obtained in an ordinary X-ray negative—that is, in localizing the foreign body in the surrounding tissues, which in the picture convey the impression of homogeneity. It is evident that if but one picture be taken, it will be impossible, without some geometrical drawing to scale, to say in what part of the path of the X-ray the foreign body casting the shadow is located. It may be very far anterior or very far posterior in the line of light, and the resulting pictures will be the same in both cases. Hence a cross photograph is necessary in order to obtain the best results with the least expenditure of time and labor. But beyond determining whether a foreign body is or is not present in the eye or orbit, the negatives tell us little. From their evidence alone it is impossible to say, even approximately, where the body is to be looked for.

There must be some means of correctly reading these pictures in order to locate the foreign body; in other words, a localizing apparatus is essential. Of several methods of localizing foreign bodies, I shall briefly describe but two. The first is included in the Transactions of the American Ophthalmological Society for 1897. Mr. Collins of the Royal Ophthalmic Hospital thus describes it: " Dr. Sweet fixes to the patient's head an indicating apparatus carrying two steel rods, each with a rounded ball at the end. These two balls are placed at a known distance from the eyeball, one pointing to the center of the cornea and the other to the external canthus, both parallel to the line of vision and perpendicular to the plate. From the relations of the images of these balls of the indicator to that of the foreign body in the skiagraph, he is able to work out on a horizontal and vertical diagrammatic section of the eyeball the approximate position of the foreign body."

The method and apparatus devised by Mr. Mackenzie Davidson of London is by far the most scientific of anything in this line we yet have.

In localizing the shadows he makes use of fine silk threads to trace the path of the Roentgen rays, which have produced two negatives at different points of view, and by their point of interception can readily calculate the exact location of the foreign body. Davidson's process is as follows: The patient sits upright with his head resting firmly against a board. The eyeball, from its extreme mobility, is exceedingly difficult to picture accurately, and unless special precautions are taken the negatives are valueless. Two knitting-needles crossed at right angles are inclosed in a square frame and brushed over with ink, in order to mark the patient's skin. The side of the head with the affected eye rests against these crossed needles. A small piece of lead wire is attached by plaster to the lower lid, and, projecting a little above, bears a definite relation to some landmark on the eyeball, such as a scar or a pigment spot.

A Crookes tube is placed vertically on the opposite side of the head at a measured distance from the point of intersection of the needles. It slides on a horizontal rod parallel with one of the wires. A photographic plate inclosed in a black envelope is applied to the temple of the affected side over the wires. The patient is directed to gaze steadily at a distant object in a line parallel with the plate —that is, straight ahead.

The tube is displaced a measured distance to one side and an exposure made, then displaced to an equal distance to the other side and another exposure made. The result is a negative that shows one image of the cross wires and two of the foreign body.

This negative is, after development, placed on the horizontal stage of the localizer. This consists, essentially, of an adjustable horizontal bar marked with a millimeter scale, starting from a central zero and notched correspondingly on the upper edge. A plate-glass stage is marked with a cross, the points of intersection of which lie exactly beneath the zero on the horizontal bar. Beneath this stage is a hinged reflector to transillumine the negative. The negative is placed on this stage film side up, with the shadows of the cross wires corresponding with the cross on the stage. The bar is raised or lowered to make it the same distance from the stage that the tube was from the plate when the original exposure was made. Two silk threads are attached to the two notches that represent the two positions of the tube when the exposures were made. The negative on the stage now occupies the same relative position to these points that it did in the original exposure to the positions of the tube.

The other end of each of these threads is fixed by a needle to a piece of lead, and represents the path of the X-ray and is movable. One of these leads is placed on any parts of the shadow of one of the foreign bodies and the other upon a corresponding part of the other shadow.

It is obvious that the point where these lines cross represents the position of the foreign body. The precise size and position can thus be ascertained and as the cross wires are marked on the patient's skin, all data for the localization are given.

A perpendicular is dropped from the intersection of the two lines to the negative below, and a mark made there. This distance is measured by a pair of compasses, and indicates the distance of the foreign body inward from the temple. The distance of the mark under the intersection from the cross lines, gives the distance of the foreign body, posteriorly, from the lines on the patient's skin. In Mr. Davidson's own words : " The height of the point where the threads cross gives one co-ordinate—that is, the depth of the foreign body below the skin on which rested the photograph plate. The other two measurements give the other two co-ordinates. As the mark of the wires is left on the patient's skin, all that is required is to measure the two co-ordinates on the skin that give the point below which the foreign body will be found, at the depth given by the third co-ordinate."

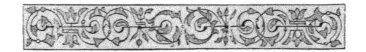

THE POINT OF VIEW.

BY JOHN L. MOFFAT, M. D., O. ET A. CH., NEW YORK,
BROOKLYN BOROUGH.

NOTWITHSTANDING the opposition usual to all advances in the world's progress, the makers of microscopes were at last induced to use a common screw-thread.

It is the purpose of this paper to suggest that every illustration of the fundus oculi be accompanied by a note indicating its amplification, or, better, the distance at which it should be held from the eye in order to give the proper size retinal image.

A landscape photographed with a twelve-inch lens appears best when viewed with one eye at a distance of a foot; that taken with an eighteen-inch lens, from a foot and a half. Similarly, the student will derive most benefit from the lithographs, etc., of the fundus if they appear to him the same size as if he were looking into an eye; especially is this so when he is estimating the caliber of the blood-vessels.

Comparing half a dozen or more of our leading text-books, I found the horizontal diameter of the optic disk measuring all the way from seven mm. to thirty mm.; frequently on the same page one drawing was upon twice the scale of another. These differences are not due to physiological variations nor to the fact that the small were inverted and the large erect images, but are attributable to thoughtlessness.

Let us hereafter have uniformity; it certainly is practicable to make each drawing of the fundus appear in detail

39

and in toto the size of the inverted or of the erect image when we view it through our ophthalmoscope with its correcting lens held as during examination of the eye.

Thus would accurate uniformity in the caliber of the blood-vessels 'make the lithographs doubly valuable to the specialist, refreshing his memory for cases of doubtful dilatation or constriction.

A material help in the accomplishment of this end will be for every reviewer to commend this feature if present, and to criticise its lack, in future atlases and text-books.

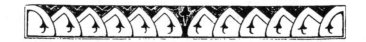

THE RESULT OF SEPTAL DEFORMITIES UPON THE UPPER RESPIRATORY TRACT.

BY E. R. JOHNSON, M. D., BOSTON, MASS.

THE quack, laity, general practitioner, and specialist have all alike been unsuccessfully seeking for a specific for that troublesome condition which they call catarrh. Of course we must admit it is an impossibility to find any one therapeutic agent or operative procedure which will cure every pathological state or every case included under the category of catarrh ; but the nearest we can attain to such a longed-for desideratum, is to first study the local pathological process, then diligently seek the cause or causes of such process, and finally consider the remedy therefor.

Such a study I hope to clearly elucidate in the following paragraphs.

For the past few years we have been making rapid strides in our knowledge of diseased conditions in all parts of the body. The nose and throat have received their share of attention. The third tonsil and its evils have been portrayed again and again. But more rarely have we heard of septal deformities and their sequelæ.

On account of the position and structure of the septum it is subject to many alternations and thereby excites many pathological conditions. It is formed by a cartilaginous portion somewhat quadrilateral in form, the perpendicular plate of the ethmoid, and the vomer. These are united at their articular borders by a fibrinous membrane, the perichondrium, forming a continuous, smooth inner

41

wall to each canal. The Schneiderian membrane covers the entire septum, thickest nearly opposite the anterior third of the middle turbinate, including at this point a small amount of cavernous erectile tissue. Thus it seems that the septum is made up of several thin perpendicular plates and covered by a vascular membrane.

Pressure at birth, traumatism, or an abnormal high arch of the roof of the mouth are the causes usually given for malformation of the septum. There may be a deflection; the septem may be thickened: curved doubly so as to cause a sigmoid flexure or corrugated appearance, with resulting exostoses or ecchondroses in the form of ridges, shelves, or spurs.

I particularly want to speak of these deformities and their effect upon the upper respiratory tract, to show how much depends upon the normal condition of the septum. I shall pass over with simply the mentioning such deformities as are due to ulceration with more or less destruction of the septum, and also deformities that are only noticeable externally.

Most authorities upon diseases of the nose and throat agree that the nasal septum should divide the nasal chamber into two cavities of equal dimensions. But this is rarely seen. A slight deviation is the rule.

Deformity of the septum may be caused by disease occurring directly in the structure or as a seconday condition depending upon some constitutional lesion. Inflammatory processes involving the mucous membrane lining the cartilage may so weaken it as to permit of a slight deflection. This is seen following purulent rhinitis of children. Superficial ulceration in syphilis, tuberculosis, and lupus without perforation may cause deflection and deformity.

By far the largest proportion of malformations of the septum are caused by traumatism. The injury may have been received in childhood, but the result not discovered until later in life. Children are especially subject to injury of the nose on account of their remarkable activity and carelessness; boys more frequently than girls. The injury is not usually recognized until the deflection, or thickening produced by the callus which is thrown out after the fracture, obstructs nasal breathing on one or both sides. The injury may be so great as to disjoint completely the cartilaginous and bony framework.

Either from disease, or more especially from injury, where the septum has been deflected there is a proliferation of cartilage cells, usually at the sutural junction of the triangular cartilage and the vomer, which results in the thickening of the septum or growth upon it. This growth, a ridge or spur, continues to increase in size, pushing out into one or both nasal cavities until it comes in contact, or nearly so, with the turbinate body. It may not necessarily come in contact with the opposite side of the cavity before nasal obstruction results. At this stage a simple cold may, by the marked hyperæmosis, bring the parts which previously have not touched into contact and result in a constant irritation of the mucous membrane lining the nasal cavities. Thus beginning, it continues and results in a chronic inflammation. In time " permanent alteration in the tissue will result from infiltration of the submucosa by leucocytes and serum. This embryonic tissue is produced by proliferation of the migrated leucocytes and fixed connective tissue cells, which, if nutrition be adequate, goes on to organization, and the formation of a fibrinous structure which alters the nutrition of the submucosa by contraction and impairs the functional activity of the mucous glands." The membrane is thickened and œdematous in the early stage. Hypertrophic rhinitis is of course the result.

Further contraction of the newly formed submucous tissue, with consequent lessening of the blood supply to the surface, and alteration of the normal function of the membrane with the shrinking of the tissues, gradually verges it from hypertrophy to atrophy. The former condition is especially annoying on account of the nasal obstruction and excessive secretion of mucus which may change into mucopurulent form ; the latter condition is especially annoying and dangerous to health on account of the fetid odor and sluggish purulent process.

Prior to an atrophic condition a myxomatous degeneration may take place, especially in the mucous membrane lining the dependent portion of the turbinate bodies, particularly the middle, resulting in a polypoid growth or growths. I do not say that a polypoid degeneration is necessarily due to the constant irritation of a spur or ridge. Although many theories have been advanced as to the cause of the polypus, I am sure that none is more reasonable than that a chronic inflammatory process, kept up by whatsoever cause it may be, will result finally in polypoid degeneration, and this chronic inflammation we most often find is due to some septal deformity. This is easily demonstrated in a large majority of cases.

The symptoms indicating myxomatous growths are similar to those of chronic rhinitis, except perhaps more marked according to the extent of the growths: nasal obstruction; nasal twang to the voice; worse in damp weather; discharge, the character of which depends entirely upon the extent of the growths and the length of time they have been pressing upon surrounding tissues; causing ozena; obstructing the lachrymal duct and the opening into the antrum with antral complications.

The myxo-fibroma and mucocele or mucous polypi have the same symptoms and appearance as the pure myoma, and these I will only mention in passing.

From the conditions which I have so far mentioned, it is very clear to be seen how naturally inflammation will extend into the accessory cavities, and especially the antrum. Closure of the antral opening often occurs, caused by inflammation in the nasal cavities, though by far the largest number of antral diseases are due to septic infection from decayed teeth, or to traumatism. There may be acute or chronic inflammation of the mucous membrane of the antrum or ozena, or there may be a purulent inflammation.

The ethmoid cells may be affected by direct extension

of inflammation from the nasal mucous membrane or by occlusion caused by turgescence or growths within the nasal cavity.   Such inflammation is easily communicated to the bony walls, with consequent caries and necroses.

Inflammatory processes of a like character and in a like manner may involve the frontal sinus and the sphenoidal cells by direct extension from the nasal membrane.

The following reflex neuroses may be wholly or in part overcome by correction of deformities of the nasal septum : sneezing, hay-fever, asthma, stammering or stuttering. And although chorea, epilepsy, and nocturnal incontinence of urine do not strictly come within the bounds of my paper, yet I mention them in passing as often caused by reflex irritation from this source.   If we accept the three conditions upon which the existence of hay-fever depends —namely : 1st, abnormally susceptible nerve-centers; 2d, hyperæsthesia of the peripheral termini of the sensory nerves, 3d, the presence of one of a large variety of irritating agents—it is easy to understand how necessary it is in the treatment of this disease to remove any local point of irritation and thereby put the mucous membrane of the nasal cavities in as healthy condition as possible.   It is a demonstrated fact that the removal of septal irregularities and breaking up of points of contact has kept under control, almost entirely the symptoms of this disease in some cases.

To briefly summarize : Slight deformity of the septum may be and often is, by a constant irritation to the nasal mucous membrane, a causative factor in the following pathological conditions of the nasal and accessory cavities:

Acute and chronic rhinitis, hyperæsthetic rhinitis or hay fever, hypertrophic rhinitis, polypoid degeneration, atrophic rhinitis, and of the accessory cavities, acute and chronic inflammation, and empyema, necroses and caries of the antrum of Highmore, ethmoid cells, sphenoid cells, and frontal sinuses.

The first indication of any abnormity of the septum would be nasal obstruction, which is brought about by most of the conditions above referred to. "One of the most important functions of the nose is to heat and moisten the inspired air. When for any reason this is interfered with, mouth breathing results," with the following consequences : irritation of the entire respiratory tract, sense of smell is retarded, dry and parched condition of the mouth, lips, and tongue, thickly coated tongue, restless sleep, snoring at night, frequent attacks of laryngitis and tonsilitis, hypertrophy of faucial and pharyngeal tonsils, coughing of retained secretions, mucous membrane of larynx and pharynx dry, voice hoarse and with nasal twang, and in children facial deformity.

All these morbid conditions may be relieved if we remove the exciting cause.

After thorough cocainization—which serves two purposes, first to anæsthetize the parts, and second to deplete the tissue —we may see clearly any deformity in the anterior nasal cavities and often see the posterior wall of the pharynx. If there is a spur, ridge, shelf, or thickening it should first be removed with the saw or knife. Such irregularities ususally develop on the convex side of the deflection. At the same time the turbinate bodies on the other side should be carefully examined for any abnormality, which should be corrected in order that there may be room enough on that side, after the septum has been straightened. After removal of such points, the tissue should be thoroughly cleansed with one of the many antiseptic washes, especially useful for the nasal mucous membrane, and the seat of such minor operations allowed to completely heal before the attempt to straighten the septum. The old method of the general surgeon indiscriminately introducing one of the various forms of punches, and breaking down the septum, cannot be too strongly condemned. It is wholly by the careful attention to the smaller details of the operation, and the following removal of redundant tissue, that assures a successful operation.

Different forms of deflection require different methods of operative procedure.

Etherization may be necessary, but the majority of cases can best be handled under cocaine. With cocaine and the addition of a solution of suprarenal capsule to make the operation bloodless, the operator can work at the best advantage ; having a reflected light and the patient in the best position, he can see clearly every step in the operation.

The bowed deflection or plain concavity on one side and convexity on the other is perhaps the simplest.

There are many methods and many modifications of the various methods. The Ash operation, which is very like the Douglas, seems to me best for the majority of cases. This consists in an incision being made parallel or nearly so with the floor of the nose, beginning at the posterior point of deflection, passing through the center of the concavity and bringing it forward completely through the triangular cartilage, another incision at right angles with this passing from the upper point of deflection, through the center to, or nearly to, the floor of the nose. If there should be a marked ridge, the incision would best be made along the line of the ridge or ridges regardless of their direction. Thus the septum is divided by several incisions, each one in turn allowing the entire septum to be forced into perpendicular line by pressure which is made by introducing the finger, well oiled, into the nostril on the convex side. It may be necessary to use the septum forceps, the blades of which are introduced on either side of the septum, and forcibly twisting by a rolling motion until the cartilaginous septum is freely movable. There is an overlapping of the edges, and this should be on the free side. The fragments are held in position by hollow malleable tubes, fitted to each particular case. It often is necessary to use two, one on either side of the septum, the larger one on the obstructed side, in order to get the best position of the fragments and a union of them in such position.

The utmost care following this operation is absolutely necessary to a favorable result. A careful examination each time the splint is removed and correction of any irregularity of the uniting fragments ; the thorough cleansing of the splints and the nasal cavities ; wearing the splint sufficiently long ; and finally, the removal of redundant tissue, which is apt to follow any injury to the septum, will result in a complete and successful restoration of the normal contour and function of the nasal cavities, and may in a measure correct external deformity. One very great advantage of the modern operation is its freedom from after-pain and discomfort.

AUTHORS REFERRED TO.

Kyle, page 57.
Kyle, page 221.
Bishop, page 232.
" American Text Book."
Ivins.
Coakley.
Brown.
Bosworth.
New York Medical Journal, August 6, 1898.
" Universal Medical Annual," Vol. IV., 1895.

TWO CLINICAL CASES.

BY J. H. BALL, M. D., ANN ARBOR, MICH.

THE following cases were presented in Professor R. S. Copeland's clinic at the University Hospital, homeopathic, at Ann Arbor.

The first case with operation is a very fine illustration of the Pagenstecher operation for cataract.

W. F. of Butternut, Mich., aged seventy-four, farmer by occupation, was admitted to the hospital November 1, 1897, and gave the following history of his condition : About nine years ago sight began to fail in the left eye. About a year after the right eye was similarly affected. Soon after this he had a fall in which he struck his head. Following this he said his sight began to fail more rapidly. Has not been able to distinguish objects for nearly eight years, but always had light perception. At present vision amounts to light projection only.

Diagnosis : Senile Cataract ; Hypermature.—Left eye was prepared for operation the evening of November 1, by being irrigated thoroughly with boracic acid, saturated solution ; a compress of moist bichloride (1–5000) gauze was bandaged over the eye and allowed to remain until patient was taken to the operating room next day. The bandage was removed and the eye again irrigated with a saturated solution of boracic acid, following which it was anæsthetized with 4 per cent. cocaine solution (sterilized).

The operation was begun with a linear incision almost entirely in the sclera, followed by a large iridectomy. The lens, with the capsule intact, was now removed by means of a lens scoop. There was little or no loss of vitreous, but some wrinkling of the cornea owing to the failure of the anterior chamber to refill and

49

lack of elasticity of its structure. This, however, passed away within twenty-four hours. The eye was dressed with a gauze pad and bandage, was redressed twenty-four hours later. At this time the anterior chamber had entirely filled. There was very little congestion and the temperature was normal. There was more congestion on dressing the eye the next day, but this passed away in a few days with no unusual complication. On the sixth day the bandage was permanently removed and patient was allowed to walk about the ward. On the eighth day he was able to read the head-lines of a newspaper by the aid of a $+13$ D. S. lens. November 15, his distant vision with $+9$ D. S. was $\frac{20}{40}$; with a $+13$ D. S. he could read No. 4 Snellen type easily.

This operation of removing lens with capsule intact is known as Pagenstecher's operation. After making a sclero-corneal incision and excising the iris, a special form of lens spoon, preferably a loop, is passed back of the lens, rupturing the suspensory ligament. Then gentle pressure is made on the lower third of the cornea, and the lens with capsule intact is removed on the loop. This operation can be of use only in hypermature cataract in which there is more or less thickening of the capsule. Otherwise there is danger of rupturing the capsule, if it be normal in thickness, as is usually the case in simple mature senile cataract. Another danger is that introduction of the loop behind the lens may cause loss of vitreous by rupture of the hyaloid membrane. This is more liable to occur if a condition of fluid vitreous be present. The chief advantage of the operation lies in the fact that after-cataract, from particles of the lens left behind or from changes in the capsule, is impossible.

The next case, though of a different character from the one just given, is of interest not only in the fact that it is a change from the usual line of treatment in the condition, but because it is a condition often met by the general practitioner as well as the specialist.

Mr. H. A. J. of West Sebewa, Mich., age thirty-six, occupation farmer. Was admitted to the hospital November 28, and gave the following history of his condition : When about five years of age he had a sudden attack of inflammation in the left eye, which was red, swollen, painful, and sensitive to light. The attack lasted nearly six months. The recovery was complete, except, as he describes it, his eyes were weak. When about fourteen years old he had a second attack of inflammation involving both eyes ; a doctor was seen who pronounced the condition granulated eyelids and treated them with the bluestone. The condition under this treatment continued about the same for nearly ten years, when he had another acute attack with marked failure of vision, brought on, he thinks, by exposure to corn-smut. The nature of the treatment at this time he does not know, except that it failed to relieve and was finally abandoned. Without treatment he gradually improved so as to be able to do ordinary farm work.

Five years after this he had another attack of inflammation and almost complete loss of vision. This, however, gradually improved to such an extent that he was finally able to read. Last October he had a fifth attack of inflammation, brought on this time too, he thinks, by corn-smut. He resorted to home treatment with the application of all the remedies suggested by neighbors and friends, such as slippery elm poultice, quinine, salt and water, sugar of lead, honey, and the various eye salves and washes suggested. Strange to say, the eyes continued to grow worse ! His vision failed rapidly, and as a last resort he presented himself at the clinic.

Upon examination the first condition seen was a narrrow and contracted palpebral opening, drawing the upper lid tightly over the cornea. Upon everting the lid it was found to be covered by a mass of granulations. The cornea was gray and hazy, with tortuous blood-vessels running through it, a very marked condition of pannus, and a marked sensitiveness to light. His vision was less than $\frac{1}{200}$; indeed, was so poor that he could hardly get about without assistance.

Diagnosis : Granular Ophthalmia with Pannus.—Treatment : Canthoplasty was performed first, to remove pressure from the cornea. As soon as the wound from this operation was healed the patient was put on euphrasia 3x internally four times a day.

A twenty-five per cent. solution of infusion jequirity was instilled into the eyes three times a day, also a lotion composed of

℞   Boracic acid.............................. .... gr. 5
     Cocaine mur .... gr. 5
     Aqua dest................................... .... oz. 1

was instilled into the eyes whenever necessary to relieve pain. This treatment was continued with gradual but marked improvement until February 24, when the patient was discharged from the hospital with instructions to continue treatment at home. At this time the sensitiveness to light had entirely passed away, the granulations had almost entirely disappeared, and the cornea was very much cleared, so much so that he was able to read large print. On March 30 the patient was again presented at clinic. The granulations had entirely disappeared from the lids, the left cornea was clear and the right practically clear except for one blood-vessel running across the cornea ; this was ligated, and April 10 the patient was discharged practically well.

As is well known, the use of jequirity bean in granular ophthalmia is not new. In fact, it is an old treatment, long since abandoned as worthless because the violent inflammation caused by it frequently left results, if not far worse, certainly as bad as the condition sought to be relieved. But the revival of its use in the form of an infusion prepared by Schieffelin & Co. has given results far in advance of all other local remedies.

The method of its application in Professor Copeland's clinic has been the instillation of a few drops of a twenty-five per cent. solution of the infusion into the eye three times a day, unless there is much irritation following the application, in which case another is not made until all irritation of the former application has subsided. The instillation of the jequirity may be somewhat painful, and it is well to instill a drop of two per cent. cocaine solution before using it.

McKinney, Richmond.—A Case of Papilloma of the Soft Palate.—*Memphis Lancet*, October, 1899.

Author reports following case :

The patient, a commercial traveler, aged thirty-two, was referred to me by Dr. Edwin Williams of Memphis for a throat examination. On first inspection, while examining his naso-pharynx, I noticed an irregularly surfaced, pinkish-white growth, about the size of a pea, attached to the soft palate at the base of the uvula. This was removed with a pair of curved scissors and a long nasal dressing forceps. On closer inspection the tumor was seen to be of the peculiar raspberry-like structure characteristic of papilloma. Its nature was further confirmed by the microscopic examination to which it was submitted. The microscopist's report is here appended :

"DEAR DOCTOR—I send herewith a section of the uvular growth, which, as you can easily see, is a hard papilloma. The most of the picture is in horizontal section, but one process is well seen in vertical section, showing the papillary ingrowth of the fibrous stroma. Some very large vessels are seen, entirely out of proportion to the size of the tumor.

"Yours truly, (signed)   "WM. KRAUSS."

PALMER.

Capps, E. D.—A Case of Complete Occlusion of the Posterior Nares.—*Texas Med. News*, October, 1899.

Mrs. M.; æt. thirty ; presented herself to me, complaining that she had nasal catarrh, and was unable to breathe through her nose. She stated that she had since a child breathed through her mouth, but thought that up to the time she was fifteen or sixteen years of age, that she could get some air through her nose. At that time (aged sixteen) she went to a physician, who told her there was an occlusion of the nares, and that he introduced his finger into her mouth and forcibly made an opening into the nose, requesting her to return again for further treatment. This she did not do, on account of the pain from the operation. For two or three years, however, she could get some air through her nose, but at no time was it free. Four or five years previous to the time I saw her, she had gone to a specialist, who had partly succeeded in opening the nose, but he had been unable to keep it open.

Examination, when I first saw her, revealed a woman in fairly good flesh, but pale and nervous. Her voice had the so-called nasal quality, as is heard in persons with obstruction in the nose. Her hearing was reduced for the want of contact in both ears ; mouth wide open all the time, the soft palate was drawn upward and backward, and attached to the post-pharyngeal wall, the posterior pillars of the former being pulled in the same direction.

From the nose there escaped a muco-purulent discharge, which was difficult for her to remove. The turbinal mucous membrane was atrophied and drawn tight over the bones posteriorly, and the inferior turbinates on either side were attached to the septum. The introduction of the finger into the mouth showed a firm attachment of the soft palate to post-pharyngeal wall, and also seemingly to the bassillar process of the occipital. In fact, the borders of the vertebræ pressed forward and the bassillar process of the occipital downward so as to materially diminish the superior pharyngeal space. A probe introduced into either nostril met a hard resistance in the posterior nares, and could not be pushed through, showing a complete occlusion. After a few days of antiseptic treatment of the nasal cavities the patient was operated on. She was first given a half grain of morphine and one-thirtieth grain of strychnine, hypodermatically, then completely anæsthetized with ether, after which the ether was dispensed with and the operation begun.

I first took a small steel sound and introduced it into the nares, and after forcing it through the tissue managed to make an opening into the pharynx. In the greater part of the space there was found to be a bony mass, the hard palate extending upward and attached firmly to the base of occipital. This was scraped and chiseled away with sharp curette and chisel. The soft palate was separated from the posterior pharyngeal wall by means of the finger and steel sound. After completion of the operation there was a good free passage, which was stuffed with iodoform gauze. The hemorrhage was very free, as one would expect, but the blood was kept out of the larynx by keeping the patient's head well over the edge of the table and at a considerably lower level than the body.

The operation occupied about half an hour's time, but notwithstanding the ether had been stopped, she complained of no pain, though sufficiently conscious to speak. Considerable shock followed the operation, but at no time was she in a dangerous condition. The gauze packing was allowed to remain in situ for forty-eight hours, when it was removed. The after treatment consisted in cleansing, antiseptic washes, and politzerization of the Eustachian tubes. Her general health improved rapidly, as did also her hearing, and she expressed herself as feeling better than she had for years. PALMER.

Jonnesco, Thos.—Resection of the Cervical Sympathetic in Glaucoma.—*Interstate Med. Jour.*, July, 1899.

This description of the above operation is taken from an article translated by James M. Ball, M. D.

The operation may be divided into four stages:

1. The cutaneous incision begins at the upper angle of the inferior maxilla and extends along the anterior border of the sterno-mastoid.

2. The anterior border of the sterno-mastoid muscle is freed. After cutting the skin, superficial cervical muscles, and superficial fascia the anterior border of the sterno-mastoid is freed by means of a grooved director and the muscle is drawn outward and backward by a retractor; by a grooved director the deep layer of the aponeurotic sheath of the muscle is cut and then a second retractor is used on the inner lip of the wound, to draw the larynx inward. This brings the operator to the bundle of vessels and nerves.

3. The identification, separation, and exsection of the superior cervical ganglion. After the anterior wall of the vascular bundle has been cut, one aims to draw the internal jugular vein outward, and the internal carotid artery and vagus nerve inward, by means of retractors. In the space thus made one finds the

superior cervical ganglion easily ; then by means of the grooved
director the deep wall of the carotid sheath and the prevertebral
fascia are opened.   Isolated by means of the director and seized
with forceps, the ganglion is followed from below upward.   Then
by means of the index finger it is carefully separated from the
surrounding structures, all afferent and efferent fibers are cut by
means of blunt curved scissors.   When this is accomplished, the
ganglion is attached only by the nerve-strand which forms its
continuation above ; a strong pull is made, and the ganglion is
torn out.   A cut is made below, and the excision is completed.

The operation described makes the complete removal of the
ganglion possible ;   it is bloodless, and permits the fibers of
the superior cervical plexus and the external branch of the spinal
accessory nerve to be spared.

4. Closure of the wound is divided into two steps :   First, the
border of the sterno-mastoid is united to the deep cellular tissue
by means of three or four catgut sutures ; the superficial part of
the wound is closed by means of fine catgut.   The wound is not
drained.

The bilateral operation can be made in fifteen minutes.   The
results of the operation are trifling ; the bandage is removed on
the sixth day.   Union is ideal only if an aseptic operation has
been made.

After the operation one observes congestion of the conjunctiva,
of the eye, the nose, lachrymation, considerable nasal secretion,
heaviness of the head, all phenomena which immediately disappear on the first day.   The remaining effects upon the eye are
contraction of the pupil, already mentioned, sinking of the eyeball in the orbit, drooping of the upper eyelid, and narrowing of
the palpebral fissure.

The therapeutic results are an immediate reduction of intra-
ocular tension ; there follows immediately, or within a few days,
an improvement in vision, which increases from day to day.
The periorbital pain and headache disappear.   Frequently after
the operation these patients complain of a heaviness in the head,
which is probably to be attributed to the removal of the ganglion
producing congestion of the brain, which should not be con-
founded with the glaucomatous pain.   In many cases a slight
dysphagia appears after this operation, and during chewing there

is pain in the cranio-mandibular articulation, which are unimportant symptoms, as they soon disappear completely.   DEADY.

The Local Treatment of Diphtheria.—*Semaine Méd.*, January, 1899. (*The Lar.*)

"The author, who finds it impossible to always obtain diphtheria serum when needed, has been so successful with the local treatment that he has only lost three patients out of 197, a mortality of 1.52 per cent.   His method is the simultaneous use of trichloride of iodine, which Behring and Kossel recommended for syringing the mouth in diphtheria, sodium sozoiodolate, sulphur and ferric chloride.   The formula for the gargle is as follows :

℞ Trichloride of iodine.......................... .... 5 gram.
 Distilled water..... .... 500 gram.
 Saccharin .... 50 gram.
 M.—Dilute with 10 parts of water and gargle ten times per day.

"Insufflate into the nose and throat, after each gargle, a powder composed of sodium sozoiodolate 5 grams, sulphur 15 grams. Administer in addition 15 to 40 drops of ethereal tincture of ferric chloride four times per day."   PALMER.

Dr. Rogers.—Tarantula in Cough.—*Am. Hom.*, July 1, 1899.

Report of Case : Symptoms—sore all over ; throat gets dry ; cough on lying down at night and in the morning after rising, dry with tearing pain in chest ; is excited by pressure of phlegm in chest ; gets short of breath for at least an hour after each coughing attack ; only relief comes from smoking ; bad taste in the morning.   Tarent. his. [30] three doses cured.   PALMER.

Close, Stuart ; Baylies, B. L.; Cardozo, A. L.; Lutze, F. H.; Lazarus, Geo. F.; Moffatt, Jno. L.—Study of Mezereum.—*N. Am. Jour. Hom.*, July, 1899.

Inasmuch as this is a drug comparatively little used in our specialties we copy in full the symptoms under these heads.

"The *tongue* is coated thick white, papillæ large, red, elevated ; fissured in the middle.   Burning on tongue, extending to mouth and throat and stomach ; but this burning is relieved sometimes by eating.

"Swelling under right side of tongue, increasing slowly to size of pigeon's egg; painless red swelling, bluish at apex, as from enlarged blood-vessels. The patient ejects a watery fluid on talking or chewing.

"*On fauces and palate.*—There is a sensation of heat and burning as from pepper, or of scraping. The saliva is increased, the breath offensive like rotten cheese.

"Flat whitish ulcers on inner side of lips and corners of mouth.

"Burning in throat and pharynx (ars., canth., caps., merc. cor.), fauces dry, causing a hacking cough, loosening but scanty mucus.

"The throat feels constricted, dry, swallowing is difficult (arum., bell., caust., ignat.).

"There is a sensation in posterior part of throat, as if it were full of mucus, which is not relieved by hawking. Swallowing fluids even is difficult (bell., ign., lach., merc. cor., stram.).

"*Respiratory Organs.*—In the larynx a burning sensation and a feeling of tightness or constriction, with tickling. These sensations produce a cough. The prominent and decided symp'toms in this connection, are, hoarseness, cough, and *rawness* of trachea (nux, caust., phos.).

"Both Allen and Farrington give the cough as dry, severe and spasmodic. Expectoration, if present at all, is tough and yellow.

"Cough is < in evening till midnight.

"Cough is < lying down (conium, puls.).

"Cough is < after meals (bry., nux., k. bich.).

"There is dyspnœa, which is due to a feeling of constriction transversely across the chest, and to stitches in chest (bry. and kali carb.).

"In the *nose* it causes dryness with blunted smell; fluent coryza with frequent sneezing; or, a discharge of acrid mucus, which may be yellow, thin, or bloody. There is a *pain in the root of the nose like pressing asunder.*

"The *throat* feels as if full of mucus; there is intense burning: dryness, scraping, and rawness, causing a dry, fatiguing cough.

"*Ear.*—Mezereum acts upon the skin, mucous membrane, and bones of the ear, same as elsewhere; we are most apt to think of it in eczema aurium, but I have had it work very satisfactorily for otorrhœa. The most marked subjective symptom is *itching* —behind or in the ears or extending to the Eustachian tube. The ears feel stopped, or distended with air; and there have been repeated confirmations of the *feeling as if the ears were too open and cold air blew into them.*

"In the eye we have still more varied symptoms, although none so important as otorrhœa, except (clinically) abscess of the cornea.

"Objectively, eczema palpebrarum is most prominent. In my experience the mezereum eczema is characterized not so much by the oft-quoted ' pus under thick crusts,' as by biting, itching, and neuralgia. The other objective symptoms are : Marginal blepharitis, congested conjunctiva or purulent conjunctivitis, lachrymation (of course) and twitches in the left upper lid.

"Subjectively, the mezereum eye *itches*; there may be smarting, biting, tearing, with a strong desire to rub the lids, or to blink or close them. There is a sensation of dryness and a pressure or pressure pain. Asthenopia is indicated by the sensation as if the eyes are *too large*, or strained, or as if drawn backward into the head. One of the characteristic symptoms is *a cold feeling in the eye as if a stream of cold air were blowing upon it.* (This symptom we also find in the ear.)

"Next to eczema, however, our drug is useful in ciliary neuralgia, especially after operations ; the pains radiate and shoot downward, they leave a numbness, and are worse by warmth ; their location is the malar bone, or over the left eye.

"Clinically, we should think of this remedy in mercurial, syphilitic, scrofulous, or rheumatic inflammation, neuralgia, or asthenopia."
PALMER.

Verbascum in Catarrhs.—*Am. Hom.*, July 15.

Verbascum thapsus is very efficacious in a hard, hoarse laryngeal and bronchial cough with hoarseness and deep bass voice. In acute cases 2 drops every hour. In chronic 3 drops three times a day. Also rub chest twice a day with the (mullein) oil.
PALMER.

White, Joseph A.—Eye Troubles Attributable to Naso-Pharyngeal and Aural Disturbances.—*Journ. Am. Med. Asso.*, November 11, 1899.

In an article on the above subject the author gives the following summary of ocular conditions so caused, collected from the records :

Blepharospasm apparently results from cerumen impaction, foreign bodies in the external ear, and syringing the ear—Rampoldi, Ziem, Buzzard, etc.; also from the presence of pus or polyps in the drum—Deleau, Duterné, Gottstein.

Blurred and double vision have also been reported as having resulted from examinations, traumatisms, and diseases of the external ear.

Lachrymation, ciliary neuralgia, and muscular disturbances have appeared as a sequence of traumatisms, causing lesions of the drum.

Amblyopia and contracted field for both light and color have seemingly been caused by obstruction of the Eustachian tube, and improved by catheterization—Kisselbach and Wolfberg. Contraction of the field was also observed by Lucae, from the use of the air douche in the external canal in perforation of the drum, probably due to irritation of the tympanic plexus.

Gervais reported strabismus with myosis from mastoid inflammation, which disappeared when the abscess was opened.

Troubles of the accommodation have been observed from irritation of the branches of the trigeminus in the organ of hearing, and cured by the improvement of the aural condition—Politzer, Wolfberg, Urbantschitcsh.

Nystagmus is probably one of the most commonly reported eye reflexes from the ear. Baginski's experiments on rabbits in this line are well known, and show the muscular disturbance to arise from water thrown into the ear, and from disease of the labyrinth and semi-circular canals—Jansen, Cohn, Kipp, Urbantschitsch.

Nystagmus should be watched for carefully, as it is sometimes so slight that it is not perceived by the patient. It is more readily noticeable when it occurs from syringing the ear in suppuration of the drum, and is nearly always from labyrinthine irritation—occasionally it accompanies meningitis of aural origin, or thrombosis about the petrous bone. Geronzi—October, 1897—reported a case from an acute non-suppurative middle ear inflammation, following influenza. There was also diplopia in outer parts of the entire field. Singer reported a case following a Stacke operation, whenever pressure was made on the drum, or the air in the external meatus was rarefied. The pupils dilated at the same time. Urbantschitsch also reported a case of aural polyp in which nystagmus was produced each time the polyp was pressed on. Pfluger had several years previously reported a similar case. Gruber has also seen such cases.

Abducens paralysis has been observed in one or two cases of intracranial involvement, and recently—German Otological Society, May, 1898—Habermann reported a case of middle-ear suppuration cured in ten days, but which relapsed in three weeks, with headache and sudden paralysis of the abducens. The dura was exposed and found hyperemic only. The paralysis, which was permanent, was supposed to be due to extension of the inflammation into the petrous and sphenoid bones. In the discussion that followed Katz stated he had seen the same thing due to meningitis caused by ear trouble. Brüger had also seen it in what was supposed to be latent meningitis of aural origin. Mann had seen it in perisinuous (?) abscess. Jansen thought it due to serous meningitis, dependent on sinus thrombosis or epidural abscess. Habermann, however, concluded that sinus trouble could be excluded, as he had seen abducens paralysis on the opposite side from the ear trouble.

Paralysis of the orbicularis has been observed as resulting from foreign bodies in the external ear—non-perforating catarrh of the drum, purulent otitis media, etc.

Hippus—alternating contraction and dilatation of the pupils—had been observed by Pisenti in a person with chronic middle ear catarrh, each time the Eustachian catheter was used, and each time air was driven into the drum. Reflex might be by three ways :

1. Irritation of the trigeminal branches in the floor of the nose, transmitted to the sensory root of the ophthalmic ganglion. 2. Irritation of the posterior and inferior ethmoidal nerves and transmitted by the ophthalmic ganglion to filaments of the oculomotor. 3. Irritation of the internal ear by dilatation of the drum and transmitted from the ampulla to Deiter's nucleus and thence to the nuclei of the sixth and third pairs.

Purulent choroido-iritis from purulent otitis is reported by Kipp and Pomeroy, either of metastatic origin from emboli, or possibly by extension to brain envelopes and along optic nerve sheaths to the eye. Panas ("L'auto-infection dans les maladies oculaire") reports a similar case in the service of Dr. Quénu, except that the metastatic panophthalmitis was on the opposite side from the diseased ear, the eye on the same side remaining intact.

Orbital cellulitis, with secondary neuritis and amblyopia, has also been observed by the same author, as the result of purulent otitis media, which was cured by injection of antistreptococcus serum when ordinary measures had failed.

Obscuration of visual field and keratitis have been observed by Knapp—mydriasis and hemiopia by Moos, in Menière's disease ; whether as a sequence or coincidence is doubtful.

Schwartze has reported a case of progressive amblyopia in a subject of an acute affection of the acoustic nerve, which was arrested and cured by leeching.

Statistics of deaf mutes show a larger number of cases of amblyopia—G. Mayer, Schermer, Gellé, Schmolz, and others.

Wyatt Wingrave—October, 1897—reported a case of tuberculosis of the ear with optic neuritis. There was a discharge from the ear, but the general health was perfect. He thought it might be due to latent meningitis or a tuberculous gumma. The good health, however, was a contra-indication of meningitis, and the age, only twenty-five, of gumma.

Optic neuritis is also frequently found in connèction with mastoid abscess, suppuration of the drum, and their intracranial complications. Exophthalmus and strabismus are also found in the same connection—Zaufal, Kipp, Schwartze, and others. Paralysis of the oculo-motor nerves and homonymous hemianopsia have also been observed from the same causation.

DEADY.

Guttmann, Jno.—Holocaine as a Local Anæsthetic. —*New York Med. Jour.*, June 17, 1899.

After giving concise history of development of the drugs of the cocaine family and experiments upon himself and four other healthy subjects, he says :

According to Traube's researches, the chemical nature of holocaine is as follows : Holocaine is a derivative of p.-phenetidine, and is in close relation to lactophenine and phenacetine. The chemical name of the latter is acetyl-p.-phenetidine. Holocaine is to be considered as formed by the union of molecular amounts of phenacetine with p.-phenetidine and the elimination of water, according to the formula :

$$C_6H_4 \left\{ \begin{array}{ll} OC_2H_5 & OC_2H_5 \\ NH.CO+ & \\ CH_3 & NH_2 \end{array} \right\} C_6H_4 = C_6H_4 \left\{ \begin{array}{ll} OC_2HO_5 & C_2H_5 \\ NHC & N \\ CH_3 & \end{array} \right\} C_6H_4 + H_2O$$

According to Schlosser, the product of this union is a beautiful crystalline, strong base, which is insoluble in water and melts at 121° C. The chloride of the substance—which is holocaine—crystallizes in white needles, which are easily soluble in hot water. The saturated solution, which contains only 2.5 per cent. holocaine, is slightly bitter, neutral in reaction, and is not changed by boiling.

It should be prepared in porcelain vessel, as it enters into a combination with the alkali of the glass, spoiling the compound. Boiling the glass vessel with muriated water obviates this difficulty.

He disagrees with other authorities, holding that in the eye it requires same time to cause anæsthesia, while in the nose it needs seven to ten minutes longer than cocaine.

Anæsthesia is produced by paralysis of the terminal nerve fibers, and not by secondary ischæma or frigidity as with other local anæsthetics.

In the following operation he considers holocaine preferable: "For the removal of a foreign body from cornea holocaine is to be preferred, for, unlike cocaine, it does not produce the subsequent disagreeable mydriasis ; also for a strabismus operation is holocaine to be preferred, for cocaine causes the muscle to shrink, and thus often permits some muscular fibers to escape the strabismus hook. In the treatment of inflammatory affections of the conjunctiva and cornea, associated with painful blepharospasm, holocaine is of great value, for it not only relieves the spasm and allays the pain, but also acts as an antiseptic, and thus as a curative agent. But, on the other hand, cocaine is to be preferred in the performance of an iridectomy where the arteries appear atheromatous and where we would avoid a considerable hemorrhage. The vasoconstrictor effect of cocaine, and the diminished tension of the eyeball, together with the subsequent deepening of the anterior chamber, are all factors in favor of using cocaine for the performance of an iridectomy under these circumstances. For the extraction of a cataract where the pupil is small, cocaine is to be preferred on account of its mydriatic action. For the many other operations on and about the eye, these two agents may be used indifferently, unless, indeed, the bactericidal action of holocaine should incline us to use it in preference to cocaine. . .

" In choosing our anæsthetic for operations on the ear, nose, and throat we must consider whether the disadvantage of the freer hemorrhage following the use of holocaine is more objectionable than the disadvantageous and undesirable shrinkage of the tissues following the use of cocaine."

In applications to the nose and throat it does not cause the disagreeable sensation of lump in and dryness of the throat, which in turn cause hawking frequently following by hemorrhage.

Author had used it upon one hundred and fifty cases without the slightest toxic or alarming manifestation.   PALMER.

Waggett, Ernest.—Cerebellar Abscess Secondary to Suppurative Otitis Media : Evacuation : Recovery.— *Brit. Med. Jour.*, October 14, 1899.

The following is a very complete report of an interesting case :

Condition when First Seen.—The patient, F. B., aged twenty-six, a young man of slender build, looking sallow and ill, presented himself at the out-patient department of the London Throat Hospital on January 24, 1899, complaining of pain in the right ear and of a slight sense of giddiness. For as long as he could remember he had been subject to a discharge from the right ear, which was totally deaf, and he had occasionally experienced pain ; but the vertigo, which had commenced some three weeks previously, was a new symptom to him. On examination I found an abundant fetid discharge and a large fimbriated polypus, which almost filled the right meatus. Evidence of mastoid disease was wanting. The polypus was removed with the snare, and proved to spring from the posterior region of the tympanum. The membrana tympani and ossicles were wanting. A routine antiseptic treatment was ordered (hydrogen peroxide, boric syringing, and boric spirit drops), and the patient sent away, to return in a few days' time with the ear in a much improved state.

Facial Palsy : Schwarze-Stacke Operation.—On February 14— that is, three weeks after the first visit—he returned in great pain. On examination I found he had thrust a plug of wood deep into the meatus, and the collection of pus pent up behind this obstruction was exceedingly foul. To avoid further indiscretion he was admitted into the wards. Two days later, when his pain had subsided under careful antiseptic treatment, he suddenly developed right facial palsy involving all branches of the nerve. Although other symptoms of deep-seated disease were wanting, an operation was undertaken on the following morning, with the purpose of preventing permanent damage to the nerve by pus infection. The ordinary Schwarze-Stacke operation was performed under ether, the patient exhibiting no unusual respiratory symptoms while under its influence. The mastoid proved to be eburnated, and the antrum, filled with pus and granulations, was no larger than a field pea. A small sequestrum was removed from the floor of the aditus and antrum, and this was taken as being an immediate factor in the causation of the facial palsy. No muscular twitchings in the face were noted during this proceeding. The operative cavity (antrum, aditus, and tympanum) was left freely exposed by the removal of a quadrangular flap from the meatus, and the operation seemed to be very satisfactory.

After-History.—The pain was relieved, the temperature was normal, and as the patient lay quiet in bed everything seemed to point to a good result, though the facial palsy showed no real sign of improvement. It was clear, however, that rapid convalescence was not taking place, in spite of the excellent condition of the ear; and on the tenth day the temperature rose to 100.5°, and some neuralgic pain was complained of behind the left ear, which was seen to be normal in appearance. The patient lost his appetite, and felt "liverish," the bowels being constipated, and the breath unpleasant. The optic disks were examined, and noted as being slightly pink, and somewhat indistinct near the edge, but the same had been observed at the routine examination on admission. For nine more days the case was watched with growing suspicion.

Onset of Vertigo and Vomiting.—At the end of that period (nineteen days from the operation) his health had clearly declined in spite of the satisfactory state of the ear, and for several days past he had been increasingly unwilling to move in his bed and to sit up, complaining that rapid movements of the head caused him to feel very giddy. On more than one occasion this vertigo had been followed by actual vomiting. Vomiting had also occurred after food on two occasions without premonitory nausea. The neuralgic pain had now become persistent, and had shifted to the right occipital region, where, however, no local tenderness could be made out. Once or twice I noticed that the right pupil was somewhat larger than the left for a few minutes at a time, and slightly sluggish in reacting to light. This phenomenon might, however, be explained by the presence of a degree of conjunctivitis on the right side, due, no doubt, to the exposure of the eyeball resulting from the facial palsy. This ocular symptom was, in fact, typical of all the symptoms present, in that some explanation other than the correct one was always forthcoming. It is clear, on revising the case, that at the period of which I am speaking (nineteen days after the mastoid operation) it was fully ripe for diagnosis and exploration, but I venture to think that no surgeon, seeing the case for the first time, would have arrived at a positive conclusion from the symptoms exhibited, and one must remember that symptoms are apt, when vague and transient, to receive a fictitious distinctness when recorded on paper. This remark does not, however, apply to the temperature and pulse-rate. The former had now, for two days, remained a degree below the normal, while the latter had fallen from about 80 a minute to between 60 and 65.

Diagnosis of Intracranial Abscess.—Two days later—March 11, the twenty-first after the operation—the diagnosis of intracranial, and in all probability of cerebellar, abscess, could be said to be definitely established. My notes for that day were to the following effect: Vomiting had become habitual after food and without premonitory nausea. Vertigo was marked even on quiet movement of the head. The gait was distinctly staggering on attempting to walk, though a tendency to fall to one or the other side could not be determined owing to the extremely weak state of the patient. The grasp of the right and left hands were equal, but some inco ordination was noted on the right side when attempts were made to bring the forefinger to the tip of the nose. The knee-jerks were exaggerated, a condition which had been present since it was first tested a week previously. The right pupil was widely dilated and very sluggish in reacting both to light and accommodation. The optic disks remained as before, slightly hyperæmic and indistinct at the edge. There was no nystagmus or diplopia. The temperature had remained for four days a degree below normal, touching 97.2 on two occasions, while the pulse-rate was at one time as low as 54 to the minute.

The bowels were very constipated and the breath foul. Cerebration was slow, but quite clear, and the slowness had been present in some degree from the onset of the case. More distinctly local evidence of disease in the posterior cranial fossa was to be found in the severe and persistent occipital pain localized in the middle line, unaccompanied by torticollis or stiffness of the back ; there was also the presence of a lesion involving the facial nerve presumably in the Fallopian canal or internal auditory meatus. It may be added that at no time since the mastoid operation had the tuning fork been heard by bone conduction, but before that operation the test had not been applied ; and I should also mention that the patient had for many days persisted in lying curled up on his left side, but this evidence of disease in the right cerebellum loses its significance when it is considered that a tender healing wound was present on the right side. No carious bone could be detected by the probe in the direction of the middle fossa or the sigmoid sinus. The *tâche cérébrale* phenomenon was present in a marked degree.

Exploratory Intracranial Operation.—The symptoms, though in some respects deficient and inconclusive, were on the whole sufficiently exact to render an exploration of the cerebellum and possibly of the cerebrum imperative. Accordingly, with Dr. Law's kind assistance, I performed Dean's operation, applying a ⅖-inch trephine immediately over the course of the lateral sinus at a point 1¼ inch behind the center of the meatus and ¼ inch above it. On removing the button the meninges were found to be bulging without pulsation both above and below the exposed lateral sinus. The latter appeared to be perfectly healthy, and on accidental puncture of its outer wall by a bone splinter the blood spurted at high pressure. In consequence of this hemorrhage I had to slit open the vessel and pack with gauze, which was left in position until the eighth day, when firm aseptic clotting was found to have taken place. I enlarged the hole in the bone upwards and downwards. On incising the dura mater the pia was found to be free from inflammation in both the middle and posterior fossæ. I then explored the cerebellum in ten different directions with Horsley's large-sized pus-seeker, attacking, as one would suppose, every part of the right lobe. The instrument was introduced as deeply as possible short of piercing the fourth ventricle, and was carried forwards and upwards to the posterior aspect of

the petrous bone 3 inches from the trephine hole on two occaisons.
No evidence of pus was obtained, and a similar thorough but
fruitless exploration was made of the temporo-sphenoidal lobe
in ten different directions.

After-History.—The patient was put back to bed to await
events, the trephine wound being merely packed with gauze.
During the next three days little change took place in his condition. The pain was slightly less evident, and he lay curled up on
his left side with the hand under the occiput. Some wandering
occurred at night, the temperature remaining subnormal, falling
on the third night to 96.8°, and remaining at that point for thirty-
six hours. On the fourth day he seemed better, the temperature
reached normal, and the pupils reacted again to light. The
brain, however, bulged into the wound and did not pulsate.
This day for the first time a complete absence of the knee-jerks,
previously exaggerated, was detected. The grasp of the right and
left hand were noted as equal.

Onset of Optic Neuritis.—On the fifth day, March 16, the
condition had undergone a marked change for the worse, and indeed the patient appeared to be dying. The optic disks had been
examined almost daily, but now for the first time marked swelling
and choking of the left disk was present. Cerebration was clear,
but the patient's memory was now a blank as to this period of his
illness. The wound of the previous operation appeared to be
quite aseptic. Pulsation was wanting over both the cerebrum
and cerebellum, but bulging was now apparent only in the cerebellar region.

Second Exploratory Intracranial Operation.—I now felt convinced of the presence of cerebellar abscess, and determined to
explore until this was found and evacuated. I enlarged the
wound and explored with the pus-seeker in all directions, but
without success. I then inserted my left index finger into the
cerebellum in the direction of the internal auditory meatus. The
œdematous tissue was no more perceptible to the sense of touch
than is warm water, and nothing was felt until the posterior
aspect of the petrous bone was reached. I withdrew the finger
and again inserted it forwards, upwards, and inwards. When the
the whole length of my finger (that is, $3\frac{1}{4}$ inches) had entered the
wound, I felt between its tip and the tentorium above it a well-
defined elastic body, of the consistency of a boiled egg with the

shell removed. It was clear from the situation that the pus-seeker must on more than one occasion have met with and displaced this compressible body. I now passed the instrument along the finger track, and on opening the blades about an ounce and a half of greenish fetid pus came away. A considerable amount of hemorrhage was taking place at the time, and the pus could not be measured. Dr. Potter, who was administering the chloroform, noted that the pulse-rate immediately rose in frequency. Two decalcified bone tubes, 3 inches long, were inserted side by side into the abscess cavity. While inserting the second of these, a gush of clear amber-colored fluid (? 2 drams) came away. The antiseptic employed throughout this and the former operation was biniodide of mercury 1 in 4000, and it is worthy of note that there was at no time any evidence that the extensive interference with both cerebral and cerebellar tissue was in any serious degree harmful to the patient.

After-History.—On March 17, the day following the operation, the outlook was very unfavorable, for the patient was very restless and irritable, and complained of very severe pain all down the back. In view of the presumed rupture of the fourth ventricle, this seemed to be as serious a symptom as one could have. A well-marked lateral nystagmus was now present for the first time, the eyes moving together slowly to the left and returning rapidly to the right. The temperature, which was at 96°, immediately before the operation, had risen in eight hours to 100°. On gently syringing the abscess cavity with boric lotion through a small tube passed up one of the drains, the patient experienced a humming tinnitus. The mental condition was that of irritation rather than torpor. In spite of this discouraging commencement, within two days of the operation the patient's general condition had very much improved, the main symptom being very great weakness, which was met by free dosing with brandy. The bowels remained constipated, but vomiting had ceased except on one or two occasions. The temperature ranged about normal and the pulse was full and 80 to the minute. The right external rectus was now found to be paralyzed, and the lateral nystagmus appeared to be no longer constant, as during the first day or two, but was always induced by attempts at fixation. The patient began to lie occasionally on his right side. On March 20, four days after the operation, the swelling and venous engorgement of the left optic disk had quite disappeared, the disk being merely red and devoid of edge ; and it may be said that this subsidence of the swelling is considered the best evidence of the successful evacuation of an intracranial abscess. During the next ten days the patient made slow progress towards recovery. The greatest difficulty experienced was with the bowels, which were difficult to move both with drugs and enemata, the evacuation having a peculiarly foul odor. On two occasions the administration of enemata was followed by a burning sensation of the skin accompanied by an evanescent crop of urticaria. The same phenomena were experienced six months previously. Vomiting occurred occasionally after drinking.

Convalescence.—During the course of convalescence the bone drain tubes became softened and collapsed more than once, causing retention of a few drops of pus ; but it was never evident that the abscess cavity secreted any great amount of pus, the discharge consisting mainly of small pieces of necrosed brain tissue which had a peculiar phosphorus-like odor. The decalcified bone tubes seemed when new to be of a very suitable consistency for the purpose in hand, not being extruded by the pulsating brain as is often the case with rubber tubes, and causing less pain during insertion than the silver tubes which at one time I employed. By March 30, a fortnight after the operation, the nystagmus had entirely ceased, except when attempts were made to look to the right. The right external rectus was again at work, and some outward movement of the eyeball beyond the middle line was possible. At the end of the third week the patient was in a fair way to complete recovery, but as a precaution I did not finally remove the drains until another ten days had passed. By April 18, a month after the operation, the patient had for some days been walking about the ward. His appetite had (as in Acland and Ballance's case) become ravenous, and he was reported as "eating seven dinners a day." He put on flesh and gained in strength, making a rapid return to good health. His general condition is now excellent, and he is at present actively engaged in his trade of harness-making.

I should mention here that thanks to the assiduous care of our house-surgeon, Dr. Lewis, and the nursing staff, the cranial wound never caused a moment's anxiety on the score of sepsis, although it was kept open for nearly a month. I subsequently closed it by a small plastic operation.

Cerebration was at no time in abeyance, though slow during the period prior to the evacuation. Three months later he complained that he was still unable to keep the attention fixed for any length of time.

Cranial pain ceased within a week of the operation. The vertigo so prominent a symptom, particularly on movement, in the early stages, practically ceased on the evacuation of the cerebellar abscess. Syringing of that cavity caused its momentary return, and was accompanied by a subjective humming sound.

Vomiting occurred on drinking fluid for some days after the operation, and constipation was prominent for several days. A slight degree of optic neuritis was present from the first, but actual swelling and engorgement only occurred a few hours before the final operation. This swelling rapidly subsided, leaving no evident impairment of vision. The right pupil remained larger than the left for two months.

Lateral nystagmus was seen for the first time on the morning following the evacuation, and the paralysis of the right external rectus was noticed two days later. The former phenomenon ceased during the first fortnight of convalescence, but the paralysis and diplopia still persist, though in a very slight and diminishing degree.

Slight ataxia of the right hand was present in the early stages, and two months after the operation slight ataxia of the right foot was detected by a skilled neurologist. A month after the evacuation there was decided weakness in the grip of the right hand, but during the early stage the condition of the patient allowed of no very satisfactory experiments in this direction. For the same reason no evidence of a tendency to fall to one or other side was forthcoming, though the gait was very staggering in character before operation.

The knee-jerks were exaggerated until the period between the two explorations, when thay suddenly became extinct. They remained so for two months, but at the end of the third month that on the left was re-established, and that on the right was with difficulty detected. At this period the plantar reflex was normal. The facial palsy remains complete in spite of galvanic treatment, but no paræsthesia of the tongue can be made out. Evidence of hearing by bone conduction on the right side has never been forthcoming. DEADY.

Peck, A. H.—Relative Toxicity of Cocaine and Eucaine.—*Jour. Am. Med. Asso.*, September 9, 1899.

The author, while extensively experimenting with some of the essential oils upon guinea-pigs, also made several with cocaine and eucaine. From the comparison, which is given in full, he deduces the following conclusions.

"1. The action of cocaine is inconstant; one never knows whether the symptoms occasioned by like quantities of the drug, in animals or individuals, under like circumstances, will be similar or dissimilar.

"2. The action of eucaine is constant. The symptoms occasioned by the use of like quantities in animals, under like circumstances, and, so far as my experiments have gone, in different individuals, are the same.

"3. The first action of cocaine on the heart is that of a depressant, and on respiration it is that of a mild stimulant, the after-effects being, on the heart, that of a decided stimulant, and on the respiration that of a decided depressant.

"4. The first action of eucaine on both heart and respiration is that of a stimulant, the after-effects being that of a decided depressant.

"5. Cocaine causes death in animals by paralyzing the muscles of the respiratory apparatus, the heart's action continuing in a feeble way for a brief period after breathing ceases.

"6. Eucaine causes death in animals by paralyzing the muscles of the heart and of the respiratory apparatus, they ceasing to operate simultaneously.

"7. Eucaine in toxic doses nearly always causes nausea and occasionally vomiting.

"8. Cocaine is much less nauseating and scarcely ever causes vomiting.

"9. Eucaine is decidedly diuretic, causing renal discharge in a majority of instances in which a toxic dose is used.

"10. Cocaine is not a diuretic to an appreciable extent, renal discharge having occurred in only one instance in connection with all my experiments.

"11. The pupils of the eyes, in nearly all cases of cocaine poison, do not respond to light and are more or less bulging from their sockets.

"12. The pupils of the eyes in most cases of eucaine poisoning, do respond feebly to light, and rarely ever bulge from their sockets.

" 13. The action of toxic doses of eucaine is more like that of a paralyzing, tetanoiding, convulsion-producing agent, than it is like an anæsthetizing one, the plantar and cremasteric reflexes nearly always respond.

" 14. Toxic doses of cocaine cause general anæsthesia in connection with the other symptoms in the majority of cases.

" 15. True tetanus of all strip muscles of the limbs and Cheyne-Stokes' breathing nearly always occur with the use of cocaine, but seldom does either occur when eucaine is used.

" 16· Cocaine is at least three times more toxic than beta eucaine, and alpha eucaine is as toxic as cocaine.

" 17. Boiling does not destroy the efficacy of cocaine, but it does modify it, and boiling in no degree lessens the efficacy of cocaine." PALMER.

Zumbroish.—So-called Acute Idiopathic Perichrondritis of the Nasal Septum.—*Wiener klin. Woch.*, May 11, 1899.

This condition was first thoroughly treated of by Clinton Wagner of New York City. It commences by a general chill with fever following ; great swelling and redness of the nose follow ; rhinological examination discloses a massive bilateral swelling of the septum ; subsequently fluctuation, evidencing the presence of pus, appears.

Every constitutional and other cause for the inflammation must be excluded before diagnosis of idiopathic is made.

PALMER.

Grindelia Robusta.—*The Am. Hom.*, June 15, 1899.

Its chief, if not its only, use in respiratory troubles is as a remedy for asthma. " The grindelia asthmatic is plethoric, there is a dusky flush upon the surface, a congestion that no doubt pervades all of the tissues. The respiration is labored, ' choky.' To this case grindelia should be given in full doses—say in from ten to twenty drops.

" In certain cases of bronchoria or bronchitis, and in pneumonia with a choking sensation—dyspnœa ; in spasmodic cough grindelia should not be forgotten. It is also recommended in heart irregularities depending upon or accompanying these symptoms. In some cases of 'hay fever' grindelia is a very efficient remedy, not in all."   PALMER.

Dewey, W. A.—Verbascum Thapsus.—*The Am. Hom.*, November 15, 1899.

"This drug belongs to the scrofula-curing order of plants. Its general action is upon (1) the inferior maxillary branch of the fifth pair of cranial nerves, (2) the ear, (3) the respiratory tract, (4) the bladder.

"The symtomatology of the 2d and 3d classes is as follows:

"Ears.—These neuralgic symptoms, rending otalgias with sense of obstruction, especially indicate the remedy.

"Neuralgic earaches are greatly benefited by its use.

"Deafness.—Instillation of mullein oil has proved useful.

"Respiratory.—The cough is of laryngeal and tracheal origin, and it is especially marked by hoarseness ; the voice is deep, harsh, and hoarse—a 'basso-profundo.' It sounds like a trumpet. The cough is worse at night. It is a useful remedy in asthma and the chronic coughs of old people when there is much hoarseness."   PALMER.

Grant, Dundas.—Nasal and Aural Diseases as a Cause of Headache.—*Jour. of Lar., Rhin., and Otol.*, September, 1889.

In searching for the cause of obstinate headaches the author urges that attention should not only be directed to the teeth the refraction of the eye, the fundus oculi, the urine, etc., but a thorough examination of the nose, throat, and ear should be made before all the causes of the cephalalgia are considered exhausted.

The following conditions in the nose, etc., are enumerated as causative of headaches : obstruction arising from naso-pharyngeal adenoids, hypertrophy of the turbinated bodies, septal outgrowths and deviation, polypi and inflammatory polypoid excrescences, and diseases of the accessory sinuses.

While the diseases of the ear causing the same result are : chronic suppuration of the attic, cholesteatoma, swelling of the epithelial tissues or a recrudescence of the purulent exudations from the influence of moisture or sepsis, respectively.

Then follow interesting clinical reports of one or more cases illustrating each course.

Finally he says headache following mastoid operations, although usually due to them, may originate from some other cause. An instance of such a case is given in which anti-uratic treatment was curative on account of it occurring in a gouty individual.

PALMER.

Gould, Geo. M.—Massage and the Relief of Eye-Strain in the Treatment of Glaucoma.—*Canadian Jour. Med. and Surgery*, November, 1899.

The author submits the following cases, with directions for the performance of massage :

CASE 4255.—A man of fifty-two consulted me on April 2, 1896, with incipient stellar cataract of both eyes, a myopia of R. E. 6 D., and L. E. 7 diopters, a visual acuity of 20/100, each eye, with correcting lenses. With the exception of pain he had the typical symptoms of glaucoma, a shallowed anterior chamber, widened and sluggish pupils, cupping of the disks, etc. The tension of the right was +1, of the left +2. I instructed his niece how to carry out massage, but it was not done so systematically and thoroughly as I wished. By earnest and thorough instructions I secured more effective exercise of massage until, by October, the tension was normal in the right and but doubtfully plus in the left. I wish particularly to note that at this time only R. E. − Sph. 4.50 D. and L. E. − 5.50 D. were required to give the man a visual acuity of 20/70, while at the first visit lenses 1.5 D. stronger were required to give 20/100. Both the patient and niece recognize that the globes soften under massage, and if it is not done at least once a day the tension is likely to rise. For three years the eyes have thus been kept normal, the vision remains 20/70, and the cataracts show no increase.

CASE 4359.—A woman of sixty-six consulted me June 4, 1896, giving a history of glaucoma during the last four years. The left eye had been operated upon nine months previously, but the operation had proved a failure in every sense of the term. The iris had been torn from about one-half of its attachment, creating a large artificial pupil on the temporal side. The disk of this eye was deeply cupped, the vision reduced to counting of fingers. The tension was +2. I was finally compelled by the confusion of the images to exclude this mutilated left eye from participating in vision by means of a ground glass. Its high tension was by massage almost immediately reduced to normal, with a tendency to rise when the massage is too long intermitted. The woman visits me about once a month ; the eye has permanently remained painless, quiet, and with a normal or slightly elevated tension. At her first visit the right eye was over tense, +1, and massage was also ordered, as also a lens correcting the ametropia + S. 1.50 + C. 0.50 ax. 140 = 20/20. At her last visit the ametropic correction was + S. 2.25 + C. 0.50 ax. 180, of course with a proper presbyopic addition. The vision remains perfect and the tension permanently and perfectly normal. She keeps up the massage every day with conscientious and intelligent accuracy.

CASE 5298.—A woman of fifty-seven consulted me June 14, 1898, who had been treated for glaucoma for two and a half years by another oculist. Sclerotomy had been performed in the right eye fourteen months previously. The vision was R. E. 20/40, L. E. 20/20 ?, with the incorrect glasses she was wearing. The field was narrowed in the right eye to an extramacular vision of from 10° to 20°. The disk was typically cupped. I at once instituted massage and soon brought the tension to normal. Two months after the first visit the tension was normal and the field doubled in extent. I now carefully tested the refraction, and found the following ametropic error :

R. + S. 4.00 D. + C. 0.75 ax. 105° = 20/30+
L. + S. 4.00 D. + C. 0.37 ax. 160° = 20/20+
Exophoria 4°.   Left hyperphoria 4°.

After the relief of the severe eye-strain by proper glasses and gymnastic exercises, the massage was discontinued, and there has since not been a symptom of glaucoma, no rise of tension, and no trouble whatever from the eyes. On July 17, 1899, the field had become much more extended.

CASE 5456.—On December 11, 1898, I was called to see a woman of fifty-two suffering from a severe attack of glaucoma of the right eye, which had appeared two weeks previously and which in the absence of a specialist had been made worse by the use of atropine. Vision was abolished, the pain intense, with the usual objective symptoms of glaucoma, except the ophthalmoscopic ones, as it was impossible to secure even a red reflex from the retina. The patient would not allow the eye to be touched or operated upon, except imperfectly palpated to gain an estimate of the tension, which I made out as between +1 and +2. By the use of eserine, leeches to the temple, etc., with appropriate general treatment, I succeeded in allaying the pain and sensitiveness, but not the tension, until in about a month after the first visit I was permitted to institute treatment by massage. This soon brought down the tension to normal or occasionally slightly above. All symptoms of pain, etc., have disappeared. The massage is continued every day. The eye is blind and without retinal reflex. As a prophylactic measure I prescribed correcting lenses for the healthy left eye, the distance refractive error being + S. 2.50 D. + C. 0.50, ax. 45°.. It would be interesting to know what it was in the ruined eye.

CASE 5498.—On January 21, 1899, a woman of fifty-nine consulted me, who had been under the care of different oculists during the last six years for repeated attacks of glaucoma. She had refused to accept their advice as to the necessity of an operation. Her daughter told me that her mother had been subject to " dizzy spells " in which she fell to the floor, but without convulsions or biting of the tongue. I found the tension of the right eye normal, the media clear, some glaucomatous cupping, and a natural visual acuity of 20/200, not improvable by glasses. I tried vainly to find any lenses that would give increased visual acuity, so noting it on my case records. This is emphasized and to be remembered. The tension of the left eye was estimated as between +1 and +2, and the vision reduced to finger-counting only. The disk was typically cupped. I at once instituted massage of *both* eyes, carrying it out myself at first, and teaching the daughter how to do it. Two days after the first visit the patient returned with the tension " hardly above normal," and improved vision. I again attacked the refractive error and to my astonishment immediately secured the following result :

R. E. + S. 2.75 = 20/40.
L. E. + S. 2.00 + C. 1.00 ax. 150° = 20/30.

With these and appropriate reading glasses the woman for a while went about in a sort of dazed amazement at her ability to see objects so plainly. When the glasses had been fitted I ordered the massage to be discontinued. Up to the present time the visual acuteness remains 20/30, and the tension normal, with no treatment whatever except the glasses.

CASE 5578 was that of a man of forty who came to me April 6, 1899, giving a history of glaucoma treated at a hospital and also by a physician at his private office during the past year. During this time the instillation of eserine had been kept up daily. The only evidence I found of the truth of the diagnosis was the cupped disk of the right eye. At the first visit there was no increased tension and the vision and fields were normal. I found his glasses did not correct his refractive error, and I was so convinced that this refractive error was the sole cause of his past attacks of glaucoma that I had the audacity to use a mydriatic and refract his eyes, finding :

R. $+$ C. 1.12 D. ax. 180° $= 20/20+$
L. $+$ S. 0.50 $+$ C. 0.25 ax. 135° $= 20/20+$
Exophoria 2°.   Hyperphoria 1°.

There was no bad result from the mydriatic ; the eserine was discontinued, proper glasses were prescribed, no massage or other treatment whatsoever was ordered, and since then there has been no trouble as regards the eyes ; the man works every day as a clerk.

CASE 5326.—A woman of fifty-two came to me September 1, 1898, having had headaches from childhood. She first began noticing blue rings about lights about three years ago. Vision had been growing dim for three months. For nine months there had been great pain in the eyes. V. $= 20/50 +$ B. E. Tn., $=$ R. $+$ 1, L. $+$ 2. The corneas were insensitive, the anterior chambers shallow, the pupils almost immobile, but undersized rather than dilated. The disks and funduses were too ill-defined to describe. Massage was at once ordered and the next day the tension was only slightly above normal in the left eye. The following refractive error was found :

R. $-$ Sp. 0.25 $-$ Cyl. 0.50 ax. 90 $= 20/40+$
L. $-$ Sp. 0.50 $-$ Cyl. 0.37 ax. 180 $= 20/50$.

Presbyopic glasses only were ordered, eserine advised in case of need or emergency, and the daughter was carefully instructed in the method of carrying out massage. Several most encouraging letters were received during the next six months, and encouraged by these eserine was ordered to be discontinued. On September 1, 1899, my assistant, Dr. Murphy, on a visit to the Catskills, called upon this patient, and writes that the tension in each eye is absolutely normal, and that massage is kept up daily without eserine. Only since this report of Dr. Murphy have I ventured to include this case-history in the present report.

The technic of massage as I advise is simple, but requires delicacy of touch and intelligence on the part of those who carry it out. If the patient have these qualities she may be instructed in the art. If not, some friend or professional nurse must be taught. The soft parts of the ends of the fingers or thumbs are used, and through the closed lids. I begin with alternate palpation (called *taxis* by Dr. Richey, of Washington, D. C., who reports his results by the method in *Annals of Ophthalmology*, October, 1896) by two fingers exactly as in estimating tension, but much more slowly. All pressures and movements should begin and proceed to the extreme, very slowly and softly ; the release or lessening of pressure may be a little more quick, but never sudden. The depth of the denting, or the force exerted will depend on the hardness of the globe. In high tensions greater pressures are safe. When the tension under massage approaches the normal, as it will do, the force exerted will be lessened to that which would produce clear discomfort if one's own or the normal eye were pressed. The patient's judgment of the matter must be consulted, and will not be far wrong—an added reason for making the patient the operator when the intelligence and self-control will warrant.

Palpation should be through the upper lid with the eyeball in the positions of extreme adduction, normal forward-looking, extreme abduction, and extreme depression. In extreme elevation the lower lid is used. Each position must be ordered systematically while massage is being carried on ; (the position of the other eye may be observed as a guide) ; in this way fully three-fourths of the globe is operated upon. The length of the sitting depends upon the time required to bring about normal tension, which is usually from three to five minutes. Sometimes normal tension will not follow so soon. I have yet to see any considerable bad results, such as conjunctival hyperemia, although patients have sometimes alluded to the fact that there was some irritation or discomfort following long-continued or too rough manipulations. I alternate the alternate palpation with two fingers with shorter rolling or rubbing movements (effleurage), carrying the lid so far as easily movable with and beneath the finger around the equatorial regions of the globe.

DEADY.

Keller (of Cologne).—The Connection between Diseases of the Lachrymal Duct and Rhinology. *Treatment.*—August 24, 1899.

Special attention is directed to the mucous valve (so called by Husner) at the lower extremity of the lachrymal duct, which is opened for evacuation by inspiration.

He considers that the origin of the majority of the cases of disease of this duct is at the nasal extremity and proceed upward.

"Nasal disease co-exists in 95 to 97 per cent. of the cases." Not only removal of nasal hypertrophies and local treatment of intranasal structures are advocated, but cleansing and treatment of the duct per narium is recommended.

PALMER.

Ball, J. H.—Atrophic Rhinitis and Its Treatment.— *The Am. Hom.*, November 15, 1899.

Will pass over good paragraphs on ætiology and pathology except to say that in this disease we have a lessening of the blood supply which results in an atrophy, more especially of the serous glands than the muciferous glands—therefore the dried crusts.

"In the treatment two ends are sought: 1st, cleanliness; 2d, stimulation."

For the first a twenty-five per cent. solution of hydrogen dioxide in water is recommended; if from this patient complains of sensation of dryness, substitute liquid petroleum for the water.

The old time-worn applications of the text-books, such as glycerin, is contra-indicated because it dehydrates the tissues. Iodine is not beneficial, as it is an irritant and astringent and not a stimulant, while nitrate of silver, weak solution, also acts as an astringent, contracting the superficial blood-vessels, coagulating the albumin of the membrane, and destroying its vitality.

Instead of the latter balsam of Peru is substituted. "It is a stimulant, and as such its properties are especially directed toward the mucous membranes and secreting organs. It is as well a detergent. And if the case be complicated with ulceration, balsam of Peru is indicated where the ulcer is large, deep, indolent, and unhealthy, does not bleed easily, and exudes a discharge which is very offensive. The balsam is not only stimulating here, but also cleansing, deodorizing, and antiseptic."

In the ozenatous ulcerations zinc-oxide ointment is beneficial. Dusting the ulcer with protonuclein is also recommended.

External irritation of the Schneiderian membrane should be removed, therefore protect it from irritating vapors, tobacco smoke, sulphur fumes, dust, etc.

The diet should be highly nourishing.

The moist climate of seacoast, etc., is preferable to the dry atmosphere of the South, West, and high altitudes.

Finally the prescription of a homeopathic remedy is recommended. This to be done before any symptoms are masked by local treatment. PALMER.

Bronner, Adolph.—The Local Use of Formalin in the Treatment of Atrophic Rhinitis (often Called Ozena).—*Jour. Lar., Rhin., and Otol*, October, 1899. (Read before the British Medical Association.)

After cleansing with an alkaline solution, he uses formal or formalin 1 to 1000 or 1 to 2000 in water in a nasal syringe, or the 1 to 500 or 1 to 1000 plus a little glycerin in a spray. If it is painful dilute. As it has a powerful effect of the glandular tissue, do not use too strong or for too long a time. He considered 25 to 30 per cent. of cases of ozena due to sinusitis. PALMER.

McBride, P. (Edinburgh).—The Treatment of Ozena, with Special Reference to Cupric Electrolysis. —*Edinburgh Med. Jour.*, March, 1899.

After making short review of the usual methods of treatment, he proceeds to give history of the development of this mode of treatment.

The strength of current used was from 3 to 10 milliamperes, rarely exceeding the latter. After cleansing the nostrils cocaine was usually employed, then the copper needle, attached to the positive pole, was introduced into the inferior or middle turbinated, sometimes into the tissues of the middle meatus, while the platinum (or steel) needle was inserted into the septum. Sitting lasted about ten minutes.

Usually the patients complained of little or no pain ; once it caused neuralgia and swelling of the eye.

Experiments were made upon eight patients. Four were practically cured for a year and a half—that is, the fetor and scurfs disappeared, although the atrophic condition of the membrane continued. In two improvement for a few weeks only. The remaining two were improved.

He concludes that cupric electrolysis "is probably the most valuable therapeutic resource that has yet been suggested."

PALMER.

Bull, Chas. Stedman.—Multiple Sinus Disease Following Influenza.—*Med. Rec.*, September 2, 1899.

A very interesting and instructive clinical record of a case of a lady fifty-eight years of age, in which developed as sequelæ of influenza a true empyema of all the nasal accessory sinuses, and two weeks after cure of nasal sinusitis by operative measures, mastoid disease developed on the right side.   PALMER.

Palmer, A. W.—The Interdependence of the Diseases of the Throat and Nose and Those of the General System.—*N. Am. Jour. of Hom.*, October, 1899.

Subject divided into (1) nasal and throat diseases dependent upon unhealthy conditions in other portions of the body, and (2) disease outside the dominion of the nose and throat caused by abnormal conditions of the upper respiratory tract.

Under the first division are considered the several catarrhal diseases and ulcerations of upper air passages which occur as sequelæ of the zymotic diseases (not those occurring during the same). Gastric disease often causes catarrh of the nares and naso-pharynx. Hepatic disorders are causative of inflammations of the adenoid tissues and turbinals. Epistaxis may be a result of alcoholic gastritis or cirrhotic liver. Menstruation or cohabitation aggravates catarrhs. Catarrhs or lymphoid hypertrophies may be caused by chronic inflammation of the sexual apparatus, —this is considered due to auto-intoxication. Uric-acid diathesis may cause inflammation of the lymphoid tissue and turbinals, quinsy, ulceration of the pharynx, anchylosis of the cryco-arytenoid articulation, or nasal sinusitis. Tophuli in the vocal cords have been observed. One authority considers hay-fever of gouty origin. Epistaxis may be an early symptom of Bright's or a precursor of a uræmic attack.

(2) may be subdivided : (a) reflex, (b) auto-intoxication, (c) interference with normal function. (a) Nasal spur, deflection, or synechiæ my cause irritating dry cough or asthma. Elongated uvula, hypertrophy of lingual tonsil, or follicular pharyngitis cause emphysema per intervention of protracted cough. Pressure of spur, polypus, or deflection has caused phlyctenular conjunctivitis, blepharitis, asthenopia, or myopia. From same irritation we m₁y have palpitation of the heart or tachycardia. (b) Chronic dyspepsia, recurrent tonsilitis, otitis media suppurativa acuta, meningitis, conjunctivitis phlyctenulosa, or bronchitis chronica may be sequelæ of catarrhalis chronica or sinusitis. Deafness may result from obstruction of nasal respiration. Otitis media suppurativa and chronica result from tonsilar hypertrophy, and insufficient lung capacity from nasal obstruction. By spreading, by contiguity of tissue, dermatitis, erysipelas, meningitis, delirium, or melancholia may follow intra-nasal or sinus disease.

PALMER.

Dr. Gilman.—Conium and Its Cough Symptoms.—*The Am. Hom.*, October 6, 1899.

The doctor, in an excellent study of this drug, refers to cough symptoms as follows :

" The cough is very persistent, frequent, and tormenting. It is periodical, dry, excited by itching, grating, tickling in the throat and behind the sternum, and is especially evoked by lying down, talking, or laughing. Old people often have a very troublesome cough at night, a dry cough seeming to originate in a small irritated or dry spot in the larynx. Expectoration only occurs after coughing a long time. The cough is apt to continue until an asthmatic attack supervenes. Hacking, almost continual, cough at night on lying down. It is one of the best remedies for the dry, teasing, continuous cough, worse on lying down at night, in old people or those prematurely old. In subacute bronchitis the cough is spasmodic, dry, teasing, worse in evening and at night, greatly fatiguing the patient. It is best adapted to old persons or those prematurely so, dried up old maids, and individuals of rigid fiber, people with yellow skin and skin lacking in action, with eruptions of a papula kind, or old ulcerations discharging

an offensive ichorous matter. The whole of the symptoms point
to the lessened vitality caused by paralysis and lack of nutrition
due to the lessened nerve supply."   PALMER.

Merry, W. J. C.—Idiopathic Perforation of the Bones of the Nasal System.—*The Lancet*, November 4, 1899.

A very interesting and full clinical history of lady forty years
old. Had deflected septa in contact with a hypertrophied right
inferior turbinated. Cauterization of the latter relieved the obstruction of which patient complained. Five months after a
severe coryza supervened, followed by purulent discharge of
about four months' duration. Then rhinoscopic examination
showed right nares completely occluded by pale, soft, friable, insensitive granulations. On removal of these with spoon a perforation the size of a shilling was found in the septum at the
articulation of the triangular cartilage, vomer, and perpendicular
plate of the ethmoid. The greatest care possible was taken to
search for symptoms or history of any syphilitic disease by the
author and a rhiniologist ; and they were satisfied that it was
not of such origin.   PALMER.

Jacques, P.—Ozena and Sinusitis.—*Rev. Herb. de Lar.* *etc.*—August 19, 1899 (per J. A. M. Assoc.).

" Idiopathic ozena is a myth," the writer declares. Ozena is
merely the secondary consequences of sinusitis of one or more of
the nasal fossæ. All therapeutic measures for ozena to date
merely respond to the symptomatic indication to combat the atony
resulting from sclerosis of the pituitary membrane due to irritations from sinusal secretions. Moure has noted 32 cases of verified sinusitis in 114 of ozena, and if we were able to examine the
spheno-ethmoidal system as easily as the fronto-maxillary, this
coincidence would probably be found the rule. Each sinus
should be minutely interrogated in turn, he concludes, in every
case of ozena.   PALMER.

Oliver, Charles A.—Traumatic Varix of the Orbit.—*Am. Jour. of Med. Sciences*, Philadelphia, March.

On July 9, 1894, T. T., a twenty-seven-year-old brakeman,
came to my clinic at Wills Eye Hospital with the history that
five days previously his left eye had been either kicked or struck

with a fist. For two days after the injury he did not notice any-thing peculiar, but on the third day the eyelids became much swollen, and on the fourth day the eyeball became prominent. This was followed by a "constant buzzing, with some pain," which the patient referred chiefly to the left temporal and audi-tory regions.

The man was in a highly nervous state, with marked tremor, especially of the extremities, he having just passed through a subacute attack of alcoholism of nearly three weeks' standing.

Examination of the affected eye and its surrounding parts showed that the upper lid was so much swollen and œdematous that it fell over in front of the eyeball. There was an intense chemosis of the ocular conjunctiva, which was so pronounced in its inferior half as to allow a broad fold of the membrane to project through the palpebral fissure and rest upon the skin of the lower lid. The globe itself, which, with the exception of a slight wheel-like motion down and in, was immobile, could be rotated a few degrees in different directions by forced palpation. The organ was proptosed directly forward. Its cornea was clear. The pupil was three millimeters in diameter. There was absolutely no movement of the iris to any form of direct or con-sensual impulse. Intraocular tension was normal, and there was not any ciliary tenderness.

Vision was reduced to one-eighth of normal, this being in a measure accounted for by a history of convergent strabismus which had existed since infancy, the sight of the left eye always having been defective.

The patient stated that when he was four years of age he was caught between two railroad cars, inflicting such an injury to his head that he bled from the mouth, the nose, and the ears.

The fields of vision for white and red of the affected eye ex-hibited decided indentations in the lower inner quadrants, with a slight enlargement of the physiological blind spot.

Ophthalmoscopic examination showed that the retinal veins were enlarged and tortuous, while the contained venous currents were so dark in places as to appear almost black. No hemor-rhage of any kind could be determined. A marked bruit in the temporal region, which was synchronous with the radial pulse, could be plainly recognized by direct auscultation. No orbital bruit or pulsation could be either heard or felt.

When the left common carotid artery during its passage through the neck was forcibly compressed for a brief period of time by the finger-tips, the affected eye slowly sank into place only to resume its former false position the moment that the pressure was removed ; while some of the palpebral and conjunctival stasis subsided.

The right eye was healthy and normal in all respects.

For the purposes of further study I immediately admitted the man into the wards of the hospital. In two days' time both the palpebral and the conjunctival chemosis had become greater and the proptosis had become more marked. Constant digital and mechanical compression upon the left common carotid artery was then decided upon and faithfully, though uselessly, persisted in for a period of eleven days, the external conditions becoming much worse and the bruit so intense as to be rendered almost unbearable to the patient. Ophthalmoscopic examination at this time showed that the retinal veins of the affected organ were much more swollen than they were when the patient was admitted into the hospital.

At this juncture, as I was about to leave the city for my summer vacation, I left the case in charge of Dr. George C. Harlan, one of my colleagues at the hospital, we agreeing that a radical operation for the relief of the condition should be tried at once.

Just before his dismissal from the hospital to go to the surgical wards of the Pennsylvania Hospital, to which institution he was sent by Dr. Harlan, he complained of pain in the left ear and upper jaw; both of which had become markedly swollen. The cornea of the affected eye was becoming hazy in its deeper layers, allowing but a dim view of the fundus. The retinal veins were enormously dilated and tortuous, while the retina itself was quite opaque in places.

On August 3 the left common carotid artery was tied by Dr. Thomas S. K. Morton of this city.

Under ether-narcosis an incision was made in the line of the sterno-mastoid muscle on the left side of. the patient's neck, and the common carotid artery was exposed at the point of election above its crossing by the omohyoid muscle. Pressure upon the elevated vessel at this point entirely controlled the bruit and pulsation. The vessel was tied by a treble ligature after the manner suggested by Ballance and Edmunds. This ligature consisted of three large strands of twisted silk being passed about the vessel. Each strand was tied tightly down by one knot, after which all six of the ends were tied in a second knot, thus cutting off and bringing into apposition almost a quarter of an inch of the coats of the vessel. The wound was closed by a continuous silk thread. No drainage was employed.

Not the slightest symptom of so large an artery having been ligated followed the procedure, there being an entire cessation of the pulsation and the bruit. The eye immediately settled back into the orbit, and nothing remained to denote the former condition save a pouch of conjunctiva which projected from the lower lid.

¶Five hours after the operation Dr. William C. Posey, my assistant at Wills Eye Hospital, kindly saw the case for me. Both the bruit and the exophthalmos had greatly diminished. The eye-ground could be more distinctly seen, the retinal veins not being so distended as they were before the operation. Uncorrected vision equaled one-tenth of normal.

Six days later the exophthalmos had much lessened and the palpebral œdema and the conjunctival chemosis had greatly subsided, allowing the patient to elevate the upper lid and to have some control over the movements of the eyeball. The retinal veins were not swollen. For the first time a few points of retinal extravasation in direct association with the veins could be determined. Vision was the same as when the patient was seen before.

On January 27, 1896, some five months after the operation for ligation, he returned to the hospital with the statement that the eye had gradually become blind, and that it took several weeks' time for the swelling of the lids and conjunctiva to disappear.

At this time it was found that the eyeball was convergent, the scleral veins were enlarged, the cornea was clear, the pupil was widely dilated, the anterior chamber was shallow with almost total obliteration of its angle, and the lens was cataractous. Intraocular tension was increased, and the eye was absolutely blind. There was no ciliary tenderness. In other words, the condition of an absolute secondary glaucoma was present. The fellow eye continued normal.

REMARKS.—The head-crush at four years of age most probably was the beginning of either an aneurismal varix situated between the petrous and the cavernous portions of the internal carotid artery and the corresponding cavernous sinus, or a varicose aneurism in which there was an intervening sac or so-called false aneurismal connection located between the two vascular channels. In either case in a well-protected situation and the connected veins subject to but little arterial pressure, it—as in all such forms of vascular disturbance—was of very slow growth and may have even terminated its extending process.

The more recent blow upon the diseased region in a debilitated subject—given to alcoholic excesses, most probably—increased the opening into the venous structures so as to give as its most prominent ophthalmic sign an orbital varix.

The cessation of the gross venous stasis of the related vascular structures of the orbit, and the eyeball and its appendages, by ligation of the main trunk supplying blood to the parts, is of interest both in regard to therapy and ætiology. The appearance of the signs of absolute secondary glaucoma as the final outcome of the condition of the ocular tissues may be in a measure understood when it is considered that the eyeball is a lymph-producing organ which is dependent upon normal blood-supply.

BOOK REVIEWS.

A MANUAL OF DISEASES OF THE NOSE AND THROAT. By COR-
NELIUS G. COAKLEY, A. M., M. D., Clinical Professor of
Laryngology in the University and Bellevue Hospital Medical
College ; Laryngologist to Columbus Hospital, The University
and Bellevue Hospital Medical College Clinic, and the Demilt
Dispensary ; Member of the New York Academy of Medicine,
Society of the Alumni of Bellevue Hospital, and Medical
Society of the County of New York. Illustrated with ninety-
two engravings and two colored plates. Lea Bros. & Co.,
New York and Philadelphia, 1899.

Dr. Coakley's Manual is a moderately small, clearly but concisely written, and, on account of the concise manner in which it
is written, a very full book for its size of 525 pages.

Every subject or disease is treated in a methodical manner—
to wit, divided into (1) Ætiology ; (2) Pathology ; (3) Symptoms ;
(4) Examination ; (5) Differential Diagnosis ; (6) Prognosis ; (7)
Treatment ; and in some cases a paragraph on Complications is
included.

The anatomy, although very tersely given, is quite full, as may be
judged by the mentioning of the occasional presence of a fourth
supernumerary turbinated bone or body in the nares.

Upon the thorough perusal of any book we can usually find a
weak point, and in this one it is the brief way in which the pathology of the different diseased conditions is treated. The author's
object throughout appears to be conciseness, and he seems to
consider this department to be one in which he could make the
most condensation while producing a practical work.

This weakness, on the other hand, is almost balanced by the
many minute directions he has given under the heading of
treatment, or, in other words, the practical suggestions in some
of the minor operative procedures. Under this head we would
call attention to his diagrams for excision of septal exostoses and

incision of peritonsilar abscess; also mention his inferred advocacy of the thorough extirpation of the faucial tonsils.

But we must admit that some of the conventional diagrams of the nasal and accessory cavities, selected from Zuckerkandl, are rather misleading.

On the other hand, the chapter on the care of instruments is very good indeed, but a little extreme in some points ; still, not only the general practitioner, but also many of the older laryngologists, would do well to peruse it and carry them out more fully in practice.

In conclusion, would indorse this book for the field in which the author in his perface says he intends it—that is, for the student and general practitioner.

CATARRH, COLDS AND GRIPPE. Including Prevention and Cure, with chapters on Nasal Polypus, Hay Fever, and Influenza. By JOHN H. CLARKE, M. D., Consulting Physician to the London Homoeopathic Hospital; Editor of the *Homeopathic World ;* Author of " The Prescriber," "A Dictionary of Domestic Medicine," " Indigestion : Its Causes and Cure, " " A Bird's-Eye View of Homeopathic System of Medicine," etc. American Edition. Revised by the Author from the Fourth English Edition. Philadelphia : Boericke & Tafel, 1899. Price, cloth, 75 cents ; by mail, 80 cents.

This little book is written in a very easy or fluent style, can probably be read from cover to cover in less than one hour, still, there is scarcely a page of the 125 that has not some little hint that will be beneficial to the physician at some time during a winter's practice.

The subject is a very commonplace, everyday one, and may be considered too much so for consideration by many of our busy medical men, and yet it seems that many of the small common-sense ideas touched upon in this monograph are too often overlooked by the hurried physician on account of having his mind occupied with more serious or weighty subjects. Although almost every doctor knows all that is in the first half of the book, it will do none of us harm (but rather benefit us) to remind ourselves of such fundamental facts.

While we can scarcely agree with the sentence, " In some instances one attack of cold appears to be protective against other attacks," and one or two other points ; still the following good advice regarding cold prevention and cure in cases of la grippe, which the author denominates epidemic influenza, would very materially reduce the frequency of these conditions and their troublesome sequelæ. "One of the chief precautions against cold is the avoidance of 'coddling.' The muffler is a great snare. It is much better to accustom the neck to bear a certain amount of exposure, giving it the protection of collar and tie, but nothing more "; and when treating of epidemic influenza he says, "What about going to bed? In a severe case this question needs no answer—the patient simply cannot stay up. . . Wherever there is the slightest doubt it should be decided in favor of bed, etc."

In the chapter on Materia Medica there are mentioned thirty-one remedies, with short but clear indications for each. This is instructive on account of including some remedies infrequently employed in this class of diseases—for instance, bapt. tinct., lemna alba, magn. mur., etc. In this chapter is the peculiarity of this book, and an exceedingly practical one, too. Not only the potency of the recommended drug is given, but also the amount of such and the frequency of administration.

In summing up we think this monograph almost indispensable to the younger practitioner and an exceedingly good reminder to the more mature one.

REFRACTION AND HOW TO REFRACT. Including Sections on Optics, Retinoscopy, the Fitting of Spectacles and Eye-Glasses, etc. By JAMES THORINGTON, A. M., M. D., Adjunct Professor of Ophthalmology in the Philadelphia Polyclinic and College for Graduates in Medicine ; Assistant Surgeon at Will's Eye Hospital ; Associate Member of the American Ophthalmological Society ; Fellow of the College of Physicians of Philadelphia ; Member of the American Medical Association ; Ophthalmologist to the Elwyn and the Vineland Training Schools for Feeble-minded Children; Resident Physician and Surgeon Panama Railroad Company, at Colon (Aspinwall), Isthmus of Panama, 1882–1889, etc. Two Hundred Illustrations, thirteen of which are colored. Octavo. 301 pp. $1.50 net, cloth. P. Blakiston's Son & Co., 1012 Walnut Street, Philadelphia, Pa.

Dr. Thorington has again placed the ophthalmic student under great obligation in this little book, which, while occupying a larger field, is equally as forcible, equally as accurate and should be equally as popular as his brochure on the shadow test. The author has the happy faculty of imparting his information in terse dogmatic sentences, which say just what they mean and mean just what they say ; not a word wasted and still the subject is adequately considered.

This book should be the standard work for the beginner in refractive work. Not that it is elementary ; far from it, on the contrary it contains much information that will be missed in more pretentious works, but it takes nothing for granted ; the subject is explained from the ground up. Taking up optics, it gives the necessary information in a nutshell, and does it well without mathematical formulæ to confuse such as are not sufficiently familiar with this branch of the subject. Then follows a description of the physiological eye and the mechanism of vision, the use of the ophthalmoscope, the various forms of ametropia ; retinoscopy ; the muscular anomalies ; a chapter (an excellent one) on cyclophysics and the examination of the eyes ; how to refract ; a a chapter of cases from practice including all forms of refractive error and the methods by which they were corrected ; concluding with the varieties of lenses, spectacles, and eyeglasses, with directions for taking measurements and fitting. There is not a word of trash from cover to cover ; everything is concise, accurate, sufficient, and up to date.

It would have seemed almost impossible to efficiently apply the author's dogmatic style to the subject of refraction, but he has done it and done it well ; and if his work fails to become *the* text-book for students in this line it will fall short of its deserts.

ANNUAL AND ANALYTICAL CYCLOPEDIA OF PRACTICAL MEDICINE. By CHARLES E. DE M. SAJOUS, M. D., and One Hundred Associate Editors, assisted by Corresponding Editors, Collaborators and Correspondents. Illustrated with Chromo-lithographs, Engravings, and Maps. Volume IV. Philadelphia, New York, Chicago : The F. A. Davis Co., Publishers, 1899, Pp. 622.

The volume of this important work under discussion takes up alphabetically the subjects from " Infants, Diarrhœal Diseases of " to " Mercury," both inclusive, and contains among other important articles those on Insanity, by the late Dr. Rohé ; Malarial Fevers, by Professor Jas. C. Wilson and Dr. Thos. G. Ashton ; Locomotor Ataxia, by Dr. W. B. Pritchard ; Intubation, by Professor F. E. Waxham ; Diseases of the Liver, by Professor

Alexander McPhedran; and Meningitis, Dr. Charles M. Hay. It also contains a paper on Leprosy by the Editor-in-chief.

The opening chapter, on Diarrhœal Diseases of Infants, by Professor Blackader of Montreal, is a valuable contribution, covering some twenty-nine pages and discussing the various forms of infantile diarrhea from the points of ætiology, pathological anatomy, diagnosis, prognosis, symptomatology, and treatment, the latter including a consideration of the various methods of feeding useful in so-called "summer complaint."

The article on Insanity, probably the last work of the late Dr. Rohé, is well written, practical both from the clinical and medico-legal aspects, and thorough so far as the seventy-five pages allotted to it will allow.

Intubation receives careful treatment at the hands of Professor Waxham, is well illustrated with cuts of the necessary instruments and the best methods of introducing the tube, and contains valuable tables of the comparative success of the method in over six hundred cases. The current volume should be of especial interest to our readers, as it contains articles on the iris, ciliary body, and choroid, on keratitis (with an illustration of a steam generator originated by Dr. E. J. Bissell of Rochester, late President of the American Homeopathic Ophthalmological, Otological, and Laryngological Society), on diseases of the lachrymal apparatus, on laryngitis (illustrated with well-executed chromo-lithographs), on diseases of the lens and of the internal ear.

About forty pages is devoted to Dr. McPhedran's excellent article on diseases of the liver, which is well worth perusal.

One of the most interesting papers in the work is that on Malarial Fevers, covering some fifty-five pages and discussing at length the malarial parasite in all its varieties (illustrated with several beautifully executed full-page chromo-lithographs containing representations of the microscopic pictures of all the known forms) and the manner of inspection, with temperature charts of the different types of the disease, and a very complete consideration of the malady in its various modes of expression.

In the present volume, as in those which preceded it, the subject matter is brought up to date by the insertion of abstracts from the current literature of the world in the body of each article, such abstracts in the present case including the year 1898.

The paper, presswork, and binding are as usual unexceptionable, and the volume is an exceedingly handsome one.

A MANUAL OF THE DIAGNOSIS AND TREATMENT OF DISEASES OF THE EYE. By EDWARD JACKSON, A. M., M. D.; Emeritus Professor of Diseases of the Eye in the Philadelphia Polyclinic, etc. With one hundred and seventy-eight illustrations and two colored plates. Philadelphia : W. B. Saunders, 925 Walnut Street, 1900. Pp. 604. Price $2.50.

As the preface states, this little book is intended for the general practitioner, and the beginner in ophthalmology, and it gives the place of first importance to the recognition and management of the conditions likely to be presented early in practice, rather than to the rarer diseases and more difficult operations that may come later. The volume before us is well adapted to the end in view. While it covers all of the important diseases of the eye, the treatment is brief, practical, easily understood, and yet sufficient for the purpose intended. Having once mastered the contents of this book, the student will find himself in possession of an excellent groundwork in ophthalmology, leaving his knowledge to be rounded out by further reading adapted to his inclinations or necessities.

Whatever is given is excellent and up to date, and in Chapter XX., treating of ocular symptoms and lesions connected with general diseases, the author has adopted the method, when speaking of the ocular manifestations of any general disease, of inserting in the body of the text the page number of the article covering such ocular affection. This is systematically carried out throughout the entire chapter, adding very much to the value of the work in the hands of the general practitioner.

Another item worth mentioning is the index, which is copious for the size of the volume, and will be appreciated by the reader.

To those acquainted with the author it is unnecessary to say that the book is well written and up to date. It is a handy little volume, and will be very useful to the class of readers for whom it is intended.

The text is interspersed with a large number of excellent cuts, and there are two full-page chromo-lithographs containing representations of certain conditions of the optic nerve and retina as seen by the aid of the ophthalmoscope.

The paper, presswork, and binding are good.

VOL. XII.   APRIL, 1900.   PART 2.

THE JOURNAL OF OPHTHALMOLOGY, OTOLOGY AND LARYNGOLOGY.

EDITOR,

CHARLES DEADY, M. D.

ASSOCIATE EDITOR,

A. W. PALMER, M. D.

A SYMPOSIUM ON ORBITAL DISEASES.*

(*In three parts :* a, *Tumors of the Lachrymal Gland ;* b, *Some Grave Lachrymal Complications ;* c, *Malignant Tumors of the Orbit.*)

a.—TUMORS OF THE LACHRYMAL GLAND.

BY DR. ROGMAN (OF GAND).

THE pathological history of tumors of the lachrymal gland is at the present time much confused. Without being numerous, observations relating to these affections are not entirely wanting. In 1868 Polaillon, in his article in the *Dictionnaire encyclopédique de Dechambre,* " Pathology of the Lachrymal Gland," recounted eighteen cases of tumors : fifteen cases of hypertrophy or adenoma (those of Gluge, Lebert, Busch, Warlomont, Fano, Rothmund, Pemberton, Berard, Halpin, Mackenzie, Todd, Anderson, Lawrence, Maslieurat-Lagemard), two cases of enchondroma (those of Busch and O'Beirne), and one case of true cancer (by Mackenzie). Pröhl[1] raised this total to 91, including the following affections : hypertrophy 20, hydatids 1, dermoid 1, lymphomata 3, myxoma 1, myx-

---

Annales d'oculistique, February, 1900. Translated by W. S. Pearsall, M. D., New York.

[1] Friedr. Pröhl.—" Zur Casuistik der Geschwulste der Thränendrüse." *Inaug. Diss.* Berlin, 1892.

adenoma 1, adenomata 7, adenoid 4, fibro-adenomata 3, fibroid 1, fibromata 4, fibro-sarcoma 1, adeno-sarcoma 1, sarcomata 12, chondromata 2, enchondro-myxo-carcinoma 1, adeno-enchondroma 1, scirrhus 8, encephaloid 1, medullary fungoid 2, carcinomata 15, chloromata 3. Through the researches of Schaeffer[2] the number of cases of tumors of the lachrymal gland reached to the number of 128, including 30 taken from ancient literature: sarcomata 21, adenomata 12, carcinomata 12, cylindromata 2. The same year Piazzi[3] mentions only 48 cases, among which he includes those of simple hypertrophy reported by Polaillon and Debierre. In his treatise, Panas,[4] confining himself only to recent cases, presents but about thirty all together.

Whatever be their number, the study of these facts, however difficult it may seem, should serve as a basis for formal, general conclusions. When, in fact, we review those that have been published, we quickly discover that in a great number the anatomical diagnosis is not rigorously fixed and that the indications of their topographical or histological origin are insufficient: noticeably, the diagnosis of endothelioma is hardly ever found clearly stated. Moreover, in 1867, Koester,[5] criticising a case of adenoid published by Becker,[6] advanced the opinion that the case of this author, like all the others, taken in connection with its own peculiarities and the qualities of hypertrophies, of adenoids or of chancroids, corresponded uniformly to those affections having their origin in the lymphatic vessels; and this view of Koester has been confirmed by the researches of Sattler[7] and of Billroth.[8] In the encyclopedia of Graefe-

[2] Schaeffer.—"Ein Fall von Sarcom der Thränendrüse." *Inaug. Diss.*, Giessen, 1895.

[3] L. Piazzi.—"Adenoma della glandola lacrimale." *Annali di Ottalmologia*, Anno XXIV., 1895, fasc. 2–3.

[4] Panas.—*Traité des maladies des yeux.* Tome II. p. 327.

[5] Koester.—"Cancroid mit hyaliner Degeneration (Cylindroma Billroth's)." *Virchow's Archiv.* Bd. LX. S. 500.

[6] Becker.—"Ueber das Adenom der Thränendrüse." *Bericht über die Augenklinik der Wiener Universität.* 1863–77, S. 162.

[7] Sattler.—*Ueber die sogenannte Cylindrome*, S. 187.

[8] Billroth.—*Chirurg. Klinik.* Wien, 1871–76. S. 102.

Saemisch, Berlin[9] recommends prudence in the diagnosis of tumors of the lachrymal gland, adding, in order to give weight to his statement, that he does not believe that a duly authenticated case of adenoma of this organ exists. And de Wecker, in his treatise,[10] does not seem less severe. Apparently these cautions received but slight consideration, since the charges were again brought forward about four years ago by Van Duyse,[11] who believes that enchondroma should be stricken definitely from the nosology of the lachrymal gland, that the existence of adenoma is uncertain, that cases of true primary carcinoma have not been incontestibly demonstrated ; almost all neoplasms will then be endotheliomata, as Koester has said. No less does Alt[12] hold the same ideas when, having had to examine seven tumors of the lachrymal gland, he says : " I believe that I am not in error in concluding that tumors of the lachrymal gland very frequently take their origin in the interstitial connective tissue and only in rare cases take on a character truly epithelial." It is to be remarked that in these later times this conception is not accepted in all its rigor by Vossius,[13] who notes most frequently sarcoma and carcinoma or mixed forms, then adenoma and cylindroma, and more rarely fibromata, enchondromata, and cysts. Fuchs[14] recognizes carcinoma, adenoma, cylindroma, lymph-adenoma, and sarcoma. Haab[15] speaks of carcinoma, of sarcoma, of adenoma, etc. Finally, less exclusively also, Axenfeld[16]

[9] Berlin.—" Die Tumoren der Augenhöhle." *Handbuch der gesammten Augenheilkunde.* Bd. VI. S. 720.

[10] De Wecker et Landolt.—" *Traité complet d'ophtalmologie.*" Tome IV. p. 1030.

[11] Van Duyse.—"Contribution à l'étude des endothéliomes de l'orbite." *Bull. de l'Acad. de méd. de Belgique.* Tome IX., 1895.

[12] Alt.—" Another Case of Tumor of the Orbital Lachrymal Gland." *Amer. Jour. of Ophth.* March, 1897, p. 72.

[13] Vossius.—*Lehrbuch der Augenheilkunde.* 1898, S. 291.

[14] Fuchs.—*Manuel d'ophtalmologie. Traduction française.* 2me edition, 1897, p. 608.

[15] Haab.—*Atlas der ausseren Erkrankungen des Auges,* 1899, S. 70.

[16] Lubarsch und Ostertag.—*Ergebnisse der speciellen pathologischen Morphologie und Physiologie der Sinnesorgane,* 1896, S. 78.

believes that, in spite of the difficulties inherent to the diagnosis of this class of tumors, there is no reason to doubt the possible existence of carcinoma and adenoma.

Under these conditions we believe it to be opportune to publish a case that we have examined, and which includes several interesting points in the subject under discussion.

H. S., aged forty-nine, custom-house officer; has noticed for two and a half or three years that his right eye was protruding from the orbit and that this deformity gradually increased up to the present time, when he presented himself for examination. Has never experienced any pain. He does not remember to have had any previous wound of the interior or about the diseased eye. The vision has not ceased to be good on both sides. The movements of the eye are free; no diplopia is apparent. The visual acuteness is normal in both eyes. The right eye is found to be considerably pushed forward and inward. The spontaneous closure of the lids is complete. Palpation gives evidence of a tumor about as hard as contracted muscle at the superior external angle of the orbit in the region of the lachrymal gland. Ophthalmic examination shows the fundus of the eye to be entirely normal. There was no induration of the glands. Before his arrival at our clinic the patient had already undergone an attempted puncture of the tumor, and an antisyphilitic treatment had been uselessly tried. We proposed radical surgical intervention.

The first of June, 1899, under anæsthesia, an incision was made along the external border of the superior orbital arch. We came at once upon the tumor, which was more or less adherent to the orbital vault, and its contour was easily made out and isolated from the other parts by the finger. The detachment of the tumor from the bone was accomplished with the finger nail, from before backward; and the tumor, fallen into the lower part of the orbit, was brought forward, freed of its posterior adhesions by a few strokes of the scissors, and extracted. It was the size of a chestnut, measuring three centimeters by two and a half by two. During the operation it had been somewhat maltreated : it presented the appearance of a pouch with a tough, thickened capsule, in which the more or less friable matter had been divided and softened by the manipulations.

The wound of the operation healed by first intention; the

ptosis which appeared after the operation diminished gradually for a couple of months, when it entirely disappeared. The vision and the mobility of the eye were maintained in all their integrity.

Eight months have nearly passed, and from news recently received we apprehend that the situation continues to improve.

The tumor was divided into four slices, and the segments plunged alternately into Flemming's and into Muller's fluid. I made a number of selections of each of these pieces ; the first were stained with safranine, the second with hematoxylin and with the von Gieson.

The microscopical examination demonstrated the tumor to be formed of a thick enveloping membrane composed of connective tissue of compact, dense-grown fibers, with few cellular elements, inclosing in its substance on one side little cavities filled by the normal lobules of the lachrymal gland and covered on the side corresponding to the exterior face by the same lobules. This membrane completely inclosed the tumor, through which it sent no marked prolongations or septa. The tumor itself is composed of a tissue essentially the same throughout : convoluted tubes branching upon each other, their lumen now almost nothing and again more or less large, most often empty, sometimes filled with a substance of granular appearance rarely slightly colored. These tubes are lined almost uniformly by a double row of epithelial cells ; the internal layer being small, flat, and cuboidal, the external layer cylindrical. Sometimes the cells of the inner layer become cylindrical like those of the external layer ; and, on the other hand again, the first are cylindrical and the second cuboidal. But the proximal layer always possesses a dense, more or less granular protoplasm, the distal layer a clear transparent protoplasm. More rarely, in some places the epithelial layers become more numerous and seem to invade the structure. Finally, here and there may be found structures analogous to epidermal pearls. These tubes are separated by a loose cellular tissue of delicate fibers, more abundant in some places than in others. Leucocytes are also seen in places. Outside the cylindrical cellular layer is seen a slender hyaline trail, more or less clearly separated from the sides ; and here and there appear hyaline balls, more often covered with a double cellular muff, of which we have spoken.

If we refer to the works of Koester, Billroth, etc., the presence of the balls and streaks of hyaline substance, and the establishment of the general structural characteristics, suggest at once the diagnosis of *hyaloid endothelioma* or *cylindroma*. In this respect, moreover, certain peculiarities of the anatomical picture of our case merit special attention. Almost without exception we notice an extreme regularity of structure; all the tubes lined with a cellular layer, always double, and arranged in the same way; on the proximal side with elements cubical in form, with dense protoplasm; on the distal side with elements cylindrical in form, having a clear transparent protoplasm. In no drawings of cylindromata which we have seen in literature have we found a like regularity.

This arrangement strongly suggests that there is an undeniable resemblance between the tubes of the tumor and the excretory ducts of the lachrymal gland, as we see them in the healthy parts of our sections; in both cases there is found a double layer of epithelium, the one cylindrical, the other cubical, and of respectively equal size. Their recriprocal arrangement, it is true, is inverse in almost the whole of the tumor; that is to say, the cylindrical layer, instead of being proximal, or next the lumen of the tube, is distal; but this variation is compensated by another histological characteristic: in the excretory ducts included in our sections, as well as in the tubes of the tumor, the protoplasm of the cells is invariably distributed in the same manner—in the cells of the proximal layer dense and granular, in those of the distal layer clear and transparent— whatever may be the form of the elements.

It is also to be noted that on the outer side of the double cellular layer of the excretory ducts there is seen a hyaline thread, the same as in the cellular lining of the tubes; and then, corresponding to the hyaline balls, the ducts are found to inclose, under the same conditions, a contents uncolored, or finely granular and sometimes oily.

Let us add finally that all histologists do not accord the

same value to the hyaline deposits as a pathognomonic characteristic (Ziegler,[17] Hansemann [18]).

Nevertheless, in spite of all these considerations, which seem to plead in favor of a glandular origin and especially the formation of the tumor dependent upon the excretory ducts, the diagnosis of endothelioma is irrefutably established by the presence of the endothelial pearls,[19] a similar product being only possible in glandular carcinoma.

The existing analogies to which we have believed it wise to call your attention demonstrate, on the one hand, the ease with which confusion may arise in researches of this kind, and, on the other hand, show the amount of reserve with which, according to the example of Koester, Berlin, De Wecker, Van Duyse, etc., we should approach the investigation of reports of tumors of the lachrymal gland.

We have already observed above, among other things, that in most of the published cases the anatomical facts are given with too little precision to afford a basis for a judgment as to their value. Here are some, more or less complete, which we have found in the literature of the subject during late years.

Alt.—"Ein Fall von Adenom der Thränendrüse." *Arch. f. Aug.*, X. 3, S. 319. The tumor is composed of cylinders with an endothelial lining and a lumen more or less large, sometimes much dilated with a serous exudate ; the cells are without exception in a single layer, polyhedral, often cubical, with a large round nucleus ; they are laid a short distance from a basement membrane. The tissue separating these cylinders is composed of fibrillæ, some of long fusiform cells and others star-shaped. No retrograde metamorphosis, fatty or colloid. Origin probably traumatic. Ablation piece by piece. Relapse in the brain.

Dobrowolsky.—"Neuroretinitis in Folge des Druckes der Thränendrüsengeschwulst auf den Sehnerven." *Klin. Monatsbl. f. Aug.*, 1881, April, S. 159.

[17] Ziegler.—*Lehrbuch der allgemeinen und speziellen pathologischen Anatomie.* 9te Auflage, 1898, Bd. I. S. 474.

[18] Hansemann.—*Die mikroskopische Diagnose der bosartigen Geschwulste,* 18;7, S. 160.

[19] Ziegler.—L. c., S. 440.

Harlan.—" Sarcoma of the Lachrymal Gland." *Transact. of the Am. Ophth. Soc.*, 1882, p. 404. A tumor the size of a hen's egg, the point of origin of which the author believes he was able to localize in the lachrymal gland.

Reymond.—" Limfomi voluminosi delle due orbite." *Ann. di Ottalm.*, XII. 337.

Huber.—" Klinische Beitraege zur Lehre von der Orbital-Tumoren." *Inaug. Diss.*, Zurich, 1882. Adenom (?) in der linken Orbita vermuthlich von der Thränendrüse ausgehend. The tumor, the size of an egg, contains a fibrous part, and another where are seen tubes lined with a layer of flattened endothelial cells, very rarely cylindrical, and of cysts containing a colloid mass and endothelial pearls. The author hesitates to advance the diagnosis of adenoma on account of the presence of the fibroid and colloid elements.

" Rundzellensarcom von der rechten Thränendrüse ausgehend." Tumor the size of an egg ; the connective tissue, rare, is filled with round cells, rarely fusiform ; vessels numerous ; no remnant of the lachrymal gland.

L. Tigos (Sassari).—" Adeno-enchondroma." *Amer. Med. Assoc.*, Chicago, III. p. 451.

Debierre.—" Trois cas d'hypertrophie de la glande lacrymale." *Revue générale d'ophtalmologie*, 1886, p. 145. Tumors the size of a small almond. Were removed, and there has been no relapse.

Ajevoli.—" Sul cilindroma della glandola lacrimale." *Revista delle scienze medich*, 1887.

De Britto.—" Note sur un cas de tumeur de la glande lacrymale." *Arch. d'opht.*, No. 6, 1888. Tumor of the lachrymal gland inferior, diagnosed fibro-adenoma.

Mazza.—" Klinisch-anatomische Studie eines Falles von Neoplasma der Thränendrüse. Adenom mit colloider Degeneration und von cancroidem Baue." *Internat. Ophth. Congress*, Heidelberg, 1888. *Bericht*, S. 417.

At the periphery the tumor had a structure similar to that of the healthy lachrymal gland ; elsewhere were found irregularly formed tubes, lined with a double layer of cylindrical epithelium, the lumen sometimes effaced, sometimes dilated with a colloid mass which gives it the appearance of a cyst.

Tumor the size of a small egg. The microscopic sections show culs-da-sac containing glandular epithelial cells with numerous fatty granulations.

Socor.—"Sur un cas d'adénome de la glande lacrymale gauche. Extirpation. Guérison avec conversation de l'œil et de la vue." *Bull. de la soc. des médecins et naturalistes de Jassy*, II., 1888, Nos. 9–10.

Snell.—"Two Cases of Adenoma of the Lachrymal Gland." *Ophth. Soc.*, May, 1889. *Transactions*, Vol. IX. In the first case the acini of differing forms are lined with cubical epithelium. At certain points they are enlarged to form cysts. In the second case is found more often a structure of round cells, with here and there an acinus lined with epithelium. On one side of the section the structure is distinctly glandular. A drawing accompanies these cases representing a lobule of the gland apparently healthy.

Bull.—"Contribution to the Subject of Tumors of the Orbit and Neighboring Cavities." *New York Med. Rec.*, August 24, 1889. At the center of the lachrymal gland the normal structure had been replaced by a very compact mass of cells.

Adler.—"Sarcom der Thränendrüse." *Wien. klin. Wochenschr.*, 1889, No. 21. This was a case of general sarcoma in which the mouth, throat, glands, etc., were all involved.

Goldzieher.—"Adenom der Thränendrüse extirpirt." *K. Ges. d. Aer. in Wien*, 14 März, 1890, *Wien. med. Presse*, 1890, No. 11. All the histological details found mentioned in the history of the case are comprehended in the following simple statement: The tumor is recognized microscopically as an adenoma. Through a personal communication from the author it is known that there were two relapses, and then the case was lost sight of.

Giulini.—"Ein Fall von Kleinzelligen Rundzellen-Sarkom der Thränendrüse beider Augen." *Münch. med. Wochenschr.*, 1892. He reports a case observed in the service of Professor Michel at Würzburg.

Pröhl.—"Zur Casuistik der Geschwulste der Thränendrüse." *Inaug. Diss.*, Berlin, 1892. In the first case "the microscopical examination revealed a round-cell sarcoma." In the second case both tumors of the orbit "consisted of fibrous (fibroid) tissue."

Lawford Collins.—"Two Cases of Sarcoma of the Lachrymal Gland. Removal and Microscopical Examination of the Tumors." *R. L. Ophth. Hosp. Rep.*, Vol. XIII. Part IV., 1893.

Sgrosso.—"Su di un sarcoma della glandola lagrimale e su di una speciosa alternatione delle cellule epiteliali del parenchima ghiandolare." Vol. III., *dei Lavori eseguiti nella Clinica oculistica di Napoli*, 1893, et *Archivio d'oftalmologia*, Vol. I. fasc. 3-4, 1893. He reports a case of sarcoma with fusiform cells.

Dianoux.—"Tumeurs de la glande lacrymale." *Ann. d'ocul.*, août, 1894. There were one case of tuberculosis and two cases of cylindroma, which name M. Malherbe, who made the microscopical examination, prefers to that of polymorphous epithelioma. But what, then, according to M. Malherbe, is the histological origin of the tumor? ectodermal or mesodermal?

Grünwald.—"Fibro-adenoma cysticum der Thränendrüse." *Münch. med. Wochenschr.*, 1895, No. 43, *Mediz. Verein zu Greifswald*, 6 Jul., 1895. Development of connective tissue, in the midst of which are large and small cavities, lined with cubical or flattened epithelium, which is in a state of proliferation, forming new cysts, with but little infiltration into the connective tissue.

Piazzi.—"Adenoma della glandola lacrimale." *Annali di Ottalmologia*, anno XXIV. fasc. 2-3. "Adenomatous tissue composed of a network of connective tissue and glandular tissue."

Van Duyse.—"Contribution à l'étude des endothéliomes de l'orbite." *Acad. de méd. de Belgique*, tome IX. A case of endothelioma in the region of the lachrymal gland.

Verliac.—"Des neoplasmes malins primitifs de la glande lacrymale orbitaire." *Thèse de Bordeaux*, 1896. A case of a tumor diagnosed tubular epithelioma. The epithelium of the acini of the gland composed of cubical cells, piled up, with protoplasm filled with hyaline vacuoles, the lumen rarely free, more often obstructed with blocks of broken-down epithelium. The connective tissue separating the acini is in some places entirely mucous.

Schaeffer.—"Ein Fall von Sarcom der Thränendrüse." *Inaug. Diss.*, Giessen, 1895. A sarcoma with small round cells extending into the interacinous cellular tissue. The vascular walls appear to be thickened and to have become hyaline.

Pick.—"Beiträge zu den Thränendrüse." *Centralbl. f. Aug.*, April, 1897. The first is a case of tuberculosis or chronic hyperplastic inflammation. The second a case of adeno-sarcoma of the gland, without anatomical details (Professor Neumann).

Bullard.—"Malignant Growths of the Orbit, with Report of a Case." *Ophth. Record*, July, 1897. Adeno-sarcoma.

Fromaget.—" Tumeurs malignes primitives de la glande lacry-male orbitaire." *Journ. méd. de Bordeaux*, juin, 1897. Concerns the case reported by Verliac.

Alt.—"Another Case of Tumor of the Palpebral (Accessory) Lachrymal Gland." *The Amer. Jour. of Ophth.*, March, 1897, p. 70. An adenoma in which the normal glandular tissue, solid tubes without central lumen, others with a central lumen much enlarged, becoming cystic. Almost all of the intertubular and interlobular connective tissue has disappeared ; in other parts, more healthy in appearance, it persists and is filled with round cells so numerous sometimes as to present the appearance of a microscopic abscess. In the drawings which accompany this article it is seen that the cellular lining is a simple layer of cubical elements.

Zelicka.—" Die Tumoren der Thränendrüse." *Correspondenz-blatt des Vereins deutcher Aerzte in Reichenberg und Umgebung*, 1888, No. 9. A myxomatous adenoma inclosing in certain parts, notably at the transition from degenerated glandular tissue to healthy gland tissue, cells which are epithelial in character, which would give rise upon the slightest cause to an adeno-carcinoma.

Ellis Jennings.—"A Case of Scirrhotic Carcinoma of the Orbital Lachrymal Gland." With microscopical examination and photograph by Alt. *Amer. Jour. of Ophth.*, April, 1897, p. 109.

Ellis Jennings.—" Further History of a Case of Scirrhotic Carcinoma of the Orbital Lachrymal Gland of the Right Eye." *Amer. Jour. of Ophth.*, January, 1898, p. 19. The tumor is composed of connective tissue and epithelial cylinders, the latter arranged as they are commonly found in carcinomatous tumors, with the cell nuclei very large. In places these cells are infiltrated and are undergoing retrograde metamorphosis, while others present an appearance of karvokinesis. A relapse occurs, and the new tumor differs from the first in a considerable diminution of the connective tissue. No characteristics of retrograde degeneration ; on the contrary, signs of cellular multiplication.

Werner.—" Myxosarcoma of the Lachrymal Gland." *Brit. Med. Jour.*, January, 1898. Carcinomatous sarcoma.

For the reasons given above, we have not attempted to criticise these cases, among which, outside of those designated as sarcomata, there may be easily recognized several whose mesodermal origin is by no means doubtful (the cases of Huber, Dianoux, etc.). Nevertheless, the lack of exact diagnosis ought not to prevent us from making certain deductions more or less independent of the meaning of the facts furnished, as well as the exactness of the interpretations made, although they are of considerable importance; such as the reports concerning the tissues surrounding the tumor in the orbit.

In several cases the authors have noted the presence of a capsule surrounding the tumor, sometimes soft and easily lacerated (cases of Piazzi, Bullard, Pick, Huber (2d case), Snell, Sgrosso, Verliac), at other times thickened and resisting (Alt (1st case), Socor, Grünwald, Zelicka, Jennings, our own case); at other times an intermediate state (Dianoux (2d case), Pröhl (1st case), Huber (1st and 3d cases)). In some cases the tumor was double or multiple (Goldzieher, Pröhl (2d case)).

As regards the limitation of the neoplasm, and the consequent possibility of complete, radical extirpation by simple ablation of the tumor, sufficient to prevent the danger of relapse, the presence of a capsule appears to several authors to afford a decided guarantee (Bullard, Dianoux, Verliac, etc.). "As long," says Vossius, "as the neoplasm, in its growth, does not go beyond the capsule, relapses do not generally seem to occur."

If we examine, in this respect, the cases that have been reviewed, it is remarked that absence of relapse was noted for six months after operation by Pick, for eight months by Schaeffer and by the writer, for one year by Pröhl (1st case) and by Huber (1st case), for eighteen months by Bull, for two years by Piazzi, for eight years by Huber (2d case). On the contrary, relapse occurred in the case of Goldzieher after a few months; in that of Jennings after six months; in the hands of Bullard, Huber (3d case), and Alt (1st case, the relapse in the brain) after one year.

In these last cases, in order to balance all the circumstances, it should be remarked that Goldzieher had a double tumor in a person aged thirty-two years; Jennings' patient had had his tumor for twelve years, and it had attained, at the time of operation, the dimensions of 1.5 by 1 inch; the tumor described by Huber, the size of a small egg, was present in a child of twelve years; in his operation, Alt was only able to remove it piecemeal.

Unfortunately, most of these cases have not been followed, or at least their histories have not been kept up for a sufficiently long time after publication to make it possible to arrive at satisfactory conclusions. Meanwhile the result of their examinations shows that simple ablation has an undoubtedly definite curative action (one of Huber's cases), in which the presence of a capsule ought certainly be taken into account. That the guarantee afforded by this last is not absolute is shown in Jennings' case. This case also emphasizes the importance of early intervention. Alt's cases show the advantage of preserving the integrity of the capsule during the operation.

If we refer to the statistics collated by Schaeffer, it is of importance that we should not forget that the cases of simple ablation of tumors of the lachrymal gland where relapses have been reported, often very shortly after the operations, are quite numerous. When the circumstances arising from the presence of a capsule, or the relatively short duration of the affection, do not appear sufficiently favorable, it is then time to recognize the necessity for the most radical operation possible—that is to say, the exsection of the orbit, even at the sacrifice of an eye that is in full function; the preservation of the sight on one side, especially when the second eye is still healthy, ought not to be considered in comparison with loss of life.

b.—SOME GRAVE LACHRYMAL COMPLICATIONS: ORBITAL PHLEGMON, OPTIC ATROPHY, PANOPHTHALMIA, MENINGITIS.

BY H. TRUC (MONTPELLIER).

Lachrymal complications may be divided as follows:

1. *Cutaneous:* erythema, eczema, impetigo;

2. *Nasal:* eczema, impetigo, ostitis, rhinitis, ozena ;

3. *Canalicular:* periostitis, osteitis, dàcryocystitis, fistula ;

4. *Palpebral:* blepharitis, entropion, ectropion, chalazion, abscess ;

5. *Conjunctival:* conjunctivitis, granulations, pterygion ;

6. *Keratitis:* vesicular, pustular, ulcerous ;

7. *Iritis:* serous, plastic, purulent ;

8. *Irido-cyclo-choroiditis:* synechia, hernia, atrophy ;

9. *Orbital:* tenonitis, cellulitis, phlegmon, abscess ;

10. *Intra-cranial:* phlebitis, thrombo-phlebitis, meningitis ;

11. *Functional:* irisation, photopsies, amblyopias, moth spots, asthenopias ;

12. *Operative:* keratitis, iritis, diffuse ocular or periocular suppuration.

As may be seen, these complications are numerous and varied. Ocular or periocular, anatomical, functional or operative, mild or grave, they all merit the attention of practitioners. Mackenzie, Desmarres, De Wecker, Galezowski, and especially Guemont,[1] Ferrand,[2] and my student Daniel,[3] have studied them for a long time. We ourselves have devoted a chapter of the *Nouveaux éléments d'ophtalmologie*[4] to this subject, and have since then, in view of the frequent occurrence of lachrymal affections in the region about Montpellier, emphasized several points in particular.[5]

---

[1] Guémont.—"Affections consecutives aux maladies lacrymales." *Thèse de Paris*, 1872.

[2] Ferrand.—"Affections oculaires produites des voies lacrymales." *Thèse de Paris*, 1873.

[3] Daniel.—"Les complications des affections des voies lacrymales." *Thèse de Montpellier*, 1871.

[4] H. Truc et E. Valude.—*Nouveaux éléments d'ophtalmologie.* Paris, 1896, t. II. pp. 90-97.

[5] H. Truc.—"De l'extirpation des glandes lacrymales orbitaires dans les larmoiements incoercibles chez les granuleux." *Arch. d'opht.*, 1889, p. 342.— "Quelques rapports entre les ophtalmies granuleuses, lymphatiques et lacrymales." *Montpellier-médical*, 1891, p. 293.—"Ablation de la glande lacrymal principale dans les larmoiements incoercibles." *Montp.-méd.*, 1892.—"Traite-

I propose to-day, on account of some personal information, to speak especially of the more grave of these complications: phlegmon or orbital cellulitis, optic atrophy,
panophthalmia, and meningitis. In spite of their rare occurrence, these complications are of great interest to the
patient as well as the physician, and also an undoubted
warning.

I will take up successively phlegmon and orbital cellulitis
with or without optic atrophy, then panophthalmias, of
which one case was accompanied with meningitis.

The cases are explicit and not accompanied by too long
commentaries.

I. PHLEGMON AND ORBITAL CELLULITIS.

CASE I. (unpublished).—*Left orbital phlegmon, consecutive
to an old purulent dacryocystitis ; acute optic neuritis, with
rapid and complete atrophy.*

P., twenty-three years of age, housewife. A year and a half
ago there was a normal accouchement followed by a uterine
abscess. For two or three years a chronic double purulent
dacryocystitis. On the evening of September 15, 1899, after
gathering grapes, a rapid swelling of the left ocular region, sharp
pain, diminution of vision. The condition remained unchanged
until the evening of September 19, when the patient came to the
clinic.

There was in the right eye a purulent dacryocystitis with
ocular integrity : VOG 1 ; in the left, enormous swelling with
palpebral occlusion ; an almost normal appearance of the globe,
slight exophthalmia and constraint in the movements, VOG 0.
Gastric disturbance, pulse 120, axillary temperature, 40.3.

ment des dacryocystites." *Semaine médicale*, 1892.—" Contribution clinique
à la pathogenie de certaines keratites lacrymales." *Arch. d'opht.*, 1895, p.
129.—" Quelques ablations de glandes lacrymales orbitaires et palpebrales dans
les larmoiements rebelles simples ou compliques." *Arch. d'opht.*, 1893.—
" États lacrymaux latents." *La clinique opht.*, 1895.—" Contribution clinique
à la pathogenie de certaines blepharites séches ; état lacrymal latent." *Recueil
d'opht.*, 1897.—" Ophtalmies lacrymales." *Montp.-méd.*, 1897.—" Traitement
opératoire de l'ectropion lacrymal." *Bull. Soc. fr. d'oph.*, 1898—" Extirpation du sac lacrymale dans les dacryocystites." *Montp.-méd.*, 1898.

The next day the fever fell (T. 38) and the second day it disappeared (T. 36.6).

There is a constant flow of pus, and the vision remains *nil*. With the ophthalmoscope there appears a white atrophy, with no trace of œdema nor of papillary congestion (VOG o). In a few days the purulent orbital and lachrymal discharge diminished, the œdema disappeared, the ocular mobility returned, and the orbital cure was at last complete. Complete white optic atrophy. VOG o.

The patient returned October 25.

In a recent examination the palpebral and ocular appearance of the patient is normal. Still a little dacryocystic pus on pressure. Definite white optic atrophy. VOG o.

There was orbital phlegmon with suppurative cellulitis, accompanied by subacute neuritis of a retrobulbar type. The vision rapidly diminished, and in three days had completely and definitely disappeared. A rapid retro-ocular cellular infiltration with optic compression must be recognized, but the principal rôle should be attributed to the rapid infection of the orbital tissues and the nervous cord.

It is probable that the fatigue and the inclined position of the work of grape-picking have been the occasional cause of the extension of a dacryocystitis to the orbit and optic nerve.

CASE II. (unpublished).—*Right phlegmonous dacryocystitis ; large incision, curettage, catheterization, lachrymal boric injection ; orbital phlegmon, neuritis, and complete optic atrophy. Lagophthalmic ulcer cured by median blepharorrhaphic incision.*

Madame P., forty-two years of age, housewife in Sauvegnargues (Gard). Habitual good health. Miscarriage at two months a a year ago. Frequent headache.

Vision normal ODG. Lachrymation on left side for five or six years ; being examined at this time, she refused all treatment. Chronic suppurative dacryocystitis for three years.

December 5, 1897, phlegmonous abscess of the lachrymal sac, with spontaneous rupture on the 12th ; at this time there was a persistent enormous swelling of the palpebral region and the right cheek. Entered the clinic the 13th. Intense cephalalgia, marked swelling of right lachrymal region of the lids and of the corresponding cheek, discharge of thick whitish-yellow pus from the puncta on the least pressure on the sac. Long, very sharp pain.

December 14.—Large cutaneous incision of the lachrymal sac. Curetting of the pocket revealed an osteitis; boric lavage, catheterization with No. 2 De Wecker sound, lachrymal injection, moist dressing.

The evening of the operation, diminution of the pain, diminished local swelling, dressing.

During the night great shivering, intense cephalalgia of the right side, considerable œdema toward the internal angle, the lids, and the right cheek. Exophthalmia, vision *nil.*

December 15.—Sharp pain, extreme swelling, ocular globe immovable, chemosis. Temperature 39; pulse 110, very small. Orbital puncture toward the region of the sac and vigorous deep cauterization with the thermo-cautery. Escape of sero-purulent fluid during the day, with no amelioration local or general. Examination of urine : no sugar, no albumen.

December 16.—Temperature 38.6. Persistent headache, restlessness ; exophthalmia and immobility of the globe ; preauricular and temporal œdema ; lagophthalmia. Punctures of the orbit with a large Graefe knife across the upper lid toward the median line and outward. Escape of sanguinolent fluid, but no pus. Moist dressing upon the globe.

December 17.—General condition better and periocular swelling diminished ; it seems as though the danger of inflammatory extension toward the brain may be imminent. There still remain a lagophthalmia and a large consecutive ulceration at the base of the cornea. Fresh orbital punctures and institution of drainage behind the globe. General condition better, almost no fever nor pain nor lachrymal discharge, but more extensive lagophthalmic ulceration. Median blepharorrhaphy without marginal freshening.

December 19.—Same condition. The exophthalmia still enormous and the lagophthalmia continues ; the blepharorrhaphic sutures have given way; strong indications of increased corneal ulceration. New sutures, with loosening of the external commissure.

December 20.—The local and general amelioration is very marked, but the corneal ulcer menaces destruction, the lids are much distended by œdema, and the exophthalmia can only be restrained by the sutures in front. We then made two cuts with the scissors in the inferior lid at the external and internal third through its entire thickness. There resulted a very loose median flap, with which the cornea could easily be recovered, and which was sutured to the corresponding part of the lower lid, also incised.

From this time the lagophthalmic ulceration of the cornea was ameliorated, the phlegmon diminished, the general health was re-established, and all returned to the normal. The ocular globe fell back into the orbit, and little by little recovered some mobility. The pupil large, immobile; vision *nil.* With the ophthalmoscope, papillitis with slight peripapillar œdema, tortuous veins, small arteries.

During the following weeks the cure advanced progressively. At the beginning of February it was well advanced ; not much œdema of the lids nor ophthalmia; the globe movable in every direction, although a little restricted, with external deviation and still red; corneal leucoma somewhat thick, but the pupil immovable; papillæ still a little congested and a tendency to atrophy; vision absolutely *nil.* Palpebral incisions healed. Much lachrymation.

February 23.—Returned. Cure complete. The vertical incisions in the lids are hardly visible. No deviation nor marginal notch. The ocular globe, excepting a slight diffuse leucoma, a little external deviation, and pupillary dilatation, appears normal; the vision is still *nil ;* complete white optic atrophy.

November, 1897.—Patient returned. Is very well. No lachrymation ; appearance of the eye is perfectly normal, except a little external deviation ; more apparent leucoma ; vision absolutely *nil ;* complete white atrophy.

There were here, together with the phlegmonous dacryocystitis, a violent cephalalgia and very extensive œdema. Perhaps an orbital phlegmon was imminent before the operation ; at any rate, the intervention, if it did not directly produce it, which is not demonstrated, at least hastened its appearance. The orbital phlegmon was evolved tumultuously, threatening to invade the cranial cavity by a phlebitis and even rudely compromise the life of the patient. The vigorous cauterization with the thermo-cautery seem to us the way to have prevented such a great disaster. Death escaped, the exophthalmia failed to accomplish the total loss of the organ. The optic nerve was apparently destined to complete atrophy by œdema and compression ; but while the optic globe was lost from a functional point of view, its importance was preserved from a physiognomic point of view. The occlusion by bandages and the classic blepharorrhaphies were insufficient ; hence the use of a suture with a median flap. The result was complete and the ultimate restoration perfectly spontaneous. This is a novel resource in excessive degrees of exophthalmia.

The following case, from Valude, is less dramatic, but ends also in complete white optic atrophy.

One analogous case was observed after cauterization of the sac following nasocomial gangrene. There had been little exophthalmia, but the papillar swelling was followed by optic atrophy and complete blindness.

CASE III.—Valude : *Bull. Soc. d'opht. de Paris*, 1895, t. VIII. p. 60. *Cathétérisme, amblyopie peu de jours àpres exorbitis et œdeme des paupières, nevrite puis atrophie optique.*

A man about sixty years of age, suffering from lachrymation. An incision was made, and the lachrymal catheter introduced. The pain was sharp, with a sensation of tearing. There appeared on the next day and the day following a noticeable swelling of the lachrymal portion of the cheek, with a large ecchymosis. Nevertheless, a second and then a third catheterization was made, without irrigation, at two days' interval. Valude saw the patient on the seventh day. On the next day there was amblyopia, scarcely a quantitative vision ; a little papillary congestion ; two days later, exorbitis and slight œdema of the lids ; vague ocular and orbital pain ; movements of the globe normal. Ten days later vision *nil*, papillæ dark red, veins distended, arteries small. Little by little complete white papillary atrophy.

Businelli of Rome (*La clinica moderna*, Anno IV. No.

20) has also published a case of orbital phlegmon consecutive to a dacryocystitis.

CASE IV.—Fulton (*Arch. opht. et otol.*, No. 9, 1885, XIV. 164–166) seems to have been more fortunate and to have cured his case with a puncture.

In a case according to Von Graefe there had been an infiltration of the cellular tissue of the orbit and consecutive phlegmon with loss of vision.

CASE V.—Von Graefe: *Klin. Mon. für Augenh.*, 1863, et *Ann. oc.*, 1863, t. XLIX., p. 247.

Forced injection by the interior lachrymal canal with penetration into the cellular tissue. A phlegmon of the lower lid was produced, with an infiltration of the cellular tissue of the orbit. There was an exophthalmia of only 4 millimeters, but vision disappeared entirely. With the ophthalmoscope was seen a papillary and peripapillary inflammatory swelling. Gangrene of a part of the adipose tissue of the orbit was also produced.

In a similar case, especially with injection of caustic solution, he would proceed at once to make an incision and establish drainage as is done by De Wecker. In view of the gravity of orbital infiltration and the possibility of consecutive optic atrophy, there would be reason to think of something of the sort.

CASE VI.—De Wecker: *Annales d'oc.*, 1863, t. XLIX. p. 247, note.

Injection of sulphate of zinc introduced by the inferior lachrymal canal with penetration into the cellular tissue and swelling of the lid. The writer immediately made an incision a centimeter in length along the inferior orbital border, introduced drainage, and applied a pressure bandage. Suppurative inflammation surpervened on the sixth day, without exophthalmia; the pus discharged through the operative wound, and the drainage remained in for fifteen days. No ultimate visual nor ocular accident.

The well-known observation of Leplat of a case of fatal meningitis closes directly the series of lachrymal complications.

CASE VII.—Leplat (*Bull. Soc. d'opht. de Paris*, 7 novembre, t. VII. p. 129, et t. VIII. No. 1, p. 60–64.)

Madame M., from the vicinity of Liège, operated for cataract of the left eye anterior; has had for two or three years a chronic purulent dacryocystitis of the same side. Neither collyria, section of the inferior lachrymal canal and injections of water, nor of acetate of alumina 30 per cent., modified the condition at all. The patient, very nervous and sensitive, refused curettage and the catheter. Owing to the persistence of the lesion, she finally decided to undergo catheterization on the 5th of June, 1894.

Introduction of a No. 2 Bowman, which penetrated about two-thirds of the lachrymal canal ; injection of water and then acetate of alumina ; the liquid did not pass through to the nose. The next day another incomplete catheterization and another injection of acetate of alumina ; the patient made a quick movement, which she attributed to the astringent action of the acetate of alumina in the narrow passage. Pain in the face and in the left upper gum. A little time after the patient's daughter noticed that a brown spot had appeared below and to the outer side of the region of the lachrymal sac. Then followed weakness ; pains in the head, especially the left side; this side tumefied ; the lids agglutinated by pus, although but little swollen ; the mouth, œdematous, causing difficult speech ; some nausea, but no vomiting ; pulse small, feeble, 120 ; temperature about 38. The family physician believed that it was the onset of phlegmon or facial erysipelas, and acted accordingly. Up to the 10th a slight diminution, but still a continuation of all the symptoms. On this day there was a very limited swelling in the region of the lachrymal sac and upon the left ala of the nose ; no general symptoms except a little lassitude and pains in the cheeks. But in the morning vomiting appeared; then, at 5 P. M., pulse irregular, temperature 39.1, Cheyne-Stokes respiration, delirium ; at 7 o'clock marked improvement. On the 11th condition better, temperature 38.4 to 39. On the 12th, in the morning, temperature 39, chilly feeling, vomiting, pains in the head, twitching of the limbs, balancing movements of the arms, drowsiness ; at 2 o'clock, 39.1, pulse bad, rapid, violent cephalalgia, drowsiness. Lachrymal tumor distended, a little painful on pressure, opened through the inferior canaliculus, a small quantity of pus. The face is swollen from the inferior orbital border to the upper lip, and the brown stain apparent in the beginning still remains. No fluctuation. Lids normal, conjunctiva pale ; the eye, in its normal position, is movable in all directions, the papilla presents nothing in particular. No swelling of the nasal mucous membrane, for respiration is easy. Coma at nine o'clock ; death the next day at noon. No autopsy.

I will not speak of orbital phlegmon following paralachrymal lesions, since Leplat, Dujardin, D'Arcy Power, and some others have reported examples ; and I will only call your attention to the case reported by Roure (*Ann. ocul.*, 1898, t. CXX., p. 121), in which he describes a case of purulent dacryocystitis toward the close of a maxillary and orbital osteo-periostitis. These facts, especially concerning the newborn, prove, moreover, that lachrymal lesions, like others, seem capable of extension and of orbital complications.

From all these facts it appears that affections of the lachrymal tract are susceptible of grave orbital, optic, and general complications ; that their first manifestations should be treated at once, and that, in local intervention, it is necessary to use prudence and circumspection. Phlegmonous suppurations are especially formidable, for the infectious germs are very virulent, and vascular extension seems to be particularly directed toward the cranium. Difficult catheterization, false passages. and caustic injections are especially to be distrusted. The orbital or lachrymal region is incised, and it is only after the onset of inflammation that the lachrymal tract is dealt with directly by catheterization and injections. In any case the possibility of formidable orbital, optic, and cerebral complications should never be lost sight of.

II. PANOPHTHALMIAS.

I have been able to collect but three cases of panophthalmia consecutive to lachrymal conditions. In Rokliffe's the suppuration of the globe supervened spontaneously ; in that of Hill-Griffith it seemed to be started up by an accidental erosion of the cornea; and, finally, in my own the glycosuria seemed to have played an important part.

CASE VIII.—Rockliffe (*Opht. Soc. Unit. King.* Lond., 1892–93., XIII. 24; December 17, 1892).

Panophthalmia consecutive to a purulent dacryocystitis.

A man aged sixty-three years; has had lachrymal obstruction for thirty years, but has never had a dacryocystic abscess. The suppuration of the lachrymal sac was followed by chemosis, by corneal ulceration with hypopion, and finally by panophthalmitis. Enucleation was performed. The globe was filled with inflammatory products; the orbital tissue appeared infiltrated.

CASE IX.—Hill-Griffith has observed a case of panophthalamia following a purulent dacryocystitis and an accidental abrasion of the cornea.

CASE X.—Personal résumé (*Montpellier-médical,* 1892, p. 20). Double purulent dacryocystitis, panophthalmia, glycosuria, enucleation, and évidement.

S. Julie, aged forty-one. Old epiphora and double purulent dacryocystitis dating back three years. He was unexpectedly attacked with a bad general state of health, and fever, redness of the eye and exophthalmia, swelling of the lids, total blindness of the left eye with infiltration of the whole cornea. Enucleation by my colleague Estor, who was taking my place. A few days later the same symptoms on the right. Évidement. The urine showed 24 gms. of sugar per liter, instead of 50 gms. per day. Before operation there appeared on the left side a plaque of gangrene along the margin of the upper lid, and some membranous exudation upon the conjunctiva. Later the glycosuria was intermittent.

The glycosuria, indeed, seemed to have favored the suppuration of the eyes, and Martin,[6] in his thesis, has reported some similar facts. Altogether it is probable that purulent dacryocystitis has played a prominent part in ocular suppuration, and has been at least its occasional or determining cause.

[6] Martin.—"De quelques manifestations oculaires du diabete." *Thèse de Montpellier,* 1892.

In lachrymal panophthalmia, as in other panophthalmias, enucleation is superfluous. Évidement of the globe,[1] a modification of evisceration with which I became acquainted in 1888 and have practiced since with success, fulfills all the indications and gives the most superior æsthetic results.

c.—A Contribution to our Knowledge of Malignant Tumors of the Orbit.

BY E. PERGENS.

Among the malignant tumors of the orbit which have presented themselves during the past few years, there are five that I have been able to follow for a relatively long time. The definitive result was always a relapse, often in the same place and ordinarily accompanied by metastases. The first case is remarkable for the abnormal invasion of the lymphatics, the second for the error in diagnosis through which an augmentation in the amount of stasis took place. The three other cases had the ordinary history of these neoplasms.

ANGIO-SARCOMA.

I.—Pierre Paul D., aged twenty-eight, has for some weeks been aware of the presence of a hard nodule in the orbit. The nodule was located on the supero-internal part of the orbit on the right side ; it was as hard as bone and could not be displaced. The fundus of the eye was normal, the vision 6/6 in each eye. I removed the tumor ; it was the size of a large hazel-nut ; its surface was like a raspberry ; the neoplasm was attached to the ethmoid and frontal bones ; I was obliged to remove a small longitudinal portion of the internal rectus muscle. Healing took place well ; there remained a slight divergent strabismus. The histological examination showed that it was a small round-celled

---

[1] " Les operations conservatrices du globe oculaire étant aujourd'hui en vogue, je ne suis pas fache de rappeler que je les ai toujours defendues," " Evacuation et enucleation dans la panophtalmie." *Montpellier-méd.*, 1888.—" Évidement de l'œil dans la panophtalmie." *Ann. occul.*, 1892.—" Contre-indications de l'enucleation de l'œil et opérations conservatrices." *Montp.-méd.*, 1897.

angio-sarcoma. The maximum vascularity was found in the part attached to the periosteum.

I examined the patient only a year later. Eight months after the operation he noticed that the strabismus was increased and that a relapse was becoming evident. To-day, a year after the operation, we have before us an anæmic patient, pulse 102 per minute, respiration 25. On the right side there is a well-pronounced ptosis, a marked deviation of the globe outward and downward, and a slight protrusion. Mobility is preserved ; the tumor has returned in the same place ; it has extended along the median line and has invaded the posterior part of the orbit. The vision is 6/24 ; the fundus normal, except a redness of the papilla, which is also found on the left side. On the right side the tumor has invaded the periauricular ganglia and the submaxillary, and infiltration is extending toward the supraclavicular glands. This path of extension is exceptional, for Billroth has demonstrated that in these sarcomatous tumors metastasis almost always takes places along the venous paths.

The patient does not suffer. Although the case may be operable, I do not believe that the patient would derive any permanent benefit from another operation. The patient was presented at the meeting of the Société belge d'ophtalmologie, November 16, and since then has had several attacks of colic. On the 3d of December palpation did not give any positive evidence of metastasis, but a week later I could demonstrate the involvement of the intestines and mesentery. Since the middle of January the patient has been confined to his bed, and has grown steadily weaker.

MALIGNANT FIBROMA.

II.—Maurice T., aged fifteen years, has a tumor of the left eye. It is five or six centimeters in length ; beginning at the internal angle of the eye it extends a finger's breadth along the under edge of the superciliary arch of the same side. When the patient bends his head down the tumor increases to more than double its usual size ; the same thing occurs when the jugular is compressed, except that the swelling comes on more slowly. We think of an angioma or some other sanguineous tumor : Dr. Hilson placed a ligature upon the pedicle near the internal angle and then applied a very hard bandage. For several days everything goes as well as could be wished for, and the tumor does not increase in volume when the patient bends his head over. On the fifth day the condition was the same as before the placing of the ligature. I then performed an extirpation which required two ligatures. The histological examination showed a fibroma invading the frontal and the musculus procerus ; the vessels had only developed a little in the neoplasm. The patient recovered well.

A year later the patient returned to the Ophthalmic Institute. There was considerable relapse. The tumor showed at the internal angle occupying the space to the left and front and ending in the left temporal region. There was ptosis of the left upper lid ; the eye on that side was deviated downward, and there was a vertical diplopia.

Inclination of the head and pressure on the jugular very noticeably increased the volume of the tumor. I extirpated again, which required another ligature of the vessels. It was necessary to detach the orbicularis muscle and resect its nasal portion ; the frontal portion and what remained of the musculus procerus was lifted up ; the orbicularis was replaced and sutured to the periosteum. After healing, the ptosis and vertical strabismus disappeared. In spite of the most careful investigation it was impossible for me to find sarcomatous elements in this tumor ; the parts in full proliferation presented only fibrous elements.

In about six months a second relapse occurred, occupying the supraorbital region and increased in volume by inclination of the head. The patient, I am told, is feeble and incapable of useful occupation.

The explanation of the swelling of these tumors seems to me to be as follows : when the patient is in a vertical position the inflow of blood is more difficult, its outflow easier ; inclination of the head and compression of the jugular reverses these conditions, whence engorgement by stasis.

FIBRO-SARCOMA.

III.—Pierre Van H., aged sixty-seven, became aware of a protrusion of the left globe two months previous to his visit to me. The fundus of the eye is normal, vision 6/6. I proposed Kronlein's operation, which the patient agreed to. Six months later he returned to me. The protrusion was increased, an ulceration of the cornea had begun, afterwards a panophthalmia. The cornea was perforated ; pus, with the remains of the retina and the uvea, presented themselves in the wound. I performed exenteration of the orbit; the neoplasm continued along the optic nerve toward the interior of the cranium ; there were no adhesions to the periosteum of the orbit. The tumor was a fibro-sarcoma, which probably took its origin from the sheath of the optic nerve. The motor muscles were invaded by the neoplasm ; sero-purulent infiltration had taken place in the episclera ; the conjunctiva showed a hyperplasia of epithelial cells. The cornea was gangrenous ; the interior of the globe contained pus, with staphylococci, the remains of the uvea, the crystalline lens, luxated downward and backward and still attached by a few fibers to the remains of the ciliary body ; in the interior is noticed some sarcomatous nodules with small round cells. The patient recovered, and no relapse has taken place.

Four months later he showed signs of mental alienation, which went on increasing up to the time of his death ; this occurred two years after the date on which the protrusion of the globe was noticed. The physician in charge considered the affection a meningitis produced by the development of the tumor.

EPITHELIOMA.

IV.—Florence B., aged fifty, has noticed that since the age of seven the inner side of the right eye has been the seat of repeated inflammations of short duration. During the past four months the conjunctiva on the nasal side has become red and thickened ; the neoplasm attacked successively the caruncle, both lids, and the naso-lachrymal canal. She went to the Ophthalmic Institute, where Dr. Lebrun performed exenteration of the orbit, extirpation of the naso-lachrymal canal, both lids, and the os unguis, and at the same time curetted the ethmoid cavities. After a few months there was a marked relapse, and the patient succumbed within a year. The histological examination demonstrated an epithelioma with numerous epidermoid globules ; the neoplastic tissue did not extend to the lid, and the conjunctiva was involved on the nasal side only.

FIBRO-SARCOMA.

V.—Francis P., aged twenty-seven, has for two weeks felt something hard in the supero-external portion of the right orbit.

The tumor was hard, immobile, and occupied the place of the lachrymal gland. I performed extirpation : it was a fibro-sarcoma of this gland. The fourth month after the operation a relapse took place ; little by little the tumor extended into the orbit. As the patient did not suffer, he refused another operation, and died in the course of seven months after the extirpation, having metastasis to the liver.

To sum up, out of the five cases, three are dead, two in the course of the first year, the third in the second year ; although still alive, the two remaining cases are in the second year after the established onset of the neoplasm, and will soon succumb.

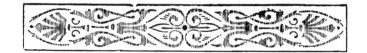

GLAUCOMA.

BY MARY E. BEALL, M. D., ST. LOUIS, MO.

OF all the afflictions to which mankind is liable none is more to be dreaded than blindness. This is frequently inevitable; nevertheless, it is the duty of the physician to be able to recognize, in their incipiency, the symptoms of the various eye diseases, lest an error in diagnosis should compel someone to spend his remaining days in darkness.

Two frequent causes of blindness are cataract and glaucoma. Though to the inexperienced observer they appear somewhat similar, to the specialist it may seem unnecessary to call attention to the differential diagnosis between cataract and glaucoma. The general practitioner, however, occasionally mistakes one for the other. In the past few years I have seen several cases where a patient has consulted his family physician about his eyes, complaining of all the initial symptoms of glaucoma, only to be told that he was suffering from cataract, that he would eventually go blind, and not until then could anything be done for him. After becoming blind he could then consult an oculist, have a cataract operation performed, and see again. This person naturally took his physician's advice, went blind, and then presented himself for operation. It was then necessary to say, "Your case is hopeless. It is not cataract, but glaucoma. Had you come in the beginning your sight might have been saved, but now nothing can be done for you." Had the general practitioner understood the symptoms of glaucoma, this person's sight might have been saved.

123

Glaucoma is the name given to a group of symptoms caused by an excess of tension.

In order to ascertain the degree of tension the patient should be directed to look toward the floor whilst the head is erect; the upper part of 'the globe is thus brought well forward, so that it can be reached by the examiner's two index fingers.

The affected eye should be compared with the other and with the normal eye of another person.

Symptoms.

In primary glaucoma, increase of tension is the first and most important symptom, from which all the rest of its phenomena arise. In secondary glaucoma, the increase of tension is only a consequence of other pathological conditions.

There is cupping of the optic disk, caused by the lamina cribrosa bulging backward as a result of the increased intra-ocular pressure.

Contraction of the visual field.

Pain is sometimes premonitory.

It nearly always accompanies the actual onset of acute glaucoma.

One of the earliest symptoms is the rapid impairment of the accommodation, rapidly increasing presbyopia.

The patient, usually middle-aged, finds that his glasses do not suit, and he gets a stronger pair, and after a while, a still stronger pair. Then he consults a physician.

Symptoms of Glaucoma Inflammatorium.

During the prodromal stage objects look misty. There will appear rainbow-like rings around the light.

Cloudiness of the cornea disturbs vision. The anterior chamber is shallower and the pupil dilated and sluggish.

An attack of this kind may last several hours and recur at intervals of weeks or months.

The second stage usually begins with an attack of acute glaucoma, occurring suddenly from some cause more or less remote and usually hard to discover. One cause which must be kept in mind is dilatation of the pupil, and for this reason atropine should not be used when there is any suspicion of glaucoma.

The onset of this attack is marked by violent neuralgic pains in the head and face and a rapid loss of vision, œdema of the lids and conjunctiva, and a discolored iris and dilated pupil.

After an attack of this kind the eye never returns to its normal condition. The tension remains permanently elevated. This inflammatory glaucoma may last several days or weeks and then improvement sets in.

The symptoms disappear and the vision may improve, but does not become as good again as it was before the attack.

The eye, after remaining in this condition quite a while, experiences another similar attack and then after a while another, each one reducing the vision until the third stage, that of glaucoma absolutum is reached. The eye is then totally blind. In glaucoma simplex the inflammatory attacks and pain are wanting, so the chief subjective symptom is disturbance of vision, which occurs gradually. It attacks both eyes and may occur in young people.

Secondary glaucoma signifies a condition of intra-ocular tension occurring as a complication of some other affection of the eye. It follows those maladies which interfere with the normal movements and position of the iris. I will only take the time to mention one and that is

Post-Iritic Glaucoma.

When an iritis is diagnosed the first step in the treatment should be dilatation of the pupil.

Failure to do this will allow the pupillary margin of the iris to become adherent to the anterior capsule of the lens.

This will arrest the passage of fluid forward, and there will be increased pressure upon the iris from behind and a secondary glaucoma may be developed.

Pathology.

The increase of tension gives rise to all the symptoms of glaucoma. The ciliary body and iris are supplied with numerous sensory nerves, and the compression of these causes the violent pain in inflammatory glaucoma.

The most important cause of the decrease of visual power is the atrophy of the nerve-fibers which they undergo by reason of the high pressure to which they are subjected, and of the flexion and interruption which they undergo at the edge of the papilla.

Theories as to causation.

There is a disturbance in the equilibrium of osmosis due either to increased secretion or decreased excretion. Primary glaucoma most likely results from the latter cause, there being some obstruction of the filtration spaces through which excretion normally takes place. Undoubtedly the principal causative factor of decreased excretion is closure of the passages at the iritic angle which may be caused by inflammation at this point, or by the lens being pressed forward and closing the angle, or by narrowing of the circumlental space. This last theory is advanced by Priestly Smith.

. The narrowing is caused by the flattening of the lens and the relaxed condition of the ciliary muscle, and the swelling of the ciliary processes partially closing the space between the lens and the ciliary processes, thus interfering with the process of osmosis so that the increase in the vitreous presses the lens and iris forward and the iritic angle is closed. The consequences of increased tension, inevitably occurring if it last a long time, are excavation of the optic nerve and ultimate annihilation of sight.

Treatment.—The instillation of eserine is frequently of service in cases where for any reason operative interference is postponed. The disease may be kept in abeyance some time, but it will nevertheless advance until operation becomes compulsory.

Glaucoma was considered incurable until Von Graefe, in the year 1856, demonstrated the curative action of iridectomy. As iridectomy reduces the tension to normal, the earlier it is performed the better. It is better to do it in the prodromal stage than to wait until the inflammatory stage has arrived, because the conditions are then more favorable for operation.

In hemorrhagic glaucoma, where the condition of the media will admit of the detection of hemorrhages in the retina, operation is contra-indicated, as the sudden lowering of the intra-ocular pressure will cause further hemorrhage.

. In inflammatory glaucoma the pain ceases and the other symptoms disappear, and these good results are generally permanent. In glaucoma simplex the result is not so pronounced, but another operation has recently been brought to the attention of ophthalmic surgeons, which is claimed to be of even more benefit in glaucoma simplex than in inflammatory glaucoma, and that is excision of the superior cervical ganglion. Professor Jonnesco first excised the superior cervical ganglion for glaucoma in September, 1897.

Dr. James Moores Ball, of St. Louis, has since performed this operation with a considerable degree of success. Through the courtesy of this gentleman I have witnessed this operation and observed the results in several cases. Jonnesco believes that the ocular sympathetic fibers from the brain and spinal cord pass through the superior cervical ganglion.

Permanent or intermittent irritation of these fibers is accompanied by dilatation of the pupil, narrowing of the intra-ocular arteries, contraction of the peri-bulbar muscular fibers, and, probably, an increased action of the elements which produce the aqueous humor.

"As a matter of fact," says Jonnesco, "any increase of the blood pressure will produce a permanent or intermittent narrowing of the arteries and cause the extravasation and increase in aqueous humor: then it is probable, although not definitely settled, that a permanent or intermittent irritation of the excito-secretory fibers is followed by an increase in the secretion of aqueous humor; the permanent or intermittent dilatation of the pupil pushes the iris into the angle, closes the canals of the filtration zone, and hinders or prolongs the exit of aqueous humor from the eye; the permanent or intermittent contraction of the unstriped peri-bulbar muscular fibers closes the efferent veins of the eyeball and hinders the venous circulation of the eye—here the dilatation of the intra-ocular veins."

He holds that excision of the superior cervical ganglion destroys all the vaso-constrictor fibers of the eye. The arteries relax, the blood pressure is lowered, and extravasation is reduced.

This operation destroys all the excito-secretory fibers of the eye, thus limiting the amount of aqueous produced.

The fibers which dilate the iris are destroyed, hence the contraction of the pupil re-opens the iris-angle and removes the obstacle to the outflow of the aqueous. The nerve-fibers supplying the unstriped muscular apparatus contained in Tenon's capsule are destroyed, hence the pressure on the efferent veins is removed and the ocular circulation is re-established.

Effects of Excision of the Superior Cervical Ganglion.—The effects of removal of this ganglion are immediate and remote. The immediate effects are relief of pain, lachrymation, and conjunctival congestion, together with a discharge from the corresponding nostril, unilateral sweating, and contraction of the pupil. Often there is immediate reduction of the intra-ocular tension. The effects are noted within five minutes after the excision.

The remote effects are ptosis, which appears on the third or fourth day, improvement of the vision, and in some instances a tardy contraction of the pupil and a tardy reduction of the intra-ocular tension. There is also a slight sinking of the eyeball into the orbit and a feeling of heaviness in the head. The slight ptosis is to be attributed to paralysis of Muller's muscle. Sinking of the eyeball is no doubt due to paralysis of the unstriped peri-bulbar fibers found in Tenon's capsule.

In one case, where I was present at the operation, the pupil was contracted within five minutes after the excision.

In unilateral glaucoma excision of the sympathetic ganglion should only be done on the corresponding side.

Conclusions.—Excision of the superior cervical ganglion is a valuable procedure in glaucoma and is more valuable. in glaucoma simplex than in inflammatory glaucoma.

In inflammatory glaucoma on which iridectomy has been done without benefit, this operation should be tried. In cases of glaucoma absolutum with pain, sympathectomy is to be tried before resorting to any operation upon the eyeball. The essential lesson to be drawn from a review of this whole subject is that operative procedures are demanded in these cases and are the only means by which a cure can be accomplished. In this affliction remedies will not avail. It is a mechanical condition and must be removed by mechanical means.

[The method of reducing tension in glaucoma by means of massage seems to promise good results. Several prominent observers have reported the successful use of this procedure. The affected eye is turned downward and slow, firm, and even pressure is made alternately on the inner and the outer side of the upper globe. The position of the eyeball is then changed to look upward, and the operation is repeated with the fingers on the lower part of the organ.

Five minutes of such massage is usually sufficient to reduce a moderate increase of tension to the normal. The process must be repeated daily, and in some cases two or three times a day, but as the patient or a member of the family can be taught to do the work, it can be attended to, at least partially, at the patient's home. The writer has had good results from this method in several cases. While the treatment must be continued for a long time, there seems to be a tendency to a gradual decrease of the tension and it is probable that after a certain period the tension would remain normal. At any rate, this means should be tried, especially in those cases where operation seems likely to be of doubtful success.—Ed.]

SPRAYS.*

FRED D. LEWIS, M. D., BUFFALO, N. Y.

IN considering the subject of sprays, it is not my intention to present to you a number of formulas that I have found useful in my practice, but to consider the matter on a broader and more general basis. That sprays have been, and are still used, in various conditions with the most gratifying results, we all know. But that they should be prescribed to a much larger extent than they now are is a fact that the physician as a rule is not aware of.

We have learned to know that the skin is one of the great vital organs of the human system ; that if its action is impeded, the kidneys and intestines are thereby given a greater amount of work to perform ; that with the morning sponge, followed by a brisk friction and an occasional Russian or Turkish bath, in chronic cases, such as rheumatism, we can expect quicker and better results from our remedies.

The public generally have been educated to that point where they recognize the importance of proper care of the teeth. They not only regularly cleanse them, but at stated intervals, usually every six months, go to their dentist and have a thorough examination to anticipate, rather than wait for, trouble.

Many persons have learned that a lavage of the stomach, in the shape of a cup of hot water, before meals, has converted a sluggish digestion into a normal one.

We are all familiar with the structure and object of the

* Read before the New York State Homeopathic Medical Society at the Annual Meeting, held in Albany, February 13 and 14, 1900.

nasal cavities. The tortuous turbinateds provide a large surface for the air to secure heat and moisture before reaching the lungs; and also remove from the air such impurities as are of a solid nature. Now we all know that the atmosphere of cities, especially where there are large manufacturing interests, is loaded with impurities, such as soot, dust, particles of pavement ground to inpalpable powder, etc., etc. This fact can easily be demonstrated when the city is on a plain or in the neighborhood of a large body of water. When in the city the air seems pure, the sky unobstructed, with no evidences of floating particles of matter; if an observation is taken from a few miles' distance, the city appears to be encompassed by a cloud.

That the deposition of foreign matter on the sensitive lining membranes of the nose should produce disturbances, there can be no doubt.

The only point I wish to bring out, and I hope it may stimulate some discussion, is this: Should not the care of the nasal mucous membranes be considered as important as the care of the skin and teeth?

In recent years I have asserted to my patients that the spray, in my opinion, is as essential on the toilet table as the toothbrush. As to the nature of the spray to be used, I think one must be guided by conditions. If there has already been a catarrhal condition established, then some remedial agent had better be employed; but if used simply as a prophylactic, then a neutral cleansing solution would be preferable.

I think this subject is deserving of profound consideration, when we know that there are establishments in most of our leading cities that advertise the cure of catarrh for so much a month. Their methods are simply to insist on the patient coming to their offices daily, and having their noses thoroughly cleansed. And they are curing many cases. Would it not be wise to educate our patients, not only to keep their own noses clean, and thus cure themselves, but by attending to themselves early enough, avoid the development of that, perhaps, most prevalent of all diseases, catarrh?

Discussion.—Dr. A. W. Palmer : Fellow members, in opening this discussion on this interesting and instructive paper I wish to remark that although every physician probably recognizes the great usefulness of sprays in the treatment of nasal diseases, the author is the first, in my recollection, to suggest the addition of the nasal spray to our usual toilet armamentarium.

Upon consideration in the brief time I've had, I wish to most heartily endorse it in the main.

I wish here just to emphasize one fact the doctor mentioned— that is—the office of cleansing which the Schneiderian membrane is provided to perform. We probably remember the corrugated form of the outer wall of each nasal cavity, produced by the turbinated bones which are covered by the moist mucosa, one of the principal duties of which is to catch any solid particles floating in the inspired air.

To convince one's self of the importance of this, one need only make a single rhinoscopic examination of a bricklayer after his day's work or of a housemaid after sweeping day.

Another mode of estimating the importance of the cleansing properties of the nasal cavities is this,—recall to your mind the dry and very dirty condition of the mucous membrane of the pharynx and naso-pharynx in cases of ozena. What is the main cause of this? The mucosa and erectile tissue of the turbinated bodies in all cases and the osseous tissue in advanced ones, are atrophied. Now, these bodies being smaller and less moist than normal, they do not sieve out the extraneous and irritating particles from the inspired air, on its passage through the nares, as they should.

Or to further recognize the deleterious effect of the continuous contact of foreign substances with the mucous membrane, one need but to recall the condition of the nasal chambers in the habitual snuff-user,—objectively we find all the tissues within the nose congested and hypertrophied, not only the mucosa, submucous cellular tissue hypertrophied, and the turbinated vascular network greatly varicosed ; but even the turbinated bones seem enlarged from a state of hypernutrition caused by the long-continued congestion superinduced by the irritation.

The nasal fossa, the care of which we are considering, is really the gate-way of the respiratory system,—one of the most important and delicate of the many interdependent divisions of which this wonderful human machine is composed. If the portal to this department of the human system is not kept normal, how can we expect to keep the remainder of the tract healthy?

One word in regard to the nasal sprays and douches. The former, in the majority of cases are preferable, because the solution in the form of a spray is less irritating to the normal sensitive Schneiderian membrane than the douche. In the normal or nearly normal condition of the nares, which is considered in this article, it is the only form of application that should be used, —vapors excepted.

On the other hand, although I am aware I differ from a number, still from clinical experience I believe the post-nasal douche far preferable in ozena and humid catarrhs with an excessive amount of discharge. It seems to need a larger amount of fluid to cleanse them than is produced by the spray.

Finally there is a caution, which I think should be taken into consideration : Can we not be too profuse in our daily ablutions? In relation to the skin, I have seen cases where I think persons have weakened themselves by taking several baths in one day for the purpose of keeping cool in hot weather.

As regards the cleansing of the normal nasal fossa, it is rather a new subject. I could only estimate .that a thorough cleansing about twice a week in persons of ordinary occupations would be sufficient, but in individuals employed in a dust-laden atmosphere, daily ablution after working hours would be advisable.

Dr. F. D. Lewis : I would like to make a few remarks. I agree with what Dr. Palmer has stated in many ways. I wish that he had given us a little more distinction between the spray and the douche. I had refrained from touching the douche, as my paper was on sprays. I believe the douche is dangerous. Where catarrhal disease is established, it may be extended into the eustachian tubes by the anterior nasal douche, producing middle-ear catarrh, but where a quantity of fluid is necessary to cleanse the cavities, I see no objection to the post-nasal douche. The cases that I spoke of in regard to the daily use of the spray were cases of chronic catarrhal conditions, treated by other physicians, without any great benefit. But where the spray was advised daily, as the bath and cleansing the teeth, the catarrhal conditions have gradually come under control ; I doubt whether any of them would have become absolutely well in the time in which they originally developed, yet they can be kept under control in comparative health.

Secretary : I have repeatedly had the experience of patients coming to me with whom I could not make out what was the matter until I discovered that they had been washing their vitality away. The tendency now is to have less and less washing of the nose with aqueous solutions. I have cases where it is necessary to wash out the nose with aqueous solution, but I direct these patients to follow that up with a spray of albolene.

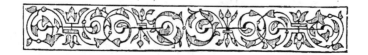

MASTOIDITIS, AND INTRA-CRANIAL COMPLICATIONS OF MIDDLE-EAR DISEASE.

BY R. G. REED, M. D., CINCINNATI, OHIO.

THESE affections are invariably secondary to suppurative disease of the middle ear, hence this is the point at which their study should begin.

An estimate made from carefully compiled statistics, from various sources, shows that at least thirty per cent. of all ear disorders are suppurative diseases of the middle ear. Five out of six of these cases come under the care of the aurist, in the chronic form. These constitute the source from which arise the secondary affections now under consideration, as they rarely follow directly in the wake of primary acute inflammation.

The structure and location of the middle ear furnish all the requisites of a well-regulated incubator ; and various forms of micro-organisms exist in the discharges, and in the lesions following them. Of these organisms, the streptococcus and staphylococcus pyogenes seem to be the most virulent—the staphylococcus being always present in cases of intra-cranial complication.

The fetor of a discharge is due to the presence of bacilli whose sole duty seems to be to furnish an aroma adequate to the occasion, hence are of little consequence, as a non-fetid discharge may be productive of results equal to that of the most fetid.

A peculiarity which has been referred to is that primary acute suppurations are less likely to be accompanied by mastoiditis, etc., than are chronic suppurations. This evidently cannot be accounted for by any lack of virulence on the part of the pathogenic elements, but rather by the resistance of the newly-invaded tissues, and the activity of the white blood-corpuscles.

The various routes by which this army of microbes seeks to invade the structures within the cranium, are : By direct continuity, as caries of the cranial walls ; or, more indirectly, through the blood and lymph channels ; or along the course of nerves entering the middle ear.

Should the discharge, by its own virulence, or on account of obstruction of the external ear, invade the accessory cavities known as the mastoid cells, an abscess is the result. This may also be produced by a careless use of the syringe, or even by the application of peroxide of hydrogen, through the external auditory canal.

The mastoid cells are frequently infected from a chronic suppuration. This infection takes place through the *aditus ad antrum*, the opening from the vault of the tympanum, or epitympanic space, into the mastoid antrum, or largest and most constant of the mastoid cells ; from whence it may involve all the other cells, and by direct continuity, the cranial cavity itself. When these cells are involved in a purulent process, we have what is known as a mastoid abscess. The form of this inflammation may be either acute or chronic. The acute form is marked by pain, redness, and swelling over the mastoid, while the auricle projects at a right angle to the side of the head. The chronic form, on the other hand, is marked by an absence of the symptoms which characterize the acute form. The inflammatory process may progress for weeks or months, without any marked symptoms to denote the serious nature of the disease. The patient complains of indefinite pain,—not headache,—but deep, persistent pain in one side of the head, which may or may not be localized. He also has attacks of vertigo, nausea, or vomiting, occasionally a slight rigor. On examination, the tongue is found to be coated ; the temperature above normal ; the symptoms, thus far, resembling those of malaria. The history of the case will show that a chronic discharge from the ear has suddenly diminished in quantity, or ceased altogether, without apparent cause. On inspection, the superior and posterior walls of the canal may be found bulging.

The danger to the life of the patient lies in the complications that may arise at any moment, from the extension of infection to other parts. For instance, pus may break into the middle cranial fossa, through the tympanic roof; or it may pass back from the cells of the mastoid and reach the lateral sinus, and even enter the posterior fossa. It may open anteriorly from the middle ear, and produce a retro-pharyngeal abscess; or passing through the lower portion of the mastoid process, may form an abscess beneath the sterno-mastoid muscle.

The complications resulting most frequently from suppurative disease are mastoiditis, meningitis, septic phlebitis, and pyæmia,—cerebral or cerebellar abscess being of comparatively rare occurrence. Two or more of these may co-exist in the same case: Sinus phlebitis and abscess may occur in the same case, and either may give rise to a fatal meningitis; while a septic phlebitis may be the direct cause of a general pyæmia. Dr. Coleman Jewell says, " In complicated cases, it is generally very difficult, or impossible, to determine which condition preceded another, or indeed, whether they were not concomitant." Pyæmia of aural origin may either set up, or be caused by, an intracranial lesion, or it may be present alone, unassociated with any such affection."

The location of secondary intracranial affections is variable, both as to position and extent. Sinus phlebitis generally occurs in that portion of the lateral sinus opposite the mastoid portion of the temporal bone, although it may extend into the internal jugular vein. It is caused by an inflammation of the adjacent bone, and gives rise to a thrombus, which may extend downward into the jugular vein, as well as upward into other sinuses. This clot may become infected, and breaking down, cause pyæmia.

Intra-cranial abscesses are either sub-dural, occurring

between the dura and the internal table of the skull; or encephalic—that is, within the brain substance.

There are two sites where sub-dural abscess is particularly liable to occur, the first and most common being about the petro-squamosal suture, while the second is that portion of the groove for the lateral sinus in closest proximity to the mastoid cells. While these are the most frequent primary sites, the pus may extend in various directions from these points, and end in a diffuse purulent meningitis.

A conservative estimate of the causes of encephalic abscess would place fully one-third as due to suppuration of the middle ear. About three-fourths of these occur in the cerebrum, while one-fourth occur in the cerebellum. While cerebral abscess, secondary to middle-ear suppuration, may occur in various situations, by far the greater number occur in the temporo-sphenoidal lobe; while abscesses of the cerebellum are most frequently found in the anterior part of the lateral lobe.

Abscess of the brain is generally single, and varies in size from a few drops of pus, to three and sometimes four ounces. It may co-exist with a sub-dural abscess, and in fact, may arise directly from it.

To diagnose these various and varying lesions is always difficult and often impossible. An exploratory operation is the most satisfactory means of arriving at a positive diagnosis. This course is justifiable, since operative measures only promise any hope of relief. However, there are symptoms which, considered relatively, are of value as indicating the nature of the lesion.

The symptoms of mastoiditis have already been referred to. Headache, rigors, vomiting, delirium, and even tenderness, while they are usual accompaniments of intra-cranial complications, give little or no information as to the nature or location of the lesion. The pulse, respiration, temperature, state of the bowels, and motor disturbances, furnish the most reliable indications of the existing condition. A pulse of moderate volume, slow and regular, with shallow, slow, and regular breathing, is suggestive of encephalic abscess; while a small, rapid, and irregular pulse, with rapid and irregular respiration, would indicate meningitis.

A temperature, sometimes below normal, and again very high, fluctuating at irregular intervals of time, indicates pyæmia; while in phlebitis, the variations are not so extreme, the fluctuations becoming less marked as the disease progresses, and gradually approaching the normal. In meningitis the temperature is high, and without marked remission. In uncomplicated brain abscess there is generally a sharp rise of temperature at the first, gradually lowering to sub-normal, and remaining so until the pus is evacuated.

Brain abscess and meningitis are generally marked by a constipated condition of the bowels, while the other complications are often accompanied by diarrhea.

When mastoiditis or signs of intracranial complication appear, the external auditory canal should be freed from all possible obstruction. Should the symptoms continue after all obstructions have been removed from the canal, the mastoid antrum should be opened, and free drainage established. By this means all the spaces of the middle ear may be reached and all dead bone removed, while the application of antiseptics is made easy.

The indications for opening the mastoid are as follows:

1. Acute inflammation of the mastoid which persists after the indicated remedy has been administered.

2. Recurrent swelling of the mastoid during a chronic suppurative otitis.

3. When there is marked tenderness and bulging of the superior and posterior walls of the external canal, with chronic suppuration.

4. When there is a fistula of the mastoid.

5. When during or following a suppuration of the middle ear, severe pains occur on the same side of the head which resist all other treatment.

Should sub-dural abscess be suspected, the opening should be continued as far as the dura-mater and the membranous sinus, and high enough to expose both situations already mentioned. In case of encephalic abscess, the opening should be made with a trephine over the suspected area, and the brain substance explored with a hollow needle. Should pus be found, the opening should be enlarged, and thorough drainage established.

The location for opening with the trephine, in suspected cerebral abscess, is over the lower and anterior portion of an area comprised within a circle with a radius of 1¼ inch, the center of which lies 1¼ inch behind, and the same distance above, the middle of the external bony meatus.

Cerebellar abscess being most frequently found in the anterior portion of the lateral lobe, the trephine should be applied at a point 1½ inch behind the center of the bony meatus, and an inch below Reid's base line.

Such are some of the troubles arising from suppurative disease of the middle ear, together with their surgical treatment. With the homeopathic remedy and cleanliness in the early stages, the cases are few, if any, that would ever need surgical interference.

POST-NASAL ADENOID GROWTHS OF CHILDREN.

ORRIN LELROY SMITH, M. D., CHICAGO, ILL.

IN some of the Eastern cities, physicians specially appointed to seek out physical handicaps among the so-called "dull children" report a large percentage to be mouth-breathers, caused by post-nasal growths, and that when so dependent, with proper curative measures, the child almost invariably gradually comes to do average class work. It is a commonly accepted clinical fact among specialists that adenoid children are *naturally* bright and only need to be freed from the incubus to demonstrate that fact. That interest in this matter in our own city is not confined to professional ranks is evidenced by the fact that public-school teachers have sought and obtained admission to my clinic for the purpose of practical information regarding symptoms, diagnosis, and treatment, and have been repaid by the satisfaction of seeing several pupils do a grade of work before impossible. The exacting nature of our profession is very apt to make us forget that we are also citizens with a paramount duty as guardians and educators in all matters that menace public health.

That heredity is one factor in the production of these growths is partially proven by the fact that frequently several children of the same family are similarly affected, and the growths date in many instances from birth.

Children of either the so-called scrofulous or lymphatic habit and boys between three and twelve years of age constitute the majority of sufferers.

Moist climates with sudden temperature variations are

blamed as prolific factors, as undoubtedly they are, yet the two worst cases I have ever seen were bred, one in the piny atmosphere of Michigan, and the other in the high dry air of Montana.

As often as diphtheria, measles, and whooping-cough are exciting causes, scarlet fever more frequently excites these growths than all three diseases combined. The mouth-breathing countenance or so-called "adenoid physiognomy" is so characteristic in children that a little practice will enable one to instantly recognize it and enumerate the child's symptoms to the parents.

In the first place the countenance is dull, sometimes almost vacant, yet not unintelligent. The child is inattentive, absent-minded, learns slowly, and seems not to have the power of mental concentration, a condition Guye aptly calls aprosexia.

The face is not only pale and elongated but also narrowed, because the air, passing through the mouth instead of the nose, has no chance of developing the supra-orbital and malar eminences. The mouth of course is usually open, the upper lip short, the lower one thickened and everted, and the chin pointed and retracted. The alæ nasi are thin, lifeless, and undeveloped, the alar fold obliterated, the nasal orifice small and narrow, while the bridge of the nose is flattened, thickened, and crossed at its root by the enlarged transverse vein.

The voice is usually distinctive, having a "deadened" quality in which the letter *b* is spoken as *p* and *m* as *b*, which is due to absence of nasal and pharyngeal resonance and lessened mobility of the soft palate. Upon examining these cases, the reflected light discloses a high nasal floor, narrow nares, catarrhal discharges, and hypertrophied turbinates, all of which at least account for the patient's loss of the sense of smell. Once in five hundred cases we have encountered the opposite conditions, atrophic rhinitis or the "dry catarrh" of the laity. Upon inspecting the mouth, the permanent teeth, sometimes already decayed, irregularly crowd and overlap each other, so that instead of the regular semicircle of the superior dental arch, we find a pointed and projecting one.. We also find the broad and low hard palate of normal childhood replaced by one very high and narrow, due of course to the unequal atmospheric pressure of mouth-breathing.

The fauces are usually narrowed by tonsillary enlargements and not infrequently you will perceive the space more narrowed from the crowding down of the soft palate by the superimposed adenoid tissue. Over the pharynx, that is so frequently granular, and the enlarged tonsils, there is ordinarily much secretion. It is difficult to make a naso-pharyngeal examination with a mirror in a child under five years of age, but I have succeeded more often since using a pivot mirror in which the shank is not set at right angles. When you do succeed you will see, as best described by Morse of Bordeaux, "a nodular irregular mass of cauliflower shape, pink color, often covered with a grayish membrane, most frequently found in the vault and on the posterior wall, where they may hang as stalactites behind the choanæ, fill up Rosenmüller's fossæ, or obstruct the orifices of the eustachian tubes." Failing in mirror examination, pass your left arm about the child's neck and press in the cheek over the teeth with the first finger of same hand, so that your examining digit cannot be bitten. Then along the teeth and over the tonsil to the posterior pharyngeal wall pass carefully the clean index finger of the right hand. At this point, incline the finger upward until it reaches the lower part of the septum which, traced up, leads you to the growth, whose peculiar spongy character, location, and extent, a little practice will enable you to instantly recognize.

Every change to moist or cold weather starts the discharges from this growth. If located well forward the trend is toward the posterior nares and into the nose, and the child constantly catches cold despite every precaution. Soon a chronic catarrh, and often nose-bleed, results. If situated laterally then the child is subject' to earache, middle-ear suppurations, impaired hearing, and frequent

attacks of tonsillitis.   The tendency of growths so placed
to occasion croup and bronchitis is greatly augmented by
the mouth-breathing habit that deprives the patient of
properly moistened, warmed, and filtered air.   In nine years
we have not seen, among children, a case of croup or bronchitis in which adenoid growths were absent.   If located
well back in the vault, the discharges gravitate downward,
collect in the pharynx with resulting dyspepsia and constipation.   This last symptom, coupled with the lack of
oxygen and consequent accumulation of carbonic acid,
culminates in Nature's antidote commonly denominated
"night-terrors," after which the child subsides into the
muscular twitchings and heavy snoring and restless sleep
of adenoid victims.

Such children are seldom robust and are usually physically below the average child of their age.   After removal of
these vegetations I have seen such nervous reflexes as
nocturnal enuresis, chorea, facial spasm, twitchings of eyelid, laryngismus stridulus, coughing, and hawking disappear
entirely.   Other observers have reported the disappearance
of stammering, stuttering, epilepsy, and convulsions after
such operations.   A reflex I have never before encountered—that of constant salivation—was present in a lad
referred by Dr. Nathan Starr of Charleston, Ill., last week,
that, however, almost disappeared four days after operation.
If the growth is recent and slight in character such remedies as sanguinaria, calcarea phos., baryta carb., or baryta
iod. will usually effect a cure.

If the growth is of such size as to mechanically interfere
with, or derange, any function, the only rational treatment
is removal by surgical means.   The attempt to remove a
portion only stimulates the remaining tissues to greater
growth and has proven wholly unsatisfactory.   A thorough
curettement should be done under an anæsthetic, preferably
chloroform, for many and good reasons.   By some the
operation is regarded as wholly devoid of dangers, but
recorded cases of sphenoidal abscess, septic meningitis,
retro-pharyngeal abscess, deafness, and fatal hemorrhage,

are unquestionably due in the majority of instances to a lamentable lack of care or knowledge, for once the proper technique is observed, the operation is a perfectly safe one.

Many children begin breathing through the nose at once, but the majority must be insistently and persistently taught to do so. In some instances a handkerchief must be tied under the child's chin and over the head, to prevent the dropping of the lower jaw while sleeping, so strong is the force of habit.

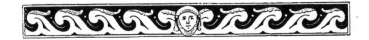

ARGENTUM NITRICUM AND OPTIC-NERVE ATROPHY.

BY ROYAL S. COPELAND, A. M., M. D., ANN ARBOR, MICHIGAN.

IN visiting the University library a few days ago I happened to examine the volume of the *Archives of Ophthalmology* for 1889. On page 123 appears a review of the then new JOURNAL OF OPHTHALMOLOGY, OTOLOGY AND LARYNGOLOGY.

The writer said: "The first (January) number of this periodical . . . . promises to become a valuable magazine of work done in its department. We welcome it so much the more as it intends to collect the researches, experience, and opinions of our homeopathic brethren, which thus far have scarcely been accessible to the profession at large . . . . Their programme is very well carried out in the first number, which contains nineteen original articles (abstracts of which will appear in our systematic report), some of considerable, other of doubtful, value, and some, in our opinion, might as well have remained unpublished. To the latter class belong the two papers on homeopathic therapeutics, in which the conscious or unconscious disregard of the natural course of disease is as conspicuous as the orthodoxy of the specific creed. On page 100, to mention but one example, are related two cases of paralysis of accommodation after diphtheria. ' I prescribed Causticum without benefit, and one week later gave Duboisin 6x, with rapid improvement, and entire cure in a short time.' The homeopathic remedy, as every physician knows, or ought to know, did exactly the same thing as nature does in every similar case without any medicine."

In this connection I wish to relate a case and inquire if "the homeopathic remedy did exactly the same thing as nature does in every similar case without any medicine."

On the 22d of March, 1898, Mrs. M. H. R., aged forty-nine, visited my clinic, complaining of asthenopia and failing vision. Her visual acuity was recorded as 20/30 for the right eye and 20/40 for the left. The field of vision of the left eye was greatly contracted and the ophthalmoscope revealed unmistakable evidence of optic nerve atrophy.

The casebook shows this diagnosis and records an unfavorable prognosis.

The patient complained also of an obstinate stomach trouble, great distentions with frequent belching. Since it is a remedy always thought of in optic atrophy, naturally these and other equally characteristic symptoms decided me to prescribe argentum nitricum, which was given in the 3d potency.

The remedy was continued up to December 30, 1899, the patient reporting occasionally for examination. On the last date vision was found to be 20/30 and field of vision practically normal in each eye, and every ophthalmoscopic evidence of atrophy had disappeared.

Now, I confess, had I read a similar report to this I should have been inclined to doubt the certainty of the original diagnosis. But feeling strongly the duty of the profession to report any progress in the treatment of the so-called incurable diseases, I am impelled to record this unusual case and to receive philosophically the criticisms of the doubters.

Contrary to the almost universal testimony of the authorities and in spite of "the natural course of the disease," to quote the writer of my introductory paragraph, I am perfectly satisfied that the homeopathic remedy has cured at least one patient of optic nerve atrophy. I doubt exceedingly if nature, unassisted, could have ended the case so happily.

MASTOID . DISEASE WITH EXTRADURAL AB-SCESS—TWO OPERATIONS; RECOVERY.

BY CHARLES DEADY, M. D.

ON March 21, 1900, Frank P., aged six years, native of New York City, presented at my clinic at the New York Ophthalmic Hospital for treatment. The mother gave the following history : Three weeks previous the child had suffered from an attack of measles, the case being well developed. During the progress of the disease, he caught cold and contracted a slight bronchitis, accompanied by a severe cough. Five days after measles was diagnosed the child complained of earache in the right ear, and within a short time a discharge appeared at the external meatus. A few days before presentation at the hospital, swelling and œdema appeared over the mastoid process.

On examination the soft parts over the mastoid process were much swollen, and there was considerable redness with tenderness on pressure. The discharge from the meatus was abundant and purulent. The face was pale and waxy, the child was restless, the pupils were slightly dilated, but showed good reaction to light. Temperature, $100\frac{6}{10}$. Patient was at once admitted to the hospital and put to bed. The ice bag was applied to the side of the head, the ear was ordered cleaned every two hours with hydrogen peroxide, and hepar 1x and capsicum 3x were given every hour in alternation. The patient was placed upon fever diet and temperature ordered to be taken every two hours.

March 22d, the temperature varied from 99.7 to 99.4, but at midnight it became subnormal, falling to 97°.

March 23, the patient was prepared for operation, and after the usual aseptic toilet he was placed upon the table. Anæsthesia being complete an incision was made through the soft parts covering the mastoid process, beginning at the tip and being carried around the insertion of the ear behind to a point directly above the organ. Pus was found immediately, and the soft parts were held aside by retractors, the periosteum stripped from the bone and, after checking the bleeding and cleaning the wound, the bony process was laid open with the chisel over the site of the antrum.

The mastoid cells were found to be infiltrated with pus, and they were broken down and removed. The wedge-shaped piece of bone between the antrum and tympanum was removed and the middle ear thoroughly cleansed.

After the parts were clean and free from blood they were examined, and a thin yellow streak was seen on the bone at the upper part of the wound, which, upon being wiped away, reappeared in a short time, showing that pus was coming down from the brain cavity. The bone was then chipped away until the dura mater was exposed over a space as large as a silver dime piece, at a point immediately above the antrum.

Pus immediately issued from this opening and after its removal the parts were irrigated, a probe being passed between the dura mater and the overlying bone for a short distance in all directions, to liberate any confined pus.

The wound was then packed with sterile gauze, a dressing applied, and the patient put to bed. Time of operation one hour and thirty minutes.

The temperature was then taken and found to be 99° at 7 P. M. Bell. 3 and Hepar 3 were prescribed, to be given every hour in alternation. On the morning of March 24 the temperature began to rise, and at 5 P. M. of that day it stood at $102\frac{6}{10}$. Pulse, 114; respiration, 22. The remedy was now changed to verat. viride φ, gtt. x. in water $\mathfrak{z}$ viii; a teaspoonful every hour.

During the night the temperature rose to $103\frac{5}{10}$ and on the morning of March 25, at nine o'clock it had dropped to

$101\frac{2}{10}$, but rose steadily during the day and at 11 P. M. it had reached $104\frac{8}{10}$, the little patient becoming more and more stupid and difficult to arouse. March 26, 9 A. M., temperature, $103\frac{6}{10}$; pulse, 128; respiration, 24.

At 1 P. M., temperature, 104; pulse, 130; respiration, 24.

On this day, at 3 P. M., the patient was again placed upon the operating table and under anæsthesia, with all aseptic precautions, the wound was opened and found to be in as good condition as could be expected.

A large probe was now inserted between the skull and the dura mater, and free excursions were made in all directions in search of pus. Nothing was found forward or directly upward, but on passing the probe posteriorly for some distance a pocket was found, and pus issued therefrom, in amount something over half a dram. The parts were then thoroughly cleansed and a fresh dressing applied.

At 7 P. M. of the same day the temperature was 102, and at 9 A. M. of the next day (March 27), it had fallen to $99\frac{8}{10}$; the patient was conscious and in good condition.

Verat. viride φ was given in alternation with sulpho-carbolate of soda in 2½ grain powders, every two hours. For the next three days the patient steadily improved, and on March 30 he was put upon silic. 3, after which date the recovery was uninterrupted.

Patient was discharged from the hospital April 22, 1900, having regained much of the flesh lost during his illness, the parts being in good condition and rapidly healing over.

Souter, Dr. J. Francis.—Ichthyol in Whooping-cough.—*Amer. Hom.*, January, 1900.

Reports very successful results with this remedy in fourteen cases of pertussis. Administered as follows,—at first give the little patient 1 grain every four hours, in a few days increase to 2 grains per dose, and proceed in like manner until 4 grain dose is reached. PALMER.

A Method for the Removal of Foreign Bodies from the Nose and Ear.—*British Med. Jour.* (*N. A. Jour. Hom.*, February, 1900).

It is based on the principle of suction. A rubber tube just small enough to be introduced either in the nares or external auditory canal is attached to the nozzle of an ordinary syringe. The stiffer the tubing the better, in order that it may not collapse when the air is withdrawn from it. The foreign body is located and the free end of the tubing introduced into the cavity in as close proximity to the body as possible, the plunger of syringe withdrawn, drawing the object into or against the end of tubing and retaining it there until the tubing itself is withdrawn from the cavity. To the better facilitate the engagement of the object into the tube it is often advantageous to dip the end of tubing in glycerin before insertion into cavity. PALMER.

Oppenheim, M. D., Seymour.—The Effect of Certain Occupations upon the Pharynx.—*Med. Record,* December 16, 1899.

The writer made a special study or investigation of this subject on fifty unselected cases in his clinic. There were twenty-nine males and twenty-one females, employed in the following occupations ; bakers, carpenters, dressmakers, dyers, firemen, hatters, laundresses, tailors, tinsmiths, and weavers. He divides the occupations into two groups in respect to their atmospheric conditions or hygienic surroundings. First, those which are distinguished mostly by having a large quantity of dirt or dust particles in the respired air and higher temperature than normal ; such as bakers, carpenters, dressmakers, firemen, portion of the hatters and weavers : and secondly, those marked by the atmosphere containing a large amount of chemical agents which are poisonous to the mucosa, such as acid fumes,—including the dyers, some of the hatters, laundresses, and tinsmiths.

The fact that the catarrhal symptoms are more amenable to treatment if the patient happens to be on a vacation during its administration, or, what is still stronger evidence, the patient frequently remarking the decided diminution of symptoms when they are laid off from work without the least treatment for the same, shows the relation of the occupation to the disease.

The patients will often date the commencement of their trouble from shortly after the beginning of their employment at such irritating occupation.

Upon examination one of three varieties of pharyngitis is found ; (a) simple inflammation without other pathological changes, in thirteen ; (b) the mucous membrane was sclerosed in fourteen, and, (c) atrophy of both the mucosa proper and the follicles in twenty-three.

Finally the author makes the following summary :

(1) The pharyngeal mucosa of the mill-hand under twenty years of age is more susceptible to unfavorable influences than is that of the individual over this age.

(2) The inhalation of dust, fibers, and chemical agents is the factor of most importance.

(3) The majority of industrial workers are affected with pharyngeal disorders, dependent to a certain extent upon their occupation.

(4) In those already affected with pharyngitis before assuming these occupations, the morbid changes are augmented by the work.

(5) The primary pharyngeal changes are those of acute congestion and inflammation. Chronic changes are the ultimate result.

(6) The pharyngitis produced in part or whole by the occupation does not differ in any respect from the ordinary forms.

(7) If the nasal chambers are in an approximately normal condition, pharyngeal affections are much less liable to occur than otherwise.

(8) Treatment bears no relation to the occupation as a factor, and the therapeutic means used will depend upon the choice of laryngologist.

(9) Prophylactic measures are very important, and much has already been done toward elevating the hygienic standard of the mill worker, by improving his daily surroundings in the way of better ventilation, the elimination or reduction of the excessive dust in the respired air, and increasing the age limit at which a youth is permitted to enter these occupations.

As regards the prevention of catarrhal affections of the upper respiratory tract, daily washing with an inexpensive alkaline antiseptic solution will be of much value ; this should be done morning and evening, and during the working hours a few drops of any of the refined petrolatum oils should be placed in each nostril. This procedure has been followed out in a number of cases among weavers, etc., and most gratifying results have been obtained.   PALMER.

Reid, A. P.—Neoplasm of Eyelid.—*Maritime Med. News*, Halifax, March, 1900.

This case is interesting from the excellent result obtained.

Mrs. E. M., aged fifty-two (in ordinary health), about five or six years ago noticed what appeared to be a wart about the center of the margin of the left lower eyelid. It gave no pain or inconvenience and was not treated in any way. For two or three years there was but little appearance of change and it was not large enough to be noticeable, but about two years ago it began to enlarge very slowly for the first year and then much more rapidly the past year, until it became from one-quarter to three-eighths of an inch wide, and one-half inch long, becoming quite prominent. Its rapid growth lately gave rise to suspicion of epithelioma, and the question of its removal was a subject of serious consideration. But how ? To use the knife meant an extensive removal of the lower lid with the surgical difficulties attending this proceeding, and as well the deformity which must result. Last fall it became painful, interfered with the comfortable closing of the eyelids, became inflamed and ulcerated. It healed partially and then it was decided to attempt its removal, and preference was first to be given to an escharotic.

There are many preparations from which to choose, but it was decided to use Bourgard's paste, as this exercises a selective affinity for neoplastic tissue and has but little effect on normal tissue other than causing a local inflammation. One of the properties of this preparation is to cause a whitish eschar of the neoplasm, leaving the normal tissue quite unaffected after its application. In addition to the local inflammation a conjunctivitis of a mild character was lighted up, owing to a portion of the paste being carried on to the conjunctiva by the upper lid. In a few days this whitish slough separated and fell off. When the local inflammation had subsided the paste was again applied ; this produced another large whitish eschar, which like the former separated in a few days, leaving a small, cupshaped ulcer, which gradually contracted and healed with scarcely an appreciable cicatrix. The paste was again applied, but it had no effect on the cicatrix. The removal of the neoplasm was complete and no appearance of its position was visible, except that the sites of lashes of the eyelids became vacant on the edge of the eyelid. The result of the treatment was very satisfactory—1st. In the complete removal of the growth. 2d. In the small amount of pain and inconvenience suffered, and 3d. Leaving no cicatrix or deformity visible.

FORMULA OF BOURGARD'S PASTE.

Wheat flour............. .... }	aa ℥ i
Starch..... .... }	aa ℥ i
Arsenious acid................................. ....gr.	viii
Hydrarg. sulph. rub...... ....gr.	xl
Ammon. muriate.... .... gr.	xl
Hydrarg. bichloride.... ....gr.	iv
Zinc chloride cryst........	℥ i
Hot water.....	℥ iss

Grind all together except the zinc chloride and water. Dissolve the zinc chloride in the water and pour on the powder, stirring all the time.

The paste, after standing twenty-four hours, is ready for use. It can be spread on linen or cotton cloth and applied to the part for twenty-four hours, and if the whole growth be not removed it can be reapplied as often as necessary. Sometimes it causes considerable pain and then cocaine may be added to the paste.

For small growths it is most readily applied by spreading on a small particle with a toothpick (wooden), and no dressing is necessary. This proceeding can be repeated as often as necessary. DEADY.

Siefert.—Diagnosis and Therapy of Diseases of the Nasal Sinuses.—*Münch. med. Wochen*, May 23, 1899 (*The Lar.*).

The author strongly recommends the employment of negative politzerization as a means of diagnosis in these cases. His manner of procedure is as follows : The nares are very thoroughly cleansed, so that no discharge of any nature is discernible in the nostrils ; the patient holds some water in the mouth, that he can swallow when directed to do so. The compressed Politzer bag is then held tightly to the nostril, and as the patient swallows it is allowed to expand. By this rarefication of the air in the nostrils, if there is any discharge in the sinuses it is drawn out in the nares. If such discharge is found on immediate inspection of nasal cavities, sinusitis is probable. He has cured seven cases of acute empyema of the frontal and four of the maxillary sinuses in this manner. PALMER.

Sachs, Dr. Richard (Hamburg).—Operation on the Pharyngeal Tonsil, Hemophilia, Death.—*Jour. of Lar., Rhin., and Otol.*, February, 1900.

A report of a case of a boy ten years old, from whom the author removed the Luschka's tonsil, the size of a walnut, with one sweep of a modified Gottstein curette. Secondary hemorrhage commenced about six hours after operation and continued intermittently till death on the fourth day, notwithstanding the following measures were employed : Tampons of iodoform gauze, plain, and others dipped in solution of ferric chloride ; the usual stimulants, camphor, etc., were administered and finally transfusion of physiological solution of sodium chloride, and also, as suggested by Heymann (Leipsig), a physiological solution of sodium chloride with $2\frac{1}{2}$ per cent. of gelatin.

Previous history of patient was: When a tooth was extracted the dentist with difficulty stopped hemorrhage four days after ;

it took long time to stop the bleeding after a slight cut of the finger. Grandfather on mother's side died of parenchymatous hemorrhage of the kidney.   PALMER.

Ziem, (Dantzig).—Trachoma of the Conjunctiva and its Relation to Diseases of the Nose.—*Annals Otol. Rhin. and Lar.*, February, 1899.

The doctor believes there is an "intimate connection between trachoma and nasal catarrh"; and is of the opinion that "many patients with one-sided trachoma will be found to have a nasal catarrh on the same side, and not unusually the localization of the trachoma in either the upper or lower fornix will be found associated with either suppuration of the frontal or superior maxillary sinus, so that the inflammation must have been extended by means of the vascular anastomosis of the naso-frontal or infra-orbital vessels to either the upper or lower lid."

PALMER.

Valentine, Ad.—The Mechanics of Coughing.—*Arch. für Laryngologie*, Band IX. Heft. 3, 1899.

The writer gives the usual explanation of the modus operandi of coughing and then gives his own.

"A sudden and very deep inspiration, with abduction of the cords, is followed by a forcible adduction of the latter, causing a firm closure and compression of the glottis. At the same time occurs an increasing compression of the chest by the muscles of expiration, the lower jaw is somewhat dropped, the mouth open, the tongue pointed and projected slightly forward. The soft palate is elevated. Then follows the real concussion of coughing. The spasmodically closed glottis is not by any means forced open by the column of expired air, but the spasm of the adductors suddenly ceases and one can see how the previously adducted arytenoids and vocal cords become abducted with lightning-like rapidity.

"The glottis opens often to the widest possible extent. After the impulse of the cough is over, the cords close again, but not so tightly as before. Of course the sudden and great expansion of the glottis is due to a reflex contraction of both postici. This contraction differs from the ordinary inspiratory contraction, mainly in the rapidity of its occurrence."   PALMER.

Hubbell, Alvin A.—The Maddox Rod or Phorometer : Which ?—*Jour. Am. Med. Assn.*, February 17, 1900.

An interesting discussion of a question exciting much attention at present.

The Maddox rod or suppressed-image or obscuration test in some of its forms, and the prism or diplopia test in some form of phorometer, are most commonly used in the determination of the co-ordination of the external muscles of the eyes. In this practice it is assumed that there is a functional position of rest for the eyes in binocular vision, and that in this position of rest, the lines of vision are both directed toward the point of fixation. It is not my purpose to discuss here the nature or limits of this co-ordination, the causes which disturb it, or the effects, or treatment of any disturbance of it. My only question is as to the comparative value of the diplopia test, by Stevens' phorometer.

Using Stevens' nomenclature I assume that orthophoria is the strictly normal condition of ocular co-ordination, although I grant that there may be, within narrow limits and in relation to unusual accommodative or other forms of innervation, a condition of "physiological" heterophoria. I further assume that the object of co-ordination tests is to determine the presence or absence of orthophoria, and if absent, the amount of variation.

During the whole period of my ophthalmic practice, I have used, more or less, the diplopia test, and for several years, as the most convenient form of it, the Stevens phorometer. Since Maddox brought forward the rod test, a number of years ago, I have also used this, and have made a large number of comparisons of the results of both.

Dissociation of the images of the two eyes is the principle governing each of these tests. In the diplopia test, the dissociation is effected by changing the visual axis of one eye by means of a prism. The displacement of one image cannot be done without associating with it, more or less, an impulse to some form of ocular effort. This may be very slight in some cases and considerable in others. It may affect one muscle or set of muscles in some, and another in others. Certainly, there is not a state of complete muscular rest.

In the obstruction or suppression test no such effort is invited, no change of innervation takes place. Binocular fixation is suspended without it, and the eyes yield to the deviation tendency in accordance with the status of innervation of the acting and governing nerve-centers. If this be true, it would seem that the Maddox rod should more correctly indicate the absence or presence and amount of heterophoria.

COMPARATIVE REPORT OF 100 CASES, SHOWING 140 MEASUREMENTS BY THE MADDOX ROD AND STEVENS' PHOROMETER.

EXOPHORIA.

MADDOX ROD.		STEVENS' PHOROMETER.							
		Same Exo.	Less Exo.		More Exo.		Lateral Ortho.	Eso.	
Degrees.	No. Cases.	Cases.	Cases.	Degrees.	Cases.	Degrees.	Cases.	Cases.	Degrees.
¼	1	1	......	......	......	......	......	......	
½	6	3	1	¼	1	1½	1	......	
¾	1	......	......	......	1	1	......	......	
1	11	5	4	¼ to ¾	1	1½	......	1	½
1½	5	1	4	½ to 1	......	......	......	......	
2	5	1	4	½ to 1	......	......	......	......	
3	1	......	4	1½	......	......	......	......	
3½	1	......	1	2½	......	......	......	......	
5	1	......	1	2½	......	......	......	......	
7	1	......	1	3	......	......	......	......	
9	1	1	......	......	......	......	......	......	
	34	12	17		3		1	1	

ESOPHORIA.

MADDOX ROD.		STEVENS' PHOROMETER.							
		Same Eso.	Less Eso.		More Eso.		Lateral Ortho.	Exo.	
Degrees.	No. Cases.	Cases.	Cases.	Degrees.	Cases.	Degrees.	Cases.	Cases.	Degrees.
½	5	1	......	......	......	......	2	2	¾ to 1
1	21	......	9	¼ to ¾	......	......	8	4	¼ to ½
1½	1	......	1	1	......	......	......	......	
2	11	......	6	¼ to 1	......	......	5	......	
2½	1	1	......	......	......	......	......	......	
3	6	1	4	½ to 1	......	......	......	1	¾
4	6	1	5	1 to 2½	......	......	......	......	
6	1	......	1	2	......	......	......	......	
9	1	......	1	1½	......	......	......	......	
	53	4	27		0		15	7	

RIGHT HYPERPHORIA.

Maddox Rod — Degrees	Maddox Rod — No. Cases	Same R.H. Cases	Less R.H. Cases	Less R.H. Degrees	More R.H. Cases	More R.H. Degrees	Vertical Ortho. Cases	Left Hyp. Cases	Left Hyp. Degrees
¼	5	1					2	2	¼
½	2				1	2½	1		
1	1						1		
2¼	1		1	1					
	9	1	1	1	1		4	2	

LEFT HYPERPHORIA.

Maddox Rod — Degrees	Maddox Rod — No. Cases	Same L.H. Cases	Less L.H. Cases	Less L.H. Degrees	More L.H. Cases	More L.H. Degrees	Vertical Ortho. Cases	R. Hyp. Cases	R. Hyp. Degrees
¼	12	7			1	½			
½	14	5	3	¼	3	¾ to 1½	4		
¾	1						1		
1	4	1	3	½ to ¾					
2	2		2	½ to 1					
	33	13	8		4		8		

ORTHOPHORIA.

Maddox Rod	Ortho. Cases	Eso. Cases	Eso. Deg.	Exo. Cases	Exo. Degrees	Right Hyp. Cases	Right Hyp. Degrees	Left Hyp. Cases	Left Hyp. Degrees
11 Cases...........	6			2	½	1	½	2	½

DEGREES SHOWN : TOTALS.

	Eso.	Exo.	Rt. Hyp.	Left Hyp.
Stevens' Phorometer..................	39¾	44¾	4¾	20¼
Maddox Rod..........	116	59½	5¼	18¾

Again, if it be contended that there is no extraneous muscular effort in the diplopia test, then, in the absence of such effort in either method, the one which, in general, shows the greater amount of heterophoria must be the most correct. Dr. Stevens and others hold that the Maddox rod does not reveal the full amount of heterophoria because of the tendency to fuse the images of the two eyes. In this case it would generally show less heterophoria than the phorometer, but the contrary has been my experience.

As an illustration of my experience, I will give the results of my measurements in 100 persons, taken consecutively as they came to my office, irrespective of conditions of general health or refraction, and without glasses. In this series I omitted cases in which vision was less than 5/12 in either eye. The comparative tests were made at the same sitting, and at a distance of 5 meters, using a gas-flame about the size of that of a common candle.

In some of them, as will be inferred, the heterophoria was mixed, so to speak ; that is, there was right or left hyperphoria with esophoria or exophoria.

In 53 cases in which the Maddox rod showed esophoria Stevens' phorometer gave an esophoria of the same degree in 4, less esophoria and lateral orthophoria in 32, exophoria in 7, and more esophoria in none. In 34 cases in which there was exophoria by the rod, by the phorometer there was the same exophoria in 12, less and lateral orthophoria in 18, esophoria in 1, and more exophoria in 3. In 9 cases of right hyperphoria by the rod, the phorometer showed the same in 1, less and vertical orthophoria in 5, left hyperphoria in 2, and more right hyperphoria in 1. In 33 cases of left hyperphoria by the Maddox rod, the phorometer showed the same in 13, less and vertical orthophoria in 16, right hyperphoria in none, and more left hyperphoria in 4. In 11 orthophoric cases by the rod, the phorometer gave orthophoria in 6, exophoria in 2, right hyperphoria in 1, and left hyperphoria in 2.

Thus it will be seen that in the 140 measurements the two tests gave the same results in 36. In the heterophoric cases there was less heterophoria or, what was the same in effect, lateral and vertical orthophoria, by the phorometer than by the rod in 71, and in 8 there was more. The opposite form of heterophoria was shown in 10, while in 7 of the orthophoric cases by the rod there were exophoria and right and left hyperphoria by the phorometer. In view of the fact that by the rod test there is introduced, absolutely, no extraneous impulse to muscular contraction, and as its findings are in the large majority of cases equal to, or in excess of, those of the phorometer, I am forced to believe that, in connection with other contributory muscular tests, it is a more precise and trustworthy guide in daily practice than the phorometer.

The foregoing table shows more fully the comparative results of the 100 cases above referred to. DEADY.

Kyle, M. D., D. Braden.—Appropriate Treatment of Certain Varieties of Nasal Deflections and Redundancy.—*The Laryngoscope*, January, 1900.

" The varieties of deflections considered in this paper are: 1, the split cartilaginous septum with bulging into both nostrils ; 2, dislocation of the columnar cartilage ; 3, simple deflection in which the cartilage is very thin ; 4, the letter S deflection ; 5, deflection of the cartilage with involvement of the bony septum ; 6, deflection due to the splitting of the cartilage with bulging on one side only ; 7, deflection in which there is redundancy of tissue overlapping the septum and extending close to the flow of the nose.

" The causes may be divided into : 1, deviation or deflection from disease ; 2, traumatic, and 3, congenital deflection. The diseases causing deviation are : (*a*) inflammation of overlying mucosa, *e. g.*, in purulent rhinitis of children, or in strumous or rachitic persons ; (*b*) dental diseases also in children ; (*c*) ulceration either simple, syphilitic, tuberculous, lupoid, post-diphtheritic or typhoid ; (*d*) perichondritis ; (*e*) encroachment of hypertrophied turbinated ; (*f*) uric-acid diathesis producing perichondritis ; (*g*) septal abscess.

2. The traumatic causes are familiar to all.

3. Congenital deflection. " I believe that many cases . . . are due to the fact that at birth during labor, owing to the position of the head in the birth canal, considerable pressure has been exerted on the soft, almost cartilaginous, bones of the nose." He also believes many heretofore considered congenital are due to the deleterious effect of mouth-breathing, through its action on the hard palate, and furthermore in the bad habit of sniffling,

the " continual drawing down of the facial muscles, while the bony union is taking place, will cause narrowing of the arch and give a peculiar fish-faced expression."

Treatment : " Each individual case, with its own peculiarities and variations, demands its own special modification of treatment." Some slight cases may be reduced merely by replacing by pressure of finger and retaining with splint.

In greater deflection confined to cartilage, after cutting through mucous membrane, he saws from the concave side at articulation with maxillary, through one-third of thickness of cartilage, and then fractures remainder with nasal forceps and applies splints.

If the deviation extends into the bony septum the aforesaid incision is extended further backward and beside, a second incision parallel to it, and about midway between it and the roof of the nares, is made ; fracture and splint as before.

"Another form of deflection occurs, in which there seems to have been splitting of the two halves, with bulging on only one side, the opposite side being almost perpendicular." (Apparently an exostosis. Editor.) For this the overlying mucosa is dissected off, the redundant tissue sawn out by V-shaped incision, and the mucosa replaced over excised cartilage and allowed to heal. Case of deflection when there is redundant tissue as also true exostosis, the author operates same as last described.

The writer requires patients to wear tubes only two or three weeks, and only from four to twelve hours per diem. After-treatment is cleansing with boracic solution, 10 grains to ounce, and advises against irritation from too frequent or strong douching. PALMER.

Dr. Lapalle.—Statistical Table of 169 Autopsies of the Accessory Sinuses.—*Jour. Lar., Rhin. and Otol.*, February, 1900. (Paper presented at the Soc. of Lar., Rhin. and Otol. of Paris.)

From the post-mortem examinations of 169 subjects he found the following conditions.

Number of cases of empyema = 55 = 32.54 per cent.
Men affected   = 43.
Women "   = 12.

" Seventeen cases of acute lung disease gave 9, or 52.94 per cent.

" Fifty-nine cases of tubercular lung disease gave 19, or 32.25 per cent.

" Sixteen cases of cancer, chiefly abdominal, gave 5, or 31.25 per cent.

" Sixteen cases of cardiac disease gave 5, or 31.25 per cent.

" Nineteen cases of brain disease gave 5, or 26.31 per cent.

" Thirteen cases of kidney disease gave 3, or 23.07 per cent.

" Among the 55 cases of empyema :

" The antrum was affected in 48 instances.

" The sphenoidal sinus was affected in 19 instances.

" The ethmoidal cells were affected in 6 instances.

" The frontal sinus was affected in 5 instances.

" Further figures are given bearing on uni- or bi-laterality, and the anatomical combinations found.

" The total percentage of empyema (32.54 per cent.) in this considerable number of unpicked cases is significant. The speaker was inclined to look upon the empyema as the cause, rather than the result of the general maladies." PALMER.

Lichtwitz, M.—Sequestration of Bone around the Lumen of the Canal Formed by Drilling the Alveolus in Antral Disease.—*Jour. Lar., Rhin. and Otol.*, February, 1900.

In several cases, after Cooper's operation with burr or trephine where the floor of antrum was thick (.75 or 1.0 centimeter), the writer found that the patient complained of severe pain followed by the throwing off of a tubular sequestrum of bone—the wall of the operative canal. The bony tissue around the canal is probably eburnated by the heat generated by the necessarily long application of the rapidly revolving drill. To obviate this he uses a special helicoid burr, and interrupts the drilling frequently.

PALMER.

Ortega, R.—Dilatation of Ophthalmic Vein : Cure.—*Jour. Am. Med. Assn.*, 1900, page 851.

I will give a brief résumé of an operation which I was called on to perform in a case of dilatation of ophthalmic vein, and which, to my gratification, proved successful.

My patient was a resident of Eagle Pass, Tex., a woman of thirty-two years of age, married, vigorous, and the mother of five children. The first of these died at the age of five months, of hydrocephalus, the second at two months, of " fever," and the third at seventeen months, also of " fever." The fourth and fifth, both girls, aged respectively four years, and five months, are now living and in good health.

The patient, referring to the illness in which my services were solicited, stated that on December 21, 1898, she was attacked by la grippe; from this date a humming began in her left ear; January 1, 1899, she noticed that the sight of her left eye was becoming weak, and shortly succeeding that time the affection of the conjunctiva of that eye commenced.

I first saw her on January 18, and after obtaining from her the data given above, I proceeded to the thorough examination which the case demanded, finding a noticeable exophthalmic tumor of the eyelids and neighboring regions, accompanied by immovability and lividity, with the conjunctiva strongly congested, and forming a burning wheal between the eye and the lower eyelid, which was so depressed as to prevent its elevation. The tension, the cornea, and the iris were normal. (I did not make the ophthalmoscopic examination, because I had not the instruments with which to do so with me, nor, indeed, did I intend doing so afterward, because of the patient's delicate condition, and the lack of proper surroundings.) This, in addition to the very intense pain which she complained of, stating that it extended to the whole side of the head and face, and even to the nape of the neck, explained to me the insomnia, want of appetite, etc., from which she was suffering, and convinced me of the existence of a tumor back of the eye.

Suspecting that it might be a retro-ocular abscess, I proposed an examination under the influence of chloroform, to which, however, she would not accede. I then prescribed iodide of potassium, two grams daily, and bichloride of mercury in lukewarm applications, myself administering an injection of morphine with atropine.

On the next day, the 19th, her condition was worse. I was then compelled to say that if they persisted in refusing to agree to the operation I had proposed, I would feel it incumbent on me to withdraw from the case. They agreed, therefore, to come to some conclusion in the matter within twenty-four hours. In the meanwhile I prescribed a continuation of the treatment then being tried, with the addition of two portions of chloral of two grams each, to be used in case the pain became intolerable. On the 20th, Dr. Duggan administering the chloroform, I introduced the bistoury in the external angle of the eye, coasting the surface of the socket as far as the caruncle, which resulted in the flow of about sixty grams of blood. Next I made a careful examination with a blunt stiletto, but found no pus, and then made some shallow incisions in the conjunctiva, ordering the continuation of the former treatment.

When the patient recovered consciousness she expressed great relief, which improvement was maintained for two days, when her condition became worse than it had been before. Suspecting, then, a venous dilatation, and, also, as the vision of that eye was lost, a hypopyon having appeared with the additional symptoms of sympathy in the other eye, I proposed enucleation, which was agreed to.

On January 30 Dr. Duggan again administered the chloroform, and I availed myself of the Volkmann spoon No. 1, to load and overset the ocular globe, because the nippers failed to grasp either conjunctiva or the tendon which was tearing it, and the spoon enabled an easier enucleation. I next proceeded to the examination of the cavity, and ascertained that there was dilatation of the ophthalmic vein of about one centimeter. I then abandoned the idea I had of binding the vessel that formed the aneurism, as, having been prevented from giving the other treatment proposed by the authors, I was forced to leave matters as they were, which I particularly regretted, because, not only would the dilatation increase greatly through need of compression, but also the troubles consequent thereupon would follow, and probably result in the need of a further posterior operation. Fortunately, however, both for my patient and myself, I remembered the advice of Dr. G. Laurens, when the lateral breast comes open when ascending the mastoid prominence, and this seemed to be a similar case, notwithstanding the fact that he referred to the opening of the breast by accident, while in this instance it was through intent, besides which I had the advantage of being able to compress it by reason of a bony surface behind the vessel. The resolution was quickly followed by the operation. With a compress of bichloride gauze in my left hand, and the spoon in my right, the dilatation was pulled out, producing a copious flow of blood. This, however, did not alarm me, as I expected and was prepared to control it, and did immediately, by compression with the gauze I held in my left hand. I immediately requested Dr. Duggan to assume charge of the compression, while I proceeded to thoroughly clean the operated part. I then raised the level of the compression above the borders of the orbit, placing over these a silver dollar to equalize the pressure at the center, and admit of free circulation in that locality. I then placed a thick wrapper of cotton and antiseptic bandage thereon.

After twelve days I removed these appliances, which had been retained all the while without producing any disagreeable odor, through my having kept them dampened with a solution of formol. There was a sudden hemorrhage, caused by the tearing of some fleshy blood clots. I applied a little glutol with fresh wrappers of gauze and cotton to the outside, which I held in place with a tight bandage. On February 17 I again removed this, without further flow of blood, applying a little glutol as before in the socket of the eye, with a gauze covering, but without a compressing bandage.

On February 20 I was again called in, the patient complaining of a slight pain, which she feared would increase. With the object of relieving this, and hastening the cicatrix retraction, I prescribed the insertion of fifteen to twenty drops of a weak solution of tannic acid and cocaine. On the 28th I found everything progressing excellently, the patient informing me that she had discontinued the use of my last prescription after two days, because she had ceased to experience the trouble. Not a drop of pus was found after the removal of the bandages.

There remains at present, as the only trace of the severe illness, a slight humming noise in the ear, which she states has already greatly diminished, and during a good portion of the day disappears entirely, enabling her to sleep without difficulty.

As another incident, which may be of interest, I would mention the following: On October 17, 1896, two partners and myself were called into consultation with Dr. Duggan, who was attending a brother of the patient referred to above. Having discovered that he was suffering from venous varices of the floor of the mouth, we suggested intervention, to which the family would not agree. He died the following day of asphyxia. He was thirty-two years of age.

Deductions.—It is undoubtedly true that the members of this family are predisposed to vascular dilatations. It is probable that the dilatation of the vein was somewhat lengthened in the interior of the skull, which produced the humming of the ear mentioned before. The cure was doubtless due to the suppression of the more extended part of the vein, and the formation of coagulated blood in the balance of the dilatation, and the presence of the gauze in the open extreme, and the lengthening of the coagulation to the walls of the vessel, which was proved by the complete cessation of the humming noise.   DEADY.

Poole, W. H.—Beta Eucaine as an Anæsthetic in Eye, Nose, and Throat Work.—*Med. News*, October 21, 1899.

The writer deduces the following conclusions after using beta eucaine in such operations as furuncle of the auditory canal, paracentesis of the drum, hypertrophy of the turbinateds, galvano-cautery, polypi, enchondroma and foreign bodies.

"1. Eucaine is decidedly less toxic than cocaine, therefore superior to it.

"2. Its aqueous solutions keep well and can be sterilized by boiling without destroying the activity of the drug.

"3. It produces anæsthesia equally well and sometimes better than cocaine.

"4. It is superior to cocaine in that it does not cause heart depression or other unpleasant effects.

"5. It does not cause mydriasis or disturbances of accommodation, which is an advantage in some cases.

"6. It is less dangerous to the cornea than cocaine, inasmuch as it does not cause desquamation of the superficial epithelium."
    PALMER.

Misenheimer, Dr. C. A.—Foreign Bodies in the Air Passages.—*North Carolina Med. Jour.*, February, 1900.

The author, after giving the pathology and symptomatology of this condition taking place in any of the air passages down to the larger bronchi, strongly opposes the use of emetics, sternutatories, inversion of the body, etc., but recommends operative procedures exclusively. The clinical histories of six cases occurring under his care are appended with the mode of treatment.   PALMER.

Rumex Crispus.—*The Critique*, February 15, 1900.

Rumex crispus has proven curative in a number of cases
where after a cold there was a continual desire to clear the
throat.   It has also been a valuable remedy in consumptives
where sulphur is ordinarily indicated by the morning diarrhea, a
dry cough with nightly aggravation.   In colds it is adapted to
where the catarrhal discharge is very profuse and thin, and is
followed by a thick, yellowish or whitish, tenacious mucus,
almost impossible to blow from the nose or to cough up.   It has
frequently been prescribed where the discharge was excessive in
amount, starting the patients on the road to recovery, and often
bringing them back to a normal condition of health without the
use of other remedies.   Secure the proper start and nature will
usually finish the cure for you.

Cowgill, Warwick M.—Why the Negro does Not Suffer from Trachoma.—*Jour. Am. Med. Assn.*, February 17, 1900.

Below will be found an interesting theory to account for the
immunity of the negro in the United States to trachoma.   The
theory is further borne out by the fact that in the West Indies,
where social conditions are different, no such immunity exists.

It is a coincident observation among oculists practicing in our
Southern States, where the larger proportion of our negro population lives, and where trachoma is a very prevalent disease, that
the negro, except very rarely, is not affected with trachoma.
Why the negro does not have it has been largely theorized on.
Probably the explanation most largely entertained is that he is
immune to the disease, that the conjunctiva of the negro does
not present a soil suitable for the development of trachoma.
To my mind this theory is untenable.   The reasoning is loose
and not based on facts to guarantee a correct conclusion.   There
is a rational, plain, scientific, and simple explanation for the fact
that negroes do not suffer from this disease; an explanation that
does not call for some unique quality of construction in the
negro ; an explanation based on a line of reasoning, concurrent
with that used in the development of facts in connection with
other diseases, viz. : trachoma is a contagious disease, and the
negro escapes it because he does not come in contact with the
contagium.

The question as to whether trachoma is a contagious disease or not is one that, I know, is in dispute. Either side can boast of able supporters. Several have announced to the world that they have discovered the germ of trachoma, but none have presented such conclusive proofs that their findings have been accepted by the profession. From my clinical experience I believe that it is contagious in the same way as gonorrhea and syphilis are contagious, and I will assume, for the sake of my argument, that such is the fact, and on this base my reasonings in support of my second proposition, that the negro does not have trachoma because he does not come in contact with the contagium.

I draw my conclusion from the study of this disease as it occurs among the people of western Kentucky, southern Illinois, and a portion of western Tennessee, from which sections my patients usually come. Paducah, a place of twenty-five thousands inhabitants, is the only city, and the center of this district. The remaining portion, including the smaller towns, hamlets, and villages, I include with the rural districts.

In Paducah, with a negro population of probably one-fifth, trachoma is not often seen. In the surrounding country, where the negro population is one in eight or one in ten, trachoma is very prevalent. In fifteen years of practice I have seen no case occurring in a negro. Nor do I find this disease among the well-to-do class of whites. But it is extremely common among the poorer class of whites in the country districts.

With these facts before us, if we look into the social relations and customs of the people, I think we can see a solution to our problem. It is a well-known fact that the negro in our Southern States comes in contact with only the upper and well-to-do class of whites, in the position of servants. And as trachoma is but rarely seen among the upper class of whites, the negro has but little chance to come in contact with the germ from this source.

It is also a well-known fact that between the negro and the poorer class of whites there is a wide gulf fixed. They do not come in immediate contact with each other at all. This fact bars the negro from contracting the disease from this most prolific source. With the lower class of whites there is a custom of having one towel, which is used in common by all the members of the family, and also by the neighbors that visit them. The-one towel used in common is the medium of conveyance of the trachoma germ from one to the other.

Burnett, in his article on trachoma, in the "System of Diseases of the Eye," by Norris and Oliver, mentions the fact that among the laborers on a railroad in east Tennessee, where Irish and negroes worked under the same hygienic surroundings, the Irish were much afflicted with trachoma, while the negroes were entirely free from this disease. I venture to assert that there was no immediate contact, in this instance, between the Irish and the negroes. I feel safe in saying that the negroes did not use the Irishmen's towel.

Statistics would show that but an extremely small percentage of virtuous maidens have gonorrhea, because they do not come in contact with the contagium of this disease. The people of Ohio do not suffer from yellow fever. Not because they are immune to this disease, for the cases in Gallipolis, in 1878, proved the contrary, but simply because they do not come in contact with the germs of yellow fever. The Hawaiians did not have syphilis until it was introduced among them by immediate contact with foreigners. I think the same line of reasoning holds good in regard to the negro and trachoma.

In order to transmit trachoma from one eye to another, the secretions from the diseased eye must be conveyed directly, while viable, to the unaffected eye. This conveyance could not be carried out more perfectly, when done in an unintentional way, than by the use of one towel in common by those who are affected with trachoma and those that are not so affected. We find, where trachoma is prevalent, the use of a towel in common is the prevailing practice.

The negro in this country, as a slave, or now as a freedman, has never in the past, nor does he now, come in immediate contact with the whites. Therefore the negro has not contracted from the whites this disease, trachoma, which can only be transmitted through immediate contact.   DEADY.

Bosworth, F. H.—The Relation of Pathological Conditions in the Ethmoid Region of the Nose and Asthma.—*N. Y. Med. Jour.*, November 18, 1899.

He holds that there is a very intimate connection between the mucous lining of the nose and that of the bronchi ; if there is inflammation or congestion of the one it will cause the same condition of the other. Asthma is a " vasomotor paresis of the blood-vessels of the mucous membrane of the bronchial tubes,"— this condition is the cause of the " œdematous hypertrophy and polypoid degeneration," which latter is at present considered to be the cause of asthma instead of the old theory of spasm of the bronchial muscular fibers.

" Polypoid degeneration of the mucous membrane of the nose, œdematous hypertrophy of the mucous membrane of the nose, and nasal polypi all indicate and are clear symptoms of ethmoiditis.

" We have ample clinical evidence for the statement that the nerve centers which preside over the vasomotor nerves must be in close proximity to the ethmoid cells. The first thing that occurs with swelling and distention of the ethmoid cells in so many cases, especially if there is a neurotic habit, is something which disturbs that control which the vasomotor center exercises over the blood-vessels of the nasal membrane, and we have sneezing, we have asthma, we have a disturbance of that nice relation which exists between the mucous membrane of the nose and the bronchial mucous membrane, upon which the integrity of the bronchial mucous membrane depends. However that may be, and whatever the train of symptoms that is set up by this distention of the ethmoid cells, certainly the indication is clear. We have to cure the ethmoiditis."

For this an oval burr, one-eighth to one-quarter of an inch in diameter, propelled by a dental engine or electric motor, is preferable to curettes or cutting forceps, as the trabeculæ separating the cells can be removed with more precision with the former instrument.   PALMER.

Fisher, Herbert, and Box, Chas. R.—Pigmented Tumor of the Eyeball : Death from Multiple Pigmented Carcinoma nearly Fourteen Years after Excision of the Eye.—*British Medical Journal*, report of the meeting of the Ophthalmological Society, March 8, 1900.

This was a case of primary pigmented tumor of the eyeball, for which the eye was excised in 1885, the patient being a man at that time aged forty-two. In 1899 he was readmitted into St. Thomas' Hospital with great enlargement of the liver, accompanied by jaundice, abdominal pain, sickness and diarrhea, and œdema of the lower extremities. For fifteen months the abdominal swelling had been progressing, accompanied by general weakness and loss of flesh. The patient died, and a post-mortem examination showed that the liver was almost replaced by a nodular mass of melanotic growth weighing 12 lb. 6 ozs. There were also a few pigmented growths in the left parietal pleura. A small pigmented growth the size of a pea sprang from the myocardium and projected into the right ventricle. Microscopic examination of the growths in the liver proved them to be melanotic carcinoma, and not sarcoma, as had been expected. Mr. Treacher Collins reported that the growth had originated in the ciliary processes, and extended thence into the iris and through the sclerotic. The cells were pigmented to a varying degree ; they were small, polygonal, and of an epithelial type, and from their arrangement in rows Mr. Collins gave it as his opinion that this growth was carcinomatous in character. It was decided to submit the sections to a pathological committee of the society for further examination and report. Mr. Devereux Marshall, while expressing no opinon as to the nature of the primary growth, said he had never heard of a case in which a true cancer had remained dormant for fourteen years, though he had seen and published a case in which a patient had died of metastatic sarcoma eleven years and five months after an eye had been removed for sarcoma. DEADY.

Warthin, Alfred Scott.—A Primary Polymorphous-cell Sarcoma of the Nose (With Universal Metastasis and Formation of a Free Sarcomatous Mass in the Right Ventricular Cavity).—*N. Y. Med. Jour.*, June 24, 1899.

A very exhaustive article, especially regarding the pathological aspect, from which we give the clinical history and summary of autopsy.

" Mr. F. E., aged thirty-nine years, was admitted to the University Hospital on the 1st of April, 1897. He was a lumberman, single, and gave a negative family history. Previous to the beginning of the present condition his health had been good. A year and a half before admission his right nostril became partially occluded. By blowing his nose with some violence he could force out large ' scabby, flaky masses.' This condition lasted for a year, when a vesicular eruption, becoming pustular, gradually spread over the right side of the nose, extending to the left. Three months before admission he had had a number of 'polypoids' removed from his right nostril. The patient did not know whether a microscopical examination of these had been made, but was told that they were ordinary nasal polypi. From the treatment of the case it is evident that the operator had . regarded them as benign growths, as when the patient entered the hospital no suspicion had been raised as to the malignant nature of his disease.

"He had been under treatment with a number of physicians who had diagnosticated his condition as eczema, syphilis, and lupus. He had no history of acquired syphilis, and under specific treatment his condition had grown steadily worse.

"A month before admission he had noticed numbness over the left side of the nose, left cheek, upper lip, and forehead to the median line. Diplopia, left-sided ptosis, and dilatation of the left pupil soon followed.

"On admission the general condition of the patient appeared fair. He complained of weakness, nervousness, insomnia, and of dull pain in his forehead. His appetite was poor, and bowels were constipated. He passed about one liter of urine daily, very highly colored, and with specific gravity of 1024. His nostrils were completely occluded, his breathing being entirely by the mouth and very.shallow in character. His nose was symmetrically enlarged ; the skin covered with yellowish, opaque crusts, with scattered pustules. Around this and extending slightly into the skin of each cheek there was redness with firm induration. The nostrils were filled with grayish-red masses. There was no odor.

"The sense of smell was entirely lost. There was complete anæsthesia over the distribution of the supraorbital and infraorbital branches of the fifth nerve. There was some atrophy of the muscles in this area. Ptosis of the left lid was present, with complete paralysis of the muscles of the left eyeball. Sight was diminished in the left eye. The retinal examination showed a marked degree of choked disk. The patient's mind was clear.

"A clinical diagnosis was made of malignant tumor of the nose with secondaries at the base of the brain, involving the first, second, third, fourth, and the first and second branches of the fifth motor fibers of the fifth and the sixth cranial nerves. The condition of the patient gradually became worse. No operation was attempted. On the 11th of May he had attacks of nausea and vomiting, followed by great disturbance of respiration and circulation. The extremities became œdematous, the patient sank into coma and died on the 17th of May. The necropsy was performed by me in the university laboratory of pathology, four hours after the patient's death." . . .

The Autopsy.—" The nasal fossa is completely filled with a soft tumor mass, showing extensive mucous degeneration. This mass is directly continuous with tumor masses filling up the frontal sinus, the sphenomaxillary fossa, and with the mass in the nostrils." . . .

" Heart : Of about twice the normal size, and very irregular in shape. The surface is irregularly nodular, the nodules appearing yellowish as seen through the epicardium." . . .

" The right ventricle contains some fluid blood and a large firm mass, about the size and shape of a large English walnut. It is grayish-red in color, and has a ribbed and furrowed surface suggesting the appearance of brain coral. Its surface presents no appearance of any previous union with the heart wall, nor can any evidence of such connection be found in the endocardium of the right heart." . . .

Summary.—"All of the growths are of the nature of sarcoma. The majority of the smaller nodules and the periphery of all the larger ones are made up of small, round, deeply-staining cells having but little intercellular substance and lying in intimate contact with the blood-vessels. In the central part of all the larger nodules, and in some of the smaller ones, the cells are larger, polymorphous, and there is an increase in the intercellular substance, which is myxomatous in character. In many of the nodules the entire central part of the growth has undergone a mucous degeneration, and early stages of this degeneration are seen in all of the growths. The tumors are further characterized throughout by the number and size of the blood-vessels. From the structure of the growth the diagnosis of the tumor as a myxomatous polymorphous-celled sarcoma would seem most appropriate.

" That the growth in the nasal fossa is the primary one there can be no reasonable doubt. The history of the case, the development of the symptoms, the size and structure of the nasal growth all support this view. The exact site of origin cannot be determined. The patient affirmed that it appeared first in the right nostril upon the right side of the septum. Moreover, the relation of the sarcoma to the polyps stated to have been removed cannot be settled in the absence of any definite microscopical evidence concerning their structure. The fact that the tumor everywhere shows a marked tendency to a mucous degeneration of its cells and the formation of a myxomatous intercellular substance might be taken as an evidence of an inherited tendency on the part of its cells tending to show a descent from a myoxmatous polyp. This, unfortunately, will not admit of further confirmation.

" The points of special interest in this case are the widespread metastases and the intracardiac growth. Secondaries are found in the dura, pineal body, hypophysis, cavernous sinus, lungs, pleura, heart, liver, spleen, kidneys, pancreas, stomach, intestines, peritoneum, testicles, prostate, and the cervical, bronchial, retroperitoneal, and mesenteric lymph glands. The richness of the growth in cellular elements, the scanty stroma, the numerous large thin-walled blood-vessels, the smallness and shape of the cells, all contributed to the facility of the rapid dissemination of the tumor. The numerous metastases throughout both venous and arterial systems are easily explained by the above-mentioned factors.

" The free sarcomatous body in the right ventricular cavity forms the most important feature of the case.

" The probable origin in my case is that suggested above— namely, the breaking loose of a polypoid nodule from the endocardium, its retention in the ventricle, and its subsequent growth." PALMER.

Gibbon, John H.—Report of a Case of a Foreign Body in the Esophagus, Located by Means of the X-Rays and Removed with a Swivel Coin-Catcher.—*North Carolina Med. Jour.*, July, 1899.

Interesting history, a clear skiagraph, and description of treatment. It was a campaign-button lodged in esophagus opposite the first and second dorsal vertibræ. Also relates a similar case of Mr. Roxburgh reported in the *Brit. Med. Jour.* PALMER.

Wright, Dudley, F. R. C. S., Eng.—Epithelioma of the Larynx :—Successful Removal of the Disease by the Operation of Laryngo-Fissure.—*Monthly Homeopathic Review.*

Mr. A. S., aged fifty-three years, first consulted me on October 26, 1898, complaining of hoarseness, which had been present five months. He had always been a healthy man, and the present trouble had attracted the notice of his friends more than his own. He had been a great cigarette smoker. There was no history of venereal disease, and no alcoholism. During the last two years he had lost about fourteen pounds in weight.

Besides the hoarseness, the presence of the following symptoms was elicited : Slight soreness in region of the thyroid cartilage ; occasional cough, with very little expectoration, and peculiar attacks of what appeared to be laryngeal spasm, in which he would have great difficulty for a few seconds in drawing a breath, and suffocation appeared imminent. These attacks were not frequent, and he had been subject to them for some years.

Examination of the throat gave no evidence of disease in the pharynx, but the larynx presented the following change. The right vocal cord showed an irregular thickening at a little posterior to its center. This thickening stood out as a somewhat distinct tumor of a nodular and sessile nature. At its base there was some redness, but the nodules on its surface were of a shining white aspect. On deep inspiration it could be seen that the thickening extended below the margin of the cord. Finally, the movement of the cord was impaired slightly, in that it did not move toward the middle line on phonation so rapidly as its fellow.

The whole condition was one suggestive of malignant disease ; at the same time I thought it advisable to temporise and see what internal and mild local treatment would do. The patient was ordered a spray of sulpho-carbolate of zinc, gr. iij to $\bar{3}$ j, and gr. v of iodide of potash were given internally three times daily. This was kept up for three weeks, and during this time some improvement in the local condition occurred.

Lotio thuja, 1 in 10, was now substituted for the zinc lotion, and thuja φ painted twice a week on the diseased cord. This was kept up for about three weeks, at the end of which time matters were very much at a standstill.

The patient now went to Buxton for a short holiday, returning to town on January 11. It was now seen that there was a marked increase in the size of the tumor, and the voice was distinctly more hoarse.

It was not considered wise to delay further ; so, having obtained the independent opinion of two other laryngologists, both of whom considered the growth to be epithelioma, and a week's treatment with increased doses of iodide being of no avail, arrangements were made for the removal of the diseased area.

This was done on January 26, 1899, and I had the advantage of the valuable assistance of Drs. Tilley and Vincent Green.

The patient was put under the influence of ether and the operation divided into two stages.

A long incision, reaching from the hyoid bone to the sternum, was made, and the larynx and trachea were fully exposed. A low tracheotomy was now performed, and a Hahn's tracheotomy tube with sponge tampon was inserted.

The ether was now administered through the tube, and five minutes were allowed for the sponge to swell up and close the lumen of the trachea around the tube.

During this time the anterior border of the thyroid cartilage was cleared and divided in the middle line, partly with the knife and partly with a fine saw.

The mucous membrane was now the only structure separating the wound from the interior of the larynx. This was divided in the direction of the original incision, and on holding the alæ of the thyroid cartilage aside with blunt hooks, the structures within were plainly visible.

A sponge was now pushed up into the pharynx, so as to shut that off from the area of operation, and to prevent saliva and mucus from flowing down.

It could now be seen that the disease affected not only a considerable portion of the cord, but had also crept up towards the mucous membrane covering the arytenoid, and involved a portion of the lining of the trachea below. The whole of the diseased area was surrounded by an elliptical incision wide of the tumor, which included the whole true vocal cord, the false cord and arytenoid of the same side, and also a fair-sized portion of the tracheal mucous membrane.

This was dissected up as one piece from the underlying cartilage, the latter being finally well scraped. The only vessel which needed seizing was one at the posterior margin of the wound ; the rest of the bleeding was mere oozing, and was stopped by sponge pressure.

The denuded surface was now painted over with Whitehead's varnish, and the sponge was removed from the pharynx. Next, the two alæ of the thyroid were approximated by means of sutures through the perichondrium and muscles, great care being taken to see that the two portions fitted into their original positions.

The tracheal tube was now removed, and the opening in the trachea closed by sutures, and the whole skin incision likewise closed, a small gauze drain being left in at the lower extremity of the cut.

The patient rallied well from the operation, and was able to swallow liquid food in small quantities within a few hours. He was kept lying on the diseased side, so that if there were any oozing of blood, it should not fall on to the opposite side and excite cough. There was very little bleeding, however, the expectoration being tinged with blood for about five days in gradually decreasing quantity. Within a fortnight the patient had left London for Brighton, where he was under the care of Dr. Herbert Wilde.

When I saw him again on March 6, thirty-nine days after the operation, I found that the parts within the larynx had healed up, and that a strong white cicatricial band had formed on the side, replacing the vocal cord removed. This band, however, did not quite reach up to the posterior wall of the larynx, there being a gap in the position of the removed arytenoid cartilage. On phonation the sound cord approximated well to the cicatricial band ; but owing to the presence of the gap, some air escaped, and hence the voice was not a strong one—but it was distinctly audible at some distance.

The patient has presented himself for examination within the past few days. It is now fifteen months all but a few days since the date of the operation, and the parts have exactly the same appearance as they had when the foregoing note was made. Moreover, he is in robust health, and is able to stand a hard day's work.

The foregoing is an illustration of the most recent and satisfactory method of removing intrinsic laryngeal carcinoma when limited to one side of the larynx. We were fortunate in being able to attack the disease at an early period, and the outlook is decidedly hopeful.

The work of Hahn of Berlin—now particularly brought home to our recollection by the case of the late celebrated Mr. Montagu Williams—has shown how the operation as described has saved many a patient from what was fifteen years ago, and is even by some at the present day, considered an incurable disease.

More recently Sir F. Semon has published his series of cases, which, owing to a more extended knowledge and perfected technique, were even more successful than those of Hahn.

At first the laryngeal cartilages were allowed to unite by granulation, and the tracheotomy tube was worn for some time. Then, as another step, the cartilages were approximated with sutures; and finally, we see that, as in my own case, the tracheotomy tube can be dispensed with entirely after the operation has been completed.

The use of Hahn's tube is particularly important, as it entirely prevents blood going into the bronchi during the operation, an occurrence which was largely responsible for the fatal broncho-pneumonia which marred the success of the first few cases submitted to this operation.

The placing of a sponge in the pharynx, as suggested by Dr. Tilley, is also a great aid during the operation.

Lastly, it is convenient to use an electric head-lamp during the intra-laryngeal stage of the operation, as a good illumination of the parts is essential. The other steps of the operation present no peculiar features, and the rule holds good as much in this as in any other operation for malignant disease, viz., to cut wide of the growth, and remove the diseased structures in one piece.

PALMER.

BOOK REVIEWS.

NEW, OLD, AND FORGOTTEN REMEDIES. Papers by Many
Writers. Collected, arranged, and edited by E. P. ANSHUTZ.
Philadelphia: Boericke & Tafel, 1900. Pp. 386. Cloth.
Price $2.00.

This book is a sort of "Old Curiosity Shop" of materia
medica. Compiled by the manager of the publishing department
of Messrs. Boericke & Tafel, in answer, as he states in the preface, to long-continued and various inquiries from members of
the profession for information as to this, that, and the other
drug which was not to be found in the ordinary works on the
subject, it consists of provings of, papers on, and general
enlightenment concerning some ninety "new, old, or forgotten
remedies," as the title states. These have been hunted up and
gathered in from dusty pigeon-holes and all sorts of out-of-the-
way places, and collected in a very handsome book, of which it
may be said that in paper, type, execution, and binding it is first-
class.

Some of the remedies which it contains are much used clinically, although not often found in text-books ; others are new,
but none of these are the so-called "laboratory remedies"
placed before the profession by the various drug firms, the
literature of which, as the author truly says, "may be had free on
request to the laboratories." Among the remedies considered
are avena sativa, arsen. brom., aurum mur. natron., baccillinum,
calc. renalis prep., echinacea angust., fucus vesic., heloderma
horridus, lac cannium, lapis albus, lycopus virg., mullein oil,
naphthalin, onosmodium virg., passiflora incarnata, scopolendra,
skookum chuck, stigmata maidis, symphoracarpus, thallium,
thyroid, tuberculinum, viscum album, etc., etc.

The data are drawn from all schools, and the result will be found
useful many times when the physician is obliged to go out of the
beaten track to conquer a "tough" case.

REFRACTION. The Refraction of the Eye. A Manual for
Students. By GUSTAVUS HARTRIDGE, F. R. C. S., Senior Sur-
geon to the Royal Westminster Ophthalmic Hospital, London.
Tenth Edition, 1900. Illustrated. 12mo. P. Blakiston's Son
& Co., 1012 Walnut St., Philadelphia, Pa. Price $1.50 net.

The tenth edition of this thoroughly good little work comes to
us as neat as a pin. Printed on good thick paper in large clear
type, profusely illustrated, beautifully bound, and containing a
set of test-types for both distant and near vision, it is a veritable
multum in parvo which has been in the past, and doubtless will
continue to be in the future, a great favorite with all students of
ophthalmology. We have always recommended it to the classes in
the college of the New York Ophthalmic Hospital and all others
desiring to enter upon the study of refraction ; it has always been
much appreciated, and in its new and revised form it should continue to occupy a very prominent place in the list of text-books
in the department which it covers.

A POCKET MEDICAL DICTIONARY, giving the pronunciation and
definition of the principal words used in medicine and the
collateral sciences, including very complete tables of clinical
eponymic terms, of the arteries, muscles, nerves, bacteria,
bacilli, micrococci, spirillia, and thermometric scales, and a
dose-list of drugs and their preparations, in both the English
and the metric system of weights and measures. By GEO. M.
GOULD, A. M., M. D. Author of "The Illustrated Medical
Dictionary," "The Student's Medical Dictionary"; Editor of
the Philadelphia *Medical Journal;* President, 1893–94, American Academy of Medicine. Fourth edition ; revised and
enlarged. Thirty thousand words. Philadelphia ; P. Blakiston's Son & Co., 1012 Walnut Street. 1900. Pp. 837.
Price $1.00.

A somewhat remarkable fact in connection with this little
work is the statement made by the publishers that 100,000 copies
of Dr. Gould's dictionaries have been sold. As they estimate
that there are only about 175,000 English-speaking physicians in
the entire world, it would seem that they are fairly well supplied
with medical dictionaries.

This is scarcely to be wondered at, when we survey the present
volume. A small book, measuring 3½ by 6 inches, one inch
thick, it can be carried in the pocket, and there are very few
things which the average physician will look for in an emergency
that he will fail to find. The various tables are alone worth the

low price of $1.00; and when we consider that the book is well printed in good clear type, on fine paper, bound in morocco, and gilt-edged, there is little more to be said.

THE AMERICAN YEAR-BOOK OF MEDICINE AND SURGERY, being a yearly Digest of Scientific Progress and Authoritative Opinion in all Branches of Medicine and Surgery, drawn from Journals, Monographs, and Text-Books of the Leading American and Foreign Authors and Investigators : collected and arranged, with critical editorial comments, by J. M. Baldy, M. D., Chas. H. Burnett, M. D., J. Chalmers DaCosta, M. D., W. A. Newman Dorland, M. D., Virgil P. Gibney, M. D., C. A. Hamann, M. D., Howard F. Hansell, M. D., Barton Cooke Hirst, M. D., E. Fletcher Ingalls, M. D., W. W. Keen, M. D., Henry G. Ohls, M. D., Wendell Reber, M. D., J. Hilton Waterman, M. D. Under the general editorial charge of GEO. M. GOULD, M. D. In two volumes. Prices: cloth, $3.00 per vol.; half morocco, $3.75 per vol. Surgical volume, pp. 560. Philadelphia: W. B. Saunders, 925 Walnut Street. 1900.

The present edition of this valuable work has been divided into two volumes, in order, as the preface states, to make the reading less tiresome, from the reduced bulk, and for the convenience of specialists. Some changes have been made in the editorial staff, notably the addition of Drs. Reynold W. Wilcox of New York and A. A. Stevens of Philadelphia, in the department of Materia Medica, Experimental Therapeutics, and Pharmacology.

Under Anæsthetics is reported the clinical observation made by Henry J. Garrigues respecting general anæsthesia by the Schleich mixture. He has used it on patients from ten to eighty years of age, of whom three had heart disease, four had lung trouble, seven had albuminuria. None of these was made worse by the anæsthetic. He concludes, in summary, that these mixtures are easily taken ; that they may be used in all cases when general anæsthesia is not contra-indicated ; that the anæsthesia can be quickly induced, and can be maintained with small quantities of the fluid ; that there is little accumulation of mucus, little vomiting, scarcely any tendency to cyanosis, no evil effect on the kidneys ; that the heart is only slightly weakened ; that there is some change in the respiratory sphere, though not so much as from ether or chloroform. He recommends the mixture for general use. On the other hand, H. Rodman, from an experience with seven hundred cases in Mt. Sinai Hospital, claims that the method is not a success. He notes the appearance of cyanosis in many cases, and says if at this stage care is not used the cyanosis increases, the respiration becomes shallow and infrequent, the pulse rapid and of low tension, and the patient stops breathing. This was noted in six cases. He thinks that it is below ether and chloroform in value. It has been discarded in Mt. Sinai Hospital. There is certainly a wide variance of opinion here.

Robert E. Bell writes on the effect of the Mauser bullet. He saw three hundred men who had been wounded with this bullet, and but one man had died ; a case in which the subclavian artery was injured. In some of these cases the bullets passed completely through the lung, the patient being little the worse for the experience. Bullets passed through the tarsus, the femur, or the humerus, simply leaving a small hole. A bullet entered the temple in one case and came out on the opposite side ; the man recovered, losing, however, the sight of one eye.

Under Refraction, Landolt criticises Snellin's test-types because of the unequal difficulty in distinguishing certain of the letters. He proposes in their stead a black circle on a white surface, presenting in some direction a gap, which for the unit of acuteness of vision corresponds to an angle of one minute. He gives this circle the same thickness as the corresponding letters in Snellin's types. By a movement of the hand the patient can indicate the direction of the gap, thus excluding to a great degree the intellectual functions and rendering the method equally valuable for the educated and the illiterate.

Two cases are reported of rapid change in refraction of diabetics. One case was a woman of forty-five whose refraction suddenly changed from —.50 D. to —2.00 D., the patient dying three weeks later of diabetic coma. In the other case, aged forty-three, the refraction changed one diopter in six weeks ; later all sugar disappeared from the urine and the patient became emmetropic.

Coppez' experience supports Snellin's observation that follicular conjunctivitis is frequently associated with post-nasal adenoids, and that their removal not only hastens the cure of the conjunctival trouble, but is often absolutely essential to it.

Thomas reports a case of divergent strabismus and mental disturbances in a child of ten following meningitis during infancy.

After curettage of the naso-pharynx for adenoids the strabismus entirely disappeared.

E. Bock claims to have seen astonishing improvement in vernal catarrh following the use of powered xeroform in three cases. As this is a very refractory disease, the observation is worth something. Several cases of the cure or relief of glaucoma by massage are recorded by various observers.

The department of the ear is specially interesting, by reason of the presentation of numerous cases of mastoid complication in all its varieties.

It is impossible to even attempt to do justice to the innumerable interesting reports of all varieties of surgical lesions treated in this volume. No physician can fail to find something in it which will be ·of service to him in his work ; whether a general practioner or a specialist, he will find that his own particular work is abundantly noticed. The publisher's work is, as usual, very well done.

A Practical Treatise on the Disorders of the Sexual Organs of Men. By Bukk G. Carleton, M. D., Genito-Urinary Surgeon and Specialist to the Metropolitan Hospital and Polyclinic of the Metropolitan Hospital ; Consulting Genito-Urinary Surgeon to the Hahnemann Hospital, etc., New York. Second edition, revised and enlarged. Pp. 333. Price $2 50 net ; by mail, $2.67. New York : Boericke & Runyon Co. 1900.

The second edition of Dr. Carleton's work is an improvement of a good thing. Equally as concise, practical, and readable as its predecessor, it has been enlarged, rewritten in places, and it fills the requirements of a text-book on the subjects covered. Beginning with a consideration of the physiology of the parts, and chapters on the sexual instinct and the prevention of sexual disorders, it proceeds in order taking up the various anomalies, injuries, and diseases of the glans and prepuce, the urethra, the penis, the seminal vesicles and ampullations of Henel, the prostate, the scrotum, the testes, the tunica vaginalis, and the spermatic cord. The various nervous derangements, impotence, psycopathia sexualis, and sterility, all receive attention, and the book concludes with a valuable section on therapeutics in which the symptoms are given of all the drugs in the materia medica which have been found useful in these diseases.

The treatise, in line with all Dr. Carleton's work, is eminently concise and practical, and will be found very useful by the general physician.

My Smoking-Room Companions. By William Harvey King. Thomas Whittaker. New York.

Seldom do we digress from our custom of excluding from these columns all books not relating to medicine. But as the author of this spicy story is a friend of so many of our readers, we feel assured that they will be glad to hear of this light and jovial effusion of the recreation hours of our mutual professional friend. It is gratifying to find another one of our usually sober and staid fraternity emulating the example of our surgeon essayist and poet (Helmuth) by using his leisure hours in giving his friends something to rest the weary mind, to distract the worried or melancholy, and by a laugh to aid digestion. And last but not least, is it a taking little book for the physician's waiting-room table, where, by killing the time of waiting, it soothes the perturbed nerves frequently caused by a few minutes' wait for the doctor.

Well portrayed are the characters of an unsophisticated and exceedingly precise youth; a phlegmatic, common-sensed Dutchman; a jolly, practical, joking Irishman; and an egotistical, hot-blooded, verbose, ignorant professional man.

One fact is almost unique: here is a pleasing story of two-hundred and ten pages with absolutely no love in it and scarcely the mention of the charming female now apparently necessary to light, pleasure literature.

The International Medical Annual and Practitioners' Index: A Work of Reference for Medical Practitioners. By Forty-one Contributors. Eighteenth Year. 1900. E. B. Treat & Co. New York and Chicago. Price $2.75.

Another year has rolled around, and after a short period of expectancy this volume, the quintessence of a year's medical progress, has appeared for our commendation or criticism. Of the first we can give much, of the latter but little.

First we notice the addition of nine new contributors to its already representative staff, among these are the well-known names of Professor Hy. P. Loomis, M. D., Wm. Milligan, M. D., F. Richardson Cross, M. B., F. R. C. S.

If we may judge the book as a whole from the articles and paragraphs upon subjects within our own special branches, it must be instructive to all classes of medical men.

The article on the Differential Diagnosis of the Diseases of the Accessory Sinuses of the Nose is very full for the space that can be allotted to it in a book of this character. It includes the tabulated symptoms of sinusitis of each sinus under the divisions of (a) suggestive, (b) probable, and (c) certain, which were first suggested by Dundas Grant of London, and which can be borne in mind more easily than the usual form, and thereby render us much practical assistance. It is also accompanied by three fine plates portraying intricacies and important anatomical relation of these hitherto rather neglected regions.

In the discussion on the anæsthetic most applicable for adenoidectomy, Wm. Milligan strongly advocates chloroform, giving good reasons in its favor and good statistics of its employment.

One item we cannot agree with is Lichtwitz' condemnation of the nasal douche in any form for ozena, as this seems the only method that will satisfactorily cleanse the nasal chambers of the hard, tenaciously adhering crusts in this disease.

Furthermore, the papers on the experimentations with and the uses of the toxins and the antitoxins and the numerous animal extracts are interesting and instructive, though much may be unpractical. These are the fads of the present medical age.

In closing, for the publishers we would remark that they have sustained their usual good reputation in typography—the twenty plates, some colored, are exceptionally good, and the wood cuts, of which there are fifty-three, are above the average.

Vol. XII.   JULY, 1900.   Part 3.

THE JOURNAL OF OPHTHALMOLOGY, OTOLOGY AND LARYNGOLOGY.

EDITOR,

CHARLES DEADY, M. D.

ASSOCIATE EDITOR,

A. W. PALMER, M. D.

NASAL OBSTRUCTION AS A CAUSE OF HAY FEVER OR ASTHMA.

BY WM. WOODBURN, M. D., DES MOINES, IA.

I DO not propose to treat this subject technically or theoretically, further than to simply say, I consider the first a mild form of the second, and both a reflex neurosis. I shall relate my experience and treatment of some half dozen cases illustrating my subject.

CASE I.—Mrs. H., a farmer's wife, æt. thirty-five, had been troubled for a number of years with hay fever from harvest time until frost came in the fall. Inspection of the nose in June, 1899, showed the lower right and both middle turbinated bodies greatly hypertrophied. Removal of the anterior and lower half of the middle and cauterization of the lower, gave complete immunity for the entire season. This patient could not, at any time, sweep the floor or ride behind horses against the wind, without violent paroxysms of sneezing, but since the operation has had no further trouble on this score.

CASE II.—Mr. D., æt. about thirty-five, a traveling man, the patient of our secretary, consulted me on August 28 last, in the midst of his annual attack of hay fever. Examination showed the entire nasal mucous membrane greatly engorged, as it always is during an attack. On the right side of the septum, near the floor, was a sharp septal spur, projecting at right angles about three-eighths of an inch, prodding the tumefied lower turbinated body. The removal of this spur under cocaine anæsthesia

greatly modified the symptoms immediately, but a grateful frost,
following in a few days, prevented an exact estimate of the
benefit to be ascribed to the removal of this offending appendage.

This year, however, will furnish opportunity to determine how
permanent the effect will be.

CASE III.—Wm. S., æt. four years, a great sufferer from
asthma, at times when having a slight cold, to which he was very
prone, to such an extent that he could not lie down for several
days and nights. Relief had been sought in the higher altitudes
of the Rockies and a residence of one year at Denver, but none
came. I was consulted on November 25, 1899. An examination
showed the post-nasal space almost occluded with adenoid
vegetations. Of course I advised their removal, which advice
was accepted, and their thorough removal, under the local application of cocaine, accomplished the purpose. This was the
child of a brother practitioner, and in April this year I had a
letter from the doctor, in which was the very gratifying sentence,
"William has not had the asthma since you removed his
adenoids, and is much better in every way." This was especially pleasing since his suffering had always been more severe
and constant during his previous winters.

CASE IV.—Male, æt. forty-five, Swede; occupation, bridge-
builder. Had suffered annually for fifteen years with, first, hay
fever, and, later in the season, asthma. In the summer of
1899 he anticipated his attack by a trip to the mountains of
Colorado, where he found exemption and remained until the first
frosts had appeared here, and then ventured to return. Immediately on arriving at Omaha on his return, his old antagonist met
him and the battle again raged with even renewed vigor. He
consulted me a few days after his arrival home, in a frame of
mind ready to accept any suggestion which promised him
relief. I examined the nasal passages. The right lower turbinated was greatly hypertrophied, and on the application of
cocaine, 3 per cent. solution, the tumefaction largely disappeared
and great immediate, but of course, temporary, relief was experienced. On the left side an immense septal spur on the osseous
portion was found and removed. After the temporary swelling
incident to the operation had subsided, his relief was, and
remains, complete. I subsequently cauterized the enlarged right
turbinated, since which time, he informs me, he has breathed
more freely than he has done for fifteen years.

all the physicians in her home town, except the one she should have at first consulted. Finally, in desperation she went to a young up-to-date homeopathic physician, who looked into her nose and assured her he knew what caused her trouble. He made an application of a solution of cocaine, and in a few minutes her respiration became nasal and normal. "Oh, what a relief! That is the first good breath I have had for weeks," was her exclamation. Both lower turbinated bodies were immensely hypertrophied, and the doctor wisely advised their removal and referred her to me to do the work. When I first saw the patient she was a frail, pale, wan little woman, thoroughly exhausted. I saw her about six weeks subsequently, in a remarkably improved condition. Had gained about twenty pounds in weight and was plump, rosy-cheeked, and had entirely lost her distressed appearance.

The last two cases both occurred in the practice of my good friend, Dr. C. M. Harrington of Knoxville, Ia., and are all the more valuable because he is here to corroborate the fair statement of the cases I have made, and emphasize the beneficial results in a discussion of my paper.

Case VI.—An old-school physician, æt. about thirty-five, had for a number of years been troubled during the late summer months and early fall with hay fever. Had sought relief from a number of specialists in his own school of medicine as well as prominent general practitioners. By chance he was directed to me, not knowing my school of practice, in the midst of attack in 1899. No satisfactory examination could be made until a 4 per cent. solution of cocaine had been applied and caused a lessening of the engorgement. There was plainly visible a large well-organized simple polypus hanging by a distinct pedicle from the right middle turbinated body. Its removal with the cold wire snare gave prompt and permanent relief and made a lasting and loyal friend of my old-school confrère.

In none of these cases do I mention any medication. None was used except to cleanse the mucous membrane of the viscid secretion always present in such conditions, and following such operations. All of the cases reported were mechanical obstructions, and demanded mechanical treatment, and no line of medicinal treatment would have done more than temporary good.

DETACHMENT OF THE RETINA—A CASE.

BY JAS. A. CAMPBELL, M. D., ST. LOUIS.

IN May, 1885, Geo. H., age thirty-seven, came to me from Indiana, with the following history : He had been very near-sighted all his life, but had never worn glasses. His eyes had never troubled him in any other way, until a few days before he came. He then noticed a few floating white spots before his left eye. This gradually increased, and the vision of this eye, by degrees, grew less and less until after four days the sight of the left eye was gone. There was no pain in either eye.

Examination showed vision of the right eye was 4/200 ; with a — 13 Ds. glass, 15/200. With the left eye he could just distinguish light in the outer upper field of vision. With the ophthalmoscope only the lower fundus of the left eye could be made out, where the retinal vessels were seen up to the lower edge of the optic disk. The disk itself could not be made out, but above it a bulging, detached retina was prominent, with a hemorrhagic spot at its inner margin. In the upper outer fundus another separate bulging detachment of the retina could be plainly seen.

The right eye was highly myopic, with a myopic arching around the disk, and the entire fundus was mottled with small choroidal pigmentation spots, clearly of long standing.

The nature of his trouble was explained to him. He was kept quiet, and all forms of tobacco and stimulants were forbidden. He was placed on kali hyd. 3d, three times daily. In one week's time a remarkable change for the better had taken place. The detachment was much reduced. The wavy retinal vessels were seen climbing over its edges. The optic disk was visible. In two days more he could count fingers with the left eye at two feet. The improvement continued. On June 24 vision of the left eye was 15/200 ; right eye, 15/100. He then went home for a few days; the kali hyd. being kept up. July 13 he returned, saying that the improvement had gone on by slow degrees, until, suddenly, the vision of the left eye was again lost, on July 12. He was then placed on 5-grain doses of kali iod. 3d, three times daily, which was followed by very slow improvement, so that in three weeks he could again count fingers with the left eye at two feet, and the detachment, which had resumed its former dimensions, was somewhat reduced. I then went back to kali hyd. 3d, three times daily, which was again followed by improvement for some months after his return home. This, with some intercurrent medication, was kept up from time to time for a year, gradual improvement being reported until the sight of both eyes seemed about as it was in former years.

May 3, 1899, fourteen years after his first visit, he again came to me, reporting that his eyes had gotten along very well, with no particular trouble until in 1897, when he took a severe cold, which settled in his left eye, which became badly inflamed. He went to St. Louis, but did not find me, as it was during my summer vacation. Returning home, he consulted Dr. Knapp of Vincennes, Ind., who advised the removal of the left eye, as it seemed hopelessly involved by that time. This was done, and he progressed nicely, the vision of the right eye remaining about the same, though occasionally its vision seemed not quite so clear.

This was the situation until two weeks before his visit, when the sight of the eye began to grow dimmer. There was no pain present at any time, but vision gradually grew worse and worse.

Examination: V. R. = 8/200; where it had before been 15/100. Ophthalmoscope revealed some increase of the old choroidal atrophic mottling, with a red blurry optic disk.

He was placed on gels. θ, three times daily, for a few days, with evident improvement of the optic nerve congestion. He was then given kali hyd. 3d, four times daily. He returned home in a week, keeping up the same remedy. In three weeks he returned to me again, when examination showed decided improvement; with — 13 Ds., V. = 15/100 once more ; still keeping up the kali hyd. 3d. ; thus having been brought back to the condition which followed the treatment in 1885, and which had remained in *statu quo* for fourteen years.

Detachment of the retina is always a serious condition. It is not an unfrequent complication in high degrees of myopia. In three hundred cases collected in Horner's clinic, 48 per cent. were in myopic eyes. Its progress is generally unfavorable. It is usually treated by perfect quiet, rest of patients, after confining them to bed for some weeks, giving infusions of jaborandi and hypodermics of pilocarpin mur. Puncture through the sclera at the points of detachment, allowing escape of the fluid, has been advocated and performed by various well-known authorities, but has not been successful enough to ensure its general adoption. In rare cases spontaneous recovery has been observed, but I cannot think that the case here presented belongs to this class, for the original attack was in 1885, and was of such a degree that the vision of the left eye was reduced to mere perception of light in the outer upper field of vision. Under kali hyd. 3d, remarkable changes and rapid improvement took place. A relapse followed on his return home, after a couple of weeks. This again yielded to the same treatment, the vision of the left eye regained what it had lost, and remained in this condition for twelve years, when a severe general inflammation of the left eye necessitated its removal. Then, in a couple of years, the vision of the right eye became suddenly involved. Rapid improvement again followed the same remedy, and it was restored to its original condition. Hence, I cannot regard the improvement as either spontaneous or a coincidence, but think I am justified in attributing it to the direct result of the remedy given.

In the old school iodide of potash, in large and repeated doses, is a very common remedy in all intraocular diseases, and the more obscure the case, the more frequently and persistently it is used. Some cases are benefited by it, others not. The points I wish to make are, first to demonstrate the homeopathic possibilities of treatment in this serious disease; that when you have a homeopathic kali hydriodicum case, kali hyd. will probably help it, whether you give it in the third trituration or in more appreciable doses. In the case here reported kali hyd. 3d was certainly more potent than the 5-grain doses used for one week and then changed to the 3d trituration again.

CLINICAL CASES.

BY C. GURNEE FELLOWS, M. D., CHICAGO.

CASE I.—Early in 1899, Mrs. H. B., age forty-nine, presented herself for an opinion as to her condition. She had been hoarse for three or four weeks, and had a little inconvenience in swallowing, with no cough, but she complained of ordinary sore throat such as would follow an everyday cold. The main symptom was an excessive amount of mucus from the nose, naso-pharynx, and pharynx.

Examination revealed a large pharyngeal ulcer on the left side, with enlarged cervical glands on the same side, and my suspicions were aroused as to its malignancy. Upon expressing such a fear the patient admitted that she had been examined by a surgeon who likewise had suspected carcinoma and advised its removal. She absolutely refused to think of operation at anybody's hands, and insisted upon my giving it the best treatment possible.

I cleansed it with the usual antiseptic solutions, and applied orthoform and other well-known and everyday methods for a week or two with a fair amount of relief, but the ulcer continuing, I applied specific treatment in the hope of clearing up the diagnosis, and, much to my delight as well as to the patient's comfort, the ulcer healed, the induration disappeared and the patient was, to all intents and purposes, well. After a number of weeks the external glands even diminished in size, so that I rather felt that the diagnosis of cancer was wrong and that it must be specific in character.

The patient ceased her visits, but returned in a few more weeks with a condition as at first, but upon the opposite side of the pharynx. Same treatment and everything else I could suggest did absolutely nothing for her relief, and I felt that the diagnosis this time must be carcinoma, but she refused even to have a small section taken for the purpose of diagnosis. Consultation agreed with me as to the malignancy of the growth, but operation was refused. She died in another month, practically from starvation.

I report this case after having read the article by A. Worrall Palmer upon cancer of the larynx, in the January number of this journal, because in the prelude, this method of diagnosis, and the application of this specific mixed treatment is advised, and because in this case it was followed by apparently successful results with what seemed to be an entire cure of the case, and therefore a clearing up of the diagnosis, but which, on the other hand, was followed by a return of the same condition, but upon the other side of the throat. The second point in the case is the great relief of all symptoms following the iodide of potash and merc. administered internally, and the administration of kali bi. and arsen., which most certainly had in the early part of the disease a very satisfactory effect. I believe that this case was cancer from the first, but that, contrary to expectations, it yielded beautifully to internal treatment.

CASE II.—Mrs. M. E. C., age fifty-six, presented herself with a sensation of swelling in the throat accompanied by stinging pain, and with a history of from one to a dozen attacks of suffocation each twenty-four hours, much worse at night ; otherwise no soreness of the throat or special sickness preceding these attacks, but they have been fairly constant for a year. She had become suspicious of the trouble being cancer, and, after having had some months of treatment from her family physician, she was more impressed with the fact than ever.

Examination revealed nothing in the way of foreign growth, but very much enlarged varicose veins at the base of the tongue, with a granular pharynx. Prognosis was favorable and the treatment as follows :

Glycerole of iodine to the pharynx and base of tongue, following cleansing and antiseptic solutions ; galvano-cautery destroying the largest of the blood vessels, and moschus 3x internally. A complete cure resulted in less than thirty days ; complete cessation of all attacks, which, of course, proved the diagnosis to be other than any malignant trouble, and, although the local treatment was probably efficacious, I believe that much of the trouble was of a neurotic type, incident to the climacteric, and that moschus deserves a good deal of credit for the result.

THREE KALI CARBONICUM CASES.

BY THOMAS M. STEWART, M. D., CINCINNATI, OHIO.

CASE I.—Patient, a tall thin woman ; dark hair and eyes. Badly nourished as a result of mal-assimilation of food. Troubled with frequent attacks of styes on the upper right eyelid. Patient anæmic. Complained of frequent chilliness ; chilly on least exposure. Physically and mentally patient was exhausted.

Some improvement was secured by correcting an eye trouble with glasses. Nux vomica, psorinum, and hepar of course acted indifferently. On a later visit the case was cleared up by the mention of the chilly sensation and the exhaustion. Kali carbonicum began an improvement and carried the case on to a point where diet did the rest.

The woman's means were limited, but she was able to carry out the diet direction, because her principal articles of diet had been meat and eggs. She was getting too much nitrogen. A generous supply of the carbo-hydrates ; a direction to drink plenty of water, but not at meal times ; and more exercise in the open air changed the conditions to healthful ones.

CASE II.—A young woman, well nourished, but not muscularly strong. Catches cold easily and is readily exhausted by muscular exertion. Sensation of a lump in the throat, with stitching sensation at each cold. With each cold has some cough, due largely to an elongated uvula. With each cold must " hawk " a great deal in the mornings to " clear the throat." The patient was a vocalist and suffered frequently from these acute colds and hoarseness.

The case had been prescribed for by several physicians. A study of the case brought out the kali carbonicum picture of " coryza with hoarseness ; catches cold at least exposure to fresh air, and with each cold there is a stitching pain in the pharynx,"

and kali carbonicum 6x trituration cured the case, including
the relaxed uvula. The patient has frequently presented this
picture and each time kali carb. did the work.

Some additional benefit, in lessening the liability to these
attacks, has been secured by the cold sponge bath each morning. Deep inhalation of fresh air three times a day, to aid in
the oxidation of the food stuffs ; and by inculcating the habit of
daily attending to Nature's demands, whether there is any desire
or urging in that direction or not.

CASE III.—Patient a nervous woman. Suffering from mixed
astigmatism and pronounced insufficiency of the internal recti
muscles, which we oculists denominate an exophoria. Patient
suffered terribly from headaches, almost daily in their occurrence,
frequently with nausea. The muscular trouble was cured by the
use of prisms, the mixed astigmatism corrected by a glass, and
there remained a severe backache. It was located in the small
of the back as if there were a heavy weight pressing there ; worse
during menses, with bearing-down pain ; patient was obliged to
sit down frequently, on account of the ache. Her physician had
prescribed sepia, cimicifuga, and natrum muriaticum—and in
response to a question, " Could the eye treatment have had anything to do with apparently aggravating the backache ? " I
replied, " No ; I think the relief of the headache has simply
allowed the attention to be drawn to the backache." I asked for
other symptoms and one day received a little line stating that the
" backache was worse after eating, and the patient could not walk
much on account of the backache, was obliged to sit down frequently," and kali carbonicum was advised. It cured the case.

ATROPHIC RHINITIS.

BY C. R. ARMSTRONG, M. D., THORNTOWN, IND.

ATROPHIC rhinitis is that chronic disease in which there is a wasting away of more or less of the mucous membrane, glands, and turbinated bones, and is generally accompanied by some abnormal conditions of pharynx and all the sinuses connected with the nasal cavities.

This is no new disease, but one physicians have had to deal with these many years; one we meet in practice every little while, and one which we cannot study too carefully, because the treatment for the disease in many cases ends in failure to cure.

I do not know that I will be able to say anything new of this morbid condition of nose, but will state a few things as I see them in practice day by day. There is always a favorable point about having a patient with this disease, along with the unfavorable ones. That is—the physician always has plenty of time to study his case and see every minute change in the recovery ere the patient is pronounced cured. This is more commonly known as ozena, or fetid catarrh, from the odor which accompanies the trouble. However, there is a form of the disease in which the atrophy is present, but has no fetor accompanying it. The latter is a much drier form with no secretions at all.

The ætiology of this disease has been discussed pretty thoroughly. It has been a question as to just what the initial symptoms and changes really are. In a majority of cases it is a secondary disease. That is, it follows other forms of rhinitis. Some authors claim that atrophic

197

rhinitis follows the hypertrophic rhinitis. Others claim
that there may be some shrinking in hypertrophic rhinitis,
but that it does not end in atrophy, but comes from the
purulent rhinitis; I believe they both are right. Either
form I feel confident may precede atrophy. Again, I do
not think that hypertrophic or purulent rhinitis is always
followed by the atrophic form. If they were we would
have many more cases of atrophic rhinitis to treat tl an
we do at present. In my opinion this disease is brought
on directly at times from various causes. Many a case of
ozena has been brought on by the indiscriminate use of
caustics on the mucous membrane of nose. Also injudi-
cious cutting away of inferior and middle turbinated bones.
Then again there is a predisposition to disease, especially
in those people with a syphilitic and scrofulous diathesis.
Excessive drinking of alcohol, excessive smoking of tobacco,
working in poorly ventilated rooms or where there is a
great deal of dust, and where there is an impoverished condition of blood from malaria or malnutrition, all have a
tendency to set up this disease.

The name of this ailment tells much of the pathology of
the disease. As atrophy implies, there is a wasting away
of all tissues attacked. Upon examination the first thing
observed is a dry, shriveled state of the mucous membrane
of the nose and pharynx. The glands and follicles are all
obliterated, which accounts for the dryness of the mucous
membrane. The turbinated bones are dwindling away.
Frequently the whole anterior portion of the turbinated
bones is absorbed. This causes the nasal cavities to be so
enlarged that we may see the pharyngeal walls from the
anterior opening of nose. The glazed or dry appearance
extends to the pharynx and in this manner affects the
eustachian tubes. All over the nasal cavities and pharnyx
numerous granulations can be noticed. Tortuous and enlarged vessels run over the walls. As a rule there is not
that bright red congested appearance of membrane as in
other forms of catarrh.

Patients with this form of catarrh are frequently mistaken

in diagnosing their own cases. I have had them to come in my office asking me to make a prescription for biliousness. They get that idea because they have a dry and coated tongue and a very bitter taste in mouth. After an examination is made you fail to find symptoms to corroborate the patient's diagnosis, but will soon find the real cause. With the reflected light and nasal speculum it takes but a short time to satisfy your mind from conditions of nose that have all the symptoms of ozena. There is a discharge made up of mucus which is very thick, therefore not very easily expelled, and as a result finds its way into all the fossæ and crevices in the nose. It is not long until this is dried into crusts which obstruct the passages of air, and being retained, decompose, throwing off a peculiar, penetrating stench. These crusts adhere very firmly to the membranes. The patients will remove them by artificial means, owing to the uncomfortable feeling produced by them. When the scabs are torn away there may be an oozing of blood. A stuffed up and oppressed fullness in the superior and posterior portion of the nasal passages is present. In the first stages of the disease the mucus will fall down from the palate in small slugs or masses, which as the disease goes on become more and more tenacious and more of a muco-purulent nature. In the beginning this discharge can be "hawked up," but soon it becomes too thick and dry. While the membranes may be so irritated that there will be a free discharge of blood, still there is no real ulcerative process. The septum in some cases is perforated, but this is caused more by tearing away the dried-up discharge than anything else.

The sufferers from ozena are never the strong and vigorous people. They are generally anæmic and having family histories which would make a physician think that the diseases were hereditary. These discharges being retained so long the poison may be absorbed into the blood, and soon the whole system will show the effects of the poison. In children the nostrils are so filled up that they can scarcely breathe at night, and it will not be far in the future when the child will be weak, nervous, irritable, and unable to sleep well. The stomach raises a disturbance as the disease gets older, which is accompanied by an occipital headache. The food which is eaten goes for naught, because the system does not seem to get the desired nourishment. Taste is destroyed, appetite gone, loss of energy for everything is apparent.

The patients scarcely ever can detect the bad odor unless their attention is called to it. After being told a few times about the odor of the breath they will shun public gatherings. If the patient is a woman, who because of offensive breath is barred from society, she will become morbid and hypochondriacal in time. There is so much of the thick mucus hanging on the walls of the pharynx that the openings into the eustachian tubes are filled up and in a short time a certain degree of deafness appears—roaring in the head and other manifestations of ear trouble. As soon as the hearing is noticed to be abnormal the patient will be ready to consult some physician.

With these symptoms it may not require much time to make a correct diagnosis, but it may be some time ere the patient is entirely free from the trouble even if he does use good homeopathic treatment. Then it is the treatment which interests us most. The patient at the beginning will ask if you can cure him and how long it will require to do it. The physician necessarily must guard his prognosis, especially if it is a case of long standing. If there is much atrophy, which has extended over several years, a permanent cure is very doubtful. But even with these cases much can be done to make patients more comfortable. Correct the odor, the dryness, and the formation of scabs. If the case is not of too long standing, very likely you will be able to produce a healthy condition of the mucous membrane. If you are so fortunate as to produce a cure, the patient will always remember you for it, and you will or should feel proud of it yourself. Much will depend on occupation, age, and persistence with which the patient carries out treatment.

The treatment, to be beneficial, implies the discovery and removal of all predisposing and exciting causes. To do this will require both local and systemic treatment. No cure can result unless good constitutional treatment is persisted in. When taking the case it is wise to inform the patient that he must expect treatment through several months, and even then the case must be examined once in a while or there may be a recurrence of the disease.

Too much time cannot be spent in a careful examination of the patient. Be certain the cause of trouble is ferreted out. The course of treatment will depend upon the cause of the disease. After thorough examination a course of treatment is planned. As I have said before, each case must be studied. There are no specifics for the disease.

In the local treatment the important object is cleanliness. The mucous membrane must be kept in a perfectly clean condition all the time. This is the main object of all local treatment. In some cases I assist nature to heal parts by getting a slight stimulating effect of medicine.

It is not always an easy task to remove all the dry crusts, but where the scabs are very dry I use an application of peroxide of hydrogen on cotton, or with the atomizer, to soften them. When the atomizer or douches are used post-nasal injections must be given as well as through the anterior chambers of nose. Any application can be used which will soften up scabs. Can use " Dobell's Solution," solution of sea salt, listerine, or glycerine. After all the crusts have been removed, others must be prevented from forming. This I do by keeping on an application of glycerine. A very good formula to keep the nostrils free is calendula and glycerine, aa 2 drams to ounce water, and used in nebulizer or directly applied on cotton. When the odor is present after removal of scabs, I use permanganate of potash, 10 grs. to ounce in spray, or aristol in lavolene used in nebulizer.

After the cleaning process has been gone through with and all the mucous membrane is perfectly clean, naturally it is ready for some healing application. A good one to use is calendula and hamamelis in lavolene. If there should be any ulceration of septum, apply an ointment of yellow oxide of mercury, 10 grs. to the ounce. This will heal ulcer in short time.

Where membranes need some stimulation a glycerite of tar, hydrastis, or eucalyptol in nebulizer will be found to be of service.

Many times patient will complain more of the deafness than anything else. When you have this complication it will be necessary to give attention to some special treatment for the pharynx and eustachian tubes. The latter must be kept open by Valsalva's method or the Politzer air bag.

In selecting the internal remedy keep in mind the constitutional and local lesions. Often I use the internal remedy locally ; say 5 to 20 drops of tincture to ounce water. Make yourself confident that you have the indicated remedy. There are many remedies which are of service. Some of the more common ones, which have syphilitic taint are, aurum, kali iod., mercury, nitric acid, argentum nitricum, and calc. iod. In scrofulous diathesis and ill-nourished patients such remedies as aurum mur., silicea, calc. phos., sulph., phosphorus, ars., hepar sulph., alumin., kali bich., cal. carb., and graphites are useful.

All through the treatment the physician should have perfect control of patient. Should be able to direct his diet and hygiene. Use all means that will recuperate the general health. If patient is laboring day by day in dust and dirt, he may be compelled to change his occupation.

It is only by looking after the general health that the physician may expect to be rewarded with any success.

SPRAYS.*

BY FRED D. LEWIS, M. D., BUFFALO, N. Y.

IN considering the subject of sprays, it is not my intention to present to you a number of formulas that I have found useful in my practice, but to consider the matter on a broader and more general basis. That sprays have been, and are still used, in various conditions with the most gratifying results, we all know. But that they should be prescribed to a much larger extent than they now are is a fact that the physician, as a rule, is not aware of.

We have learned to know that the skin is one of the great vital organs of the human system. That if its action is impeded, the kidneys and intestines are thereby given a greater amount of work to perform. That with the morning sponge, followed by a brisk friction and an occasional Russian or Turkish bath, in chronic cases, such as rheumatism, we can expect quicker and better results from our remedies.

The public generally have been educated to that point where they recognize the importance of proper care of the teeth. They not only regularly cleanse them, but at stated intervals, usually every six months, go to the dentist and have a thorough examination to anticipate rather than wait for trouble.

Many persons have learned that a lavage of the stomach, in the shape of a cup of hot water, before meals, has converted a sluggish digestion into a normal one.

We are all familiar with the structure and object of the

* Read before the New York State Homeopathic Medical Society at the annual meeting, held in Albany, February 13 and 14, 1900.

nasal cavities. The tortuous turbinateds provide a large surface for the air to secure heat and moisture, before reaching the lungs; and also remove from the air such impurities as are of a solid nature. Now we all know that the atmosphere of cities, especially where there are large manufacturing interests, is loaded with impurities, such as soot, dust, particles of pavement ground to impalpable powder, etc., etc. This fact can easily be demonstrated when the city is on a plain or in the neighborhood of a large body of water. When in the city the air seems pure, the sky unobstructed, and no evidence of floating particles of matter, if an observation is taken from a few miles' distance, the city appears to be encompassed by a cloud.

That the disposition of foreign matter on the sensitive lining membranes of the nose should produce disturbances, there can be no doubt.

The only point I wish to bring out, and I hope it may stimulate some discussion, is this: Should not the care of the nasal mucous membranes be considered as important as the care of the skin and teeth?

In recent years I have asserted to my patients that the spray, in my opinion, is as essential on the toilet table as the toothbrush. As to the nature of the spray to be used, I think one must be guided by conditions. If there has already been a catarrhal condition established, then some remedial agent had better be employed; but if used simply as a prophylactic, then a neutral cleansing solution would be preferable.

I think this subject is deserving of profound consideration, when we know that there are establishments in most of our leading cities that advertise the cure of catarrh for so much a month. Their methods are simply to insist on the patient coming to their offices daily, and having their noses thoroughly cleansed. And they are curing many cases. Would it not be wise to educate our patients, not only to keep their own noses clean, and thus cure themselves, but, by attending to themselves early enough, avoid the development of that, perhaps, most prevalent of all diseases, catarrh?

GALVANISM IN NASAL HYPERTROPHY.*

BY JOHN B. GARRISON, M. D., NEW YORK.

HYPERTROPHIC rhinitis is one of the most frequent of the diseased conditions pertaining to the nasal cavities that we are called upon to treat, and the question of the most suitable method of treatment is to be decided with care.

We have all used, for the removal of the excess of tissue, perhaps, with more or less success, the acids, the actual cautery, or some form of cutting instrument, but the patient, at least, will welcome a method that promises a good result with the least amount of pain at the time of treatment, and the least soreness afterward.

I have found that the application of the galvanic current does, in many cases, furnish just the method desired, and I shall beg your attention for a few minutes while I speak of the method as I practice it.

I shall not burden you with my ideas of what cause most enters into the production of these nasal hypertrophies, leaving to you the perusal of the text-books that will give all the knowledge extant upon the subject. We do find an increase of the nutritive forces, and our treatment must be directed to a lessening of the blood supply in some way. Of course where there is a local source of irritation, that must be removed at once. If it is a deflected septum that is causing an irritation by contact with the opposite side, suitable means must be adopted for its repair before at-

---

* Presented at the Annual Meeting of the National Society of Electro-Therapeutists, Atlantic City, N. J., September, 1900.

tempting to treat the hypertrophies opposing the irregularities of the septum.

The hypertrophies that I shall speak of as being most amenable to treatment by means of the aid suggested in my title are mainly those of the turbinated bodies: and, of these, the inferior is the one most often enlarged. It may be confined to either extremity, or the whole body may be the subject of hypertrophy. When, as is sometimes the case, the bony portion of the turbinate has become enlarged, the saw, and not electricity, will be the best means of cure.

But when the occlusion of the nares is caused by true increase of tissue we have, in galvanic electricity, a potent agent to safely and rapidly remove the obstruction.

To prepare a case for treatment, I always first thoroughly irrigate the nasal cavities with some antiseptic fluid, using the post-nasal syringe. The solution that I most frequently use is Electrozone one part, and tepid water four parts. Then an application of a four per cent. solution of cocaine is made to the location about to be treated, simply to prevent the little pain which accompanies the introduction of the electrode.

The electrode I use is a slender needle about the size of an ordinary darning needle, of suitable length for easy use on the part selected, and I insulate it by dipping it in shellac and laying it away until it is perfectly dry, then scraping away the insulation as far from the point as it is calculated it will be impaled into the tissues. It is fastened into an ordinary needle-holder and connected with the negative pole of the battery, when it is introduced into the tissue at the point selected. The patient is then given the sponge electrode connected with the positive pole of the battery and is told to grasp it firmly, and the current is slowly turned on until the meter registers from three to five ma., which current is allowed to remain stationary for about five minutes, unless the patient is very nervous, when three minutes should be the limit.

The current is now turned off as gradually as it was

turned on and the needle carefully removed. I do not attempt a second treatment at the same point until a week has expired, and in some cases two weeks can be permitted to go by before the shrinkage due to the electrolysis has subsided. The stronger currents have been tried, but the strength I have used and given here acts much more pleasantly and gives equally good results.

During the summer just past I had the opportunity of noticing the reduction of an enormously hypertrophied inferior turbinate in a most unexpected manner, which I am glad to relate at this time.

A lady of about fifty years of age, who was stopping at the hotel at which my family and myself were located, came to me one day to ask my opinion as to her eye and nose. She had had a stricture of the nasal duct for a number of years, which had been duly dilated several times, and for a considerable time had had a dacryocystitis which annoyed her greatly, and from which she was able to press a large amount of mucus and pus from the canaliculus.

The inferior turbinate on the affected side was hypertrophied for nearly its whole length and was in contact with the septum for some distance at the anterior extremity, being of a deep red color and very sensitive to touch. I told her that I believed it would be necessary to remove the turbinate with the saw and advised its removal as soon as possible, giving it as my opinion that it would be necessary to do the operation before the condition of the eye could be relieved. The patient admitted the force of my argument, but was inclined to wait a while until she could get her courage up a little higher. Meanwhile she wanted the canal dilated and begged me to do it. Visiting New York, I supplied myself with a canaliculus syringe and a set of Bowman's probes, and on my return announced myself ready to commence treatment. I proceeded to insulate the probes in the manner alluded to for needles in nasal work, scraping the points bright for about a quarter of an inch.

Before introducing the probe I washed the sac out

thoroughly with a fifty per cent. solution of enzymol, and then, connecting the probe electrode with the negative cord of a galvanic battery by means of an artery forceps, introduced it (No. 2,—a No. I would not pass in the ordinary manner with considerable pressure) into the canal, and turned on the current until the meter registered two milliamperes. Using just enough pressure to guide the electrode, it gradually found its way along the canal, and in less than five minutes it had entered the nasal cavity without causing the loss of a drop of blood. In three days I passed a No. 4 in the same manner, and four days later a No. 6 passed easily. Three days after this a No. 7 was passed, and that size was passed three or four times afterwards at intervals three or four days. After the first passage of the No. 7, all of the solution used for the purpose of cleansing the sac passed through into the nasal cavity directly from the syringe, and there was no further collection of pus in the sac during a week in which the syringe was not used.

The point I wanted to bring out, however, is that after the second treatment by electricity, the color of the mucous membrane covering the turbinate began to grow paler, and at the end of the treatments the entire body had contracted sufficiently to permit free and easy drainage and natural respiration.

I am led, by this, to the thought that it may be good treatment in many cases of hypertrophy of the inferior turbinate, and possibly the others as well, to use the insulated probe electrodes in the lachrymal canal with the weak current, not exceeding one or two milliamperes. The careful use of this method may prove it to be a valuable addition to the present means of treating a class of cases that are troublesome to the patient and the doctor.

THE PATHOGENIC AND THERAPEUTIC ACTION OF RHUS TOX. UPON THE EYE.

BY CHARLES DEADY, M. D.

IN the collection of provings of rhus toxicodendron made by Samuel Hahnemann, and published in Vol. II. of the Materia Medica Pura, the number of symptoms relating to the eye and its neighborhood is so large as to lead to the supposition that, if the theory of homeopathy be a correct one, this drug should prove of special value in the treatment of diseases of the visual organs. Never did an hypothesis receive better support when reduced to practice ; and if the efficacy of the law of *similia similibus curentur* were compelled to rest upon a single test to demonstrate its truth, few better selections could be made than that of rhus tox. in the department of ophthalmology.

Many of the symptoms contained in the Materia Medica Pura are indefinite, and the great majority of them point to apparently superficial diseases, but when we consider the fact that at the time these provings were made the science of ophthalmology, as understood at the present day, actually had no existence, that the principle of the ophthalmoscope had not yet been discovered, and that the methods of precision in the examination and diagnosis of diseases of the eye now available were at that time unknown, this is little to be wondered at. And we are compelled to admire the industry and energy of the men, some of them of our own day and generation, whose tireless labor has sifted and arranged the numerous symptoms of this and other drugs and indicated the method of their proper application to the various pathological processes.

When the New York Ophthalmic Hospital was placed in charge of the adherents of the homeopathic school, they were confronted by the fact that no definite materia medica of diseases of the eye and ear, as such, was in existence, and in order to ascertain the remedy for a given case of disease they were obliged to take the conditions throughout the body, and by comparing these with the general materia medica find a suitable drug for the totality of the symptoms. Had they been content with simply curing their cases in this routine way little would have been gained, but they made it a rule to take down the special eye or ear symptoms in each case with great care, and when a drug had cured a certain case of disease the eye or ear symptoms which had disappeared under its use were carefully noted. With a multiplicity of cases, and a systematic verification of symptoms, a valuable special materia medica of these diseases was compiled, and the curative properties of drugs in the various pathological entities of the eye and ear were definitely demonstrated and their characteristic symptoms for each disease mapped out.

Under this methodical procedure the relative value of drugs apparently indicated in these diseases gradually became better known; some, although presenting many and varied symptoms, were found by experience to be superficial and evanescent in their action, while others proved of the greatest efficacy in the most serious lesions, and became indispensable in the armamentarium of the physicians of the hospital staff.

In the latter group, rhus tox. speedily assumed prominence as a drug of special value in ocular disease, and this was enhanced by such a large measure of success in its application over a wide range of affections that it came to be regarded (at least in this hospital) as a veritable sheet-anchor in ophthalmological work, and as time passed it was used more or less in almost all the acute diseases to which the eye and its adnexa are subject.

A prominent symptom of rhus is great swelling of the eyelids. This it has in common with a number of other remedies, but differentiation becomes less difficult when we remember that rhus is specially indicated when swelling and œdema of the lids are the result of the deeper and more serious lesions. After the operation for cataract, one of the first symptoms indicating danger is œdematous swelling of the lids, and no drug in the materia medica compares with rhus for insuring the safety of the eye. When the pathological process becomes advanced, even to the appearance of pus within the eyeball, still we may confidently rely on this remedy, which has cured many such cases when they were apparently hopeless. In all post-operative complications it is of the greatest value, and too much emphasis cannot be placed upon this statement.

When a sound eye takes on sympathetic irritation from its diseased fellow, the fact is first manifested by a certain amount of swelling of the lids and more or less profuse lachrymation, the latter another valuable indication for rhus tox. In this condition I have personally used it many times with complete success, and it is the first drug to be thought of in this extremely dangerous complication.

It is a well-known fact at the present time that rhus is particularly applicable in rheumatic conditions, especially where these are resultant upon a wetting or exposure to dampness. This, together with its nightly aggravation, points to another sphere of usefulness in rheumatic iritis, where it will prove all-sufficient when the characteristic symptoms exist. In suppurative iritis and cyclitis it is very serviceable, no matter what the cause.

The symptom "while he turns the eye or it is pressed, the eyeball is painful, can hardly move it," indicates its use in acute retrobulbar neuritis, which causes this symptom exactly and is well known to be frequently due to a rheumatic diathesis. The same symptom may call for its use in tenonitis, in which the stiffness, difficulty of and pain on moving the eye are specially prominent and which also has swelling and œdema of the upper lid, chemosis of the conjunctiva, and protrusion of the eyeball ; all symptoms of rhus tox. The idiopathic form of this disease is almost always rheumatic or gouty in origin, furnishing still another indication for the remedy. In orbital cellulitis we have swelling of the lids, chemosis, protrusion of the eyeball, almost complete abolition of motion with pain on the attempt and also on pressure, aching in and around the eye, with the probable formation of pus in the deeper structures, all conditions curable by rhus tox., which is one of the best remedies for this disease whatever may be its origin, traumatic or otherwise, and has cured many of the most desperate cases.

In panophthalmitis, or suppurative inflammation of the eyeball, we find the swollen lids, difficulty of, and pain on motion, chemosis of the conjunctiva, severe pain in the eyeball, lachrymation, etc., again indicating the remedy.. Rhus tox. is one of the few drugs that have cured this most fatal of lesions, and its success in restoring the integrity of the eye, in some cases where this result has seemed almost impossible, is a matter of record.

The symptom "heaviness and stiffness of the eyelids, like paralysis, as if difficult to move the eyelids," would seem to indicate its use in ptosis, and this condition as well as paralysis of certain of the ocular muscles, is curable by rhus tox., especially if due to wetting or dampness. Such cures have been made frequently in the clinics of the Ophthalmic Hospital. Erysipelas of the eyelids often presents the characteristic symptoms of rhus. Of course the swelling of the lids is always present, but many of these cases have in addition the chemosis, hot lachrymation, the characteristic pains and aggravation, restlessness, vesicular eruptions, etc., and it is a valuable and efficient remedy when these exist.

Although rhus tox. is specially useful in the most serious inflammations of the deeper and more important structures of the eyeball and surrounding tissues, its sphere is not confined to these conditions alone, but seems to cover almost all the acute diseases to which the visual organs are subject. Given a rheumatic origin, especially if it be from exposure to damp or wet weather, with profuse lachrymation (pain in and about the eye) a tendency to chemosis of the conjunctiva, œdema of the lids, photophobia, and the characteristic aggravation and restlessness at night, and this valuable drug will rarely be found wanting in any of the inflammations of the conjunctiva, cornea, or lids.

I have many times cured with it acute catarrhal conjunctivitis, phlyctenular conjunctivitis and keratitis and ulcers of the cornea, and have subdued the acute aggravations of conjunctivitis trachomatosa, where the above symptoms, or some of them, were present. It is also frequently successful in the treatment of abscess of the lid, which, while not a serious, is an extremely painful disease.

Dr. W. A. Phillips, in an article published in the *Jour. of Oph., Otol. and Lar.*, July, 1899, page 224, recommends the use of rhus tox., "when the ciliary muscle itself seems to be the special seat of trouble; when its muscular tone is disturbed from previous straining, and when inability is present after using the eyes for reading any considerable time, notwithstanding optical correction."

He has had much success with the drug in these cases and considers that its action here is on a plane with that on lameness or soreness due to rheumatism. In my opinion another factor may be spoken of. One of the differential points between arsenic and rhus is that the arsenic patient is *actually* so weak that he cannot do what he would wish, while the rhus patient *feels* so weak that he cannot do it, but by making the effort he can overcome his weakness and accomplish what he desires. This seems to indicate in the rhus case an indisposition to exertion due to want of *tone* of the muscular system, and this explanation applied to the ciliary muscle would account for the successful action of this drug in the class of cases indicated.

I would not have it understood that I consider rhus tox. an universal panacea for all the inflammatory diseases of the eye; all of these affections are many times extremely variable in their presenting symptoms and other remedies are frequently called for, but the drug under consideration is one of the first importance and is most reliable and efficient when accurately prescribed.

TREATMENT OF SARCOMA WITH THE MIXED TOXINS OF ERYSIPELAS AND BACILLUS PRODIGIOSUS.

BY A. WORRALL PALMER, M. D., NEW YORK.

THE numerous modes of treating sarcoma or any other variety of cancer, and the constant experimentation on the part of the profession with new methods, only go to show how inadequate is our ability to meet this intractable disease.

These neoplasms are not so rare, as there are ninety-nine authentically recorded cases, situated within the restricted domain of the naso-pharynx and pharynx.

For these reasons, and because I have been able to find only one case of sarcoma treated with Coley's fluid reported in our homeopathic literature, do I take the liberty of occupying your time with the *résumé* of my investigations into the subject and my meager practical experience.

Although surgery is, at present, the best method to meet this condition, personally I believe that more investigation into or trials of the remedial treatment should be made, because cancer is a constitutional disease, and it so very frequently recurs after removal with the knife.

Apropos to this, C. Mansell Moullin says in the Boston *Medical Journal:* "There is at least as much hope after an internal remedy that causes disappearance by atrophy or fatty degeneration as from the most extensive removal by operation. On *a priori* grounds there may be even more."

Among the numerous drugs or substances which have been experimented with are the interstitial injection of alcohol 40 per cent., by Haase ; the injection of Pure Yeast Ferment, by De Bracher ; subcutaneous use of 50 per cent. solution of the fluid extract of chelidonium majus re-en-forced by same drug per orem ; the cataphoric diffusion of mercury from gold electrodes used by Massey ; and lastly the mixed toxins of the streptococcus erysipelas and bacil-lus prodigiosus.

From my research the last is the only one that has attained any success or wide reputation and not been rele-gated to the usual oblivion of other medical fads. The reason for this I consider to be because Dr. Coley has not only been persevering, but scientific, unbiased, and very cautious in its advocacy. At first he hoped and believed that in some form it would be beneficial in all forms of can-cer ; but he now only recommends it in sarcoma, and claims marked results only in the spindle-celled variety of this.

As in many other cases, the discovery of the influence of erysipelas on sarcomatous growths was by investigation founded upon accidental occurrences, to wit : Busch reported a case of multiple sarcoma of the face cured by an attack of facial erysipelas ; Durante, a sarcoma of the neck ; Biedert, an enormous round-celled sarcoma, including the mouth, nose, and pharynx ; Bruns, a melanotic sarcoma of the breast ; Gerster and Bull, each a recurrent sarcoma of the neck ; all cured or disappeared with no return, after an erysipelatous attack. This happy result does not always follow erysipelas, as cases of sarcoma relieved by erysipelas, and later recurring or progressing after the attack is over, are reported by Busch, Nelaton, Deleüs, Richochon, Win-slow, Powes, and Dowd.

On account of these accidental cures a few observers pro-duced erysipelas artificially by infusion with the living cul-ture, with success in many cases.

Then almost simultaneously Lassar of Berlin, Spronck of Utrecht, and Coley of New York, believing that· the curative action of erysipelas lay in the toxin of the living culture, experimented and found that they could produce equally good results with toxin, thereby avoiding both the danger and discomfort of the patient passing through an attack of erysipelas.

It has been shown by different observers that the combination of certain bacilli with disease toxins makes such toxins more potent, and Rogers of Paris demonstrated that the combination of the bacillus prodigiosus with the streptococcus of erysipelas greatly augmented the virulence of the streptococcus on rabbits. Thereupon Dr. Coley used the combination on the human subject in sarcoma with far better results than before.

Regarding this, Dr. Coley says he cannot say exactly what part the bacillus prodigiosus plays in the cure of sarcoma, but remarks that the only cases cured were treated by the combination.

This preparation, the combined toxins, had been given the name of Coley's fluid, and that used during the last seven years has been made by Dr. B. H. Buxton of Loomis Laboratory.

Until about five years ago the toxins were made from cultures from a fatal case of erysipelas, but since that, sufficient strength has been obtained by passing the cultures through about fifty rabbits. The method of the preparation is virtually this: the mixed unfiltered toxins of the streptococcus of erysipelas and the bacillus prodigiosus are made from cultures grown together in the same bouillon and sterilized by heating to 58 degrees C. and then diluted in a sterilized menstruum.

In a recent conversation with Dr. Buxton he said that at present he made a double sterilization and then added some drugs such as thymol to preserve the preparation.

Dr. Coley, in his exhaustive article in the *Jour. Am. Med. Assoc.*, August 20 and 27, 1898, affixed a table of fifty-seven cases of cancerous tumors treated with either his fluid or other preparation of erysipelatous poison with cure, or at least disappearance of the then present manifestation of the disease and lengthening of the usual period of a recurrence of the condition.

The following is a list of cases of sarcoma of the nose and throat treated by cultures of erysipelas, or Coley's fluid, the physicians in charge, and the time the patient is living after treatment at the time of the report in Dr. Coley's paper, in 1898:

(a) A spindle-celled sarcoma of the neck and tonsils, inoculated culture—patient living six years after.

(b) A spindle-celled sarcoma of the parotid; it had been extirpated twice previous to treatment—patient living one year after.

(c) A sarcoma (mixed celled) of the parotid—patient living three years after. The foregoing under Dr. Coley's care.

(d) A spindle-celled sarcoma of the palate and pharynx extending to the vocal cords—Dr. W. B. Johnson—living four and three-quarter years.

(e) A round-celled sarcoma of antrum, pharynx, and neck —Dr. L. L. McArthur—child aged five years, weight gained from 37 to 69 pounds—later, fatal recurrence.

(f) A round-celled sarcoma of parotid, size of the fist— Czerny of Heidelberg—living over a year.

(g) A spindle-celled sarcoma of the parotid—Horace Packard—living two and three-quarter years.

(h) A round-celled sarcoma of the neck—H. Montague —slight return in six months.

(i) A recurrent sarcoma of the neck and tonsil—J. O. Roe—six months after treatment died of erysipelas.

The mode of administration is cumulative. The injection is of course to be made under the most thorough antiseptic principles attainable. It is by far preferable to make the injection into the growth itself, although, if this is impossible, it may be introduced into the nearest accessible point, but in the latter case the dosage needs to be doubled.

As a rule one-half drop is the initial dose, and this is increased one-half drop each succeeding day until toleration is reached. This is evidenced by the natural reactionary fever rising to 102° or 103° F. In such case the following dose should be the same as the preceding, and if it should again go so high reduce the next dose one-half drop. The dose is increased in this manner until the maximum is attained. When applied to the neoplasm itself 8 drops is the full dose, or if elsewhere, double that amount, 16 drops.

This last amount is to be continued daily until the tumor has disappeared.

The toxin may commence to reduce the tumor in a week, but its administration should not be abandoned in less than three weeks' trial. The time necessary to effect a cure is very variable; occasionally the neoplasm will almost disappear in two weeks, while on the other hand it may take several months.

The reactionary symptoms are a chill, followed by fever, generally lasting about three hours, although occasionally it may continue twelve hours; acute transitory swelling of tissues in the immediate vicinity of injection; usually myalgic pains commencing at point of injection and radiating frequently over the whole body; in the more severe reactions there is nausea or even vomiting—in my own case it produced a weakening menorrhagia.

CASE.—Mrs. E. C., æt. thirty-four years. A tall, thin woman of neurotic temperament.

Family History.—Father had chronic bronchitis, but died of kidney disease. Mother was an invalid for seven years with rheumatism of hip and knee until death, which was caused by apoplexy; a sister died of gastric disease. The patient married eleven years; has two children living; boy at nine months died of entero-colitis; boy three and one-half years died of fall from window; two miscarriages. At ten years æt. the patient had diphtheria; at twenty-six, pleurisy; at thirty-one years, rheumatism of left shoulder and post-cervical region. It is impossible to obtain any indication of hereditary predisposition.

Subjective Symptoms.—Complains of post-nasal dropping of mucus, constant short hacking cough, malodorous breath, pain in region of spleen; aggravated when lying down and throbbing in character when walking rapidly. After discovering the swelling in the throat and speaking of it she admitted there had been a sensation of a lump in the throat for about a year, but so slight she considered it of little consequence.

Objective Symptoms.—Nares : Rhinitis sicca, covered with dry crusts, but turbinated bodies hypertrophied.

Naso-pharynx and pharynx : Mucosa slightly hyperæmic, follicles inflamed and enlarged. On the left side of these cavities is a sessile swelling, the general surface of which is much inflamed, and half of the surface is covered with varicose veins about one-eighth of an inch in diameter ; it extends more than half the width of the pharynx and vertically from the vault above to the lateral sinuses below ; is neither painful nor hyperæsthetic ; it has a boggy feel, but not as soft as an abscess. The tumor springs from the posterior wall of the pharynx, not connected with the tonsil, as the left posterior pillar lies in front of the neoplasm and can be lifted free from it. Neither of the tonsils is inflamed nor hypertrophied ; a few cervical lymphatics on the left side are slightly indurated, but slightly sensitive—if at all.

The swelling had probably existed longer than an abscess would be in forming, and there was neither pain nor fluctuation. Still an exploratory incision was made, but with the expected negative results.

Although the tumor was situated over the principal chain in lymphatics of the pharynx, it was not nodular, but smooth. Therefore the neoplasm was probably not of lymphatic origin, but an implication of the muscular tissue behind the pharynx.

A specimen was submitted by Dr. Klotz, the pathologist of the hospital, and the provisional diagnosis of angio-sarcoma made—sarcoma because it seemed to spring from the muscular tissue and apparent predominance of blood-vessels, and of the angiomatous variety because of the enlarged blood vessels on the surface.

The removal of the specimen for microscopical examination caused quite a severe hemorrhage, lasting about two hours, notwithstanding the employment of the usual hemostatics.

The microscopist pronounced it a small round-celled sarcoma.

I showed the case to the Academy of Pathological Science, where two general surgeons who examined the case advised against extirpation of the tumor, because of its close proximity to the important blood vessels and nerves of the neck, an opinion I entirely coincided with, because of seeing two similar cases before. This agreement decided me in determining to try the mixed toxins as the treatment promising the best results for the patient.

April 4. Commenced injections with one-quarter of a drop. I diminished the initial dose one-half because Dr. Coley personally advised it, as he thought the possible reactionary local swelling might seriously interfere with respiration.

April 14. The dose was increased one-quarter drop each day to date—when she took only two drops, because it was deemed advisable to omit treatment two days during menstruation on account of great weakness of patient.

April 20. Increased dose half drop per diem—on 16th and 19th treatment omitted on account of debility—dose 4 drops, which dose was continued till April 23, when on account of the temperature twice having risen to 103° F. and menorrhagia having supervened only ten days after previous regular menstruation, I thought it prudent to reduce dosage to 3½ drops, which was continued until April 26. Examination of pharynx to-day for first time showed a decided diminution in the congested appearance and size of the tumor. Formerly the tumor pushed the posterior pillar forward, so that, if the pillar could not have been lifted away from swelling by the ring probe, it would have seemed to be part of it ; while to-day a small space could be distinguished between the tumor and the pillar. Dosage 4 drops.

In *résumé*, I would call attention to the apparent susceptibility of the patient to the toxin. Because, although she never received over half the maximum dose, the following reactionary symptoms developed : Of the seventeen days on which full records were kept, on thirteen she had chills after every dose; there were muscular pains throughout the left side, occasionally extending to the right—one-third of the time the patient was nauseated, and three times vomited—the average temperature was 100.8 F.; twice it did not rise at all after injections of ½ or 2½ drops. 'Tis well to bear in mind that chills very seldom occur after the third injection.

Finally, I wish to thank Dr. Clausen, resident physician, who carried out most of the treatment while the patient was at the Ophthalmic Hospital ; also Dr. Bernard Clausen, who continued it after she returned home.

REPORT ON "HENPUYE" IN THE GOLD COAST COLONY.*

BY ALBERT J. CHALMERS, M. D., VICT., F. R. C. S. ENG.

HENPUYE, or dog nose, is a disease frequently met with in the Gold Coast Colony and in certain portions of its Hinterland. The hideous deformity of the face which it causes is very striking to anyone who has lived in this part of West Africa. It is also known on the French Ivory Coast under the name of "goundu" or "anakhre," but "henpuye" is the native name (Appolonian) for the disease on the Gold Coast. The peculiar nature of the disease and the fact that, as far as I could find, very little was known as to its nature led me to make the inquiries which are now embodied in this report. I regret very much that I am unable to refer to original papers on the subject or to be certain that I have the full literature, but my excuse is that libraries do not exist in West Africa. The only references which I have met with are those mentioned in Dr. Patrick Manson's work on "Tropical Diseases" (p. 594), and they are those of (1) Professor Alexander Macalister (Royal Irish Academy, 1882), (2) Surgeon J. J. Lamprey, A. M. S. (*Brit. Med. Jour.*, vol. ii., 1887), (3) Dr. Henry Strachan (*Brit. Med. Jour.*, vol. i., 1894), and (4) Dr. Maclaud (Archives de Médecine Navale, 1895). It is by the kind permission of the Governor of this colony, Sir Frederick Hodgson, K. C. M. G., that I am allowed to publish this report. I am much indebted to Captain Armitage for

* Published by the permission of Sir Frederick Hodgson, Governor of the Gold Coast Colony.

his kindness in giving me information with regard to the
different places in which he has noticed this disease in his
travels, for drawing my attention to notes of the late
Mr. Ferguson on the presence of the disease in Akim and
Kwahu, and for making a painting of an advanced case of
the disease; also to Dr. Henderson, the chief medical
officer of the colony for many kind suggestions: and, lastly,
to Mr. Crowther, draughtsman in the Public Works Department, for supplying me with a map of the colony and its
Hinterland. The description of the disease will be divided
into the following headings: (1) the General Description of
the Disease; (2) the Description of Cases of the Disease; (3) the Treatment; (4) the Morbid Anatomy; (5) the
Ætiology; and (6) the Geographical Distribution.

THE GENERAL DESCRIPTION OF THE DISEASE.

Henpuye starts in a native of West Africa during or soon
after an attack of yaws in which there is a history of the
nasal mucous membrane being attacked as a small bony
swelling symmetrically placed on either side of the nose.
This swelling, which is generally oval with the long axis
directed downwards and outwards, is attached to the nasal
bones, the nasal process of the superior maxilla, and also
to the superior maxilla in the more advanced cases. It is
produced by the deposition of new bone under the periosteum on the external aspect of these bones and grows
slowly in all directions. It in no way affects the mouth or
the orbital or nasal cavities in any case which I have seen,
and the nasal ducts are quite unaffected. Rarely the
growth is asymmetrical, being situated only on one side of
the nose. Pain in the nose and the presence of a sore in
that organ are the symptoms complained of at the commencement of the disease; later headache is sometimes
felt, and pain in the swelling during wet weather. As the
growth becomes larger it seriously interferes with the sight
by growing up in front of the eyes and even hiding them,
but I have never seen it cause destruction of the eyeball.
In many cases the patient has to bend his head downwards

in order to be able to see over the tops of the swellings. The skin over the tumor is normal and is freely movable. The course of the disease is that the swellings may cease to grow at any period of their existence or may continue to grow for years—that is to say, they may remain quite small or may grow to be large lumps, in the latter case giving rise to the deformity and the interference with the sight, but I am unacquainted with any case in which they break down or ulcerate. Finally, the disease is much more common, in my experience, in men than in women.

DESCRIPTION OF CASES.

The following cases will be described: (1) slightly developed cases; (2) moderately developed cases; (3) an advanced case; and (4) an asymmetrical case.

Slightly Developed Cases.—CASE I.—The patient, a boy of about seventeen years of age, said that about seven years ago he noticed two small lumps on the nose which began after yaws in which there was a sore in the nose. They increased slightly in size, but soon ceased to grow and have been in their present condition for some years. He never felt any discomfort or pain in them. The two lumps had their long axis directed downwards and outwards, the measurements being half an inch by a quarter of an inch. They were attached to the nasal bones just above the cartilages and the nasal process of the superior maxilla, and were firm, smooth, bony tumors. The skin over them was quite normal and they did not in any way project into the nasal cavity or affect the line of vision, being too small for the latter purpose. There was very little deformity and no treatment was necessary. In this case the lumps soon ceased to grow.

CASE II.—A small Grunshi girl from Kumassi, about seven years of age, who had had yaws some time previously, felt pain in the nose a few months ago and noticed a small swelling on each side of the nose, and this gradually increased in size till it reached its present condition. Her mother was most anxious to have it removed on account of the deformity. On inspection there was found to be an oval swelling on each side of the nose, attached to the nasal bones and the nasal process of the superior maxilla. The long axis of the swelling was directed downwards and outwards—an inch in length and half an inch in breadth. The nasal cartilages were not affected and the interior of the nose was normal. The orbital cavity, the mouth, and the nasal ducts were quite unaffected. The skin over the swelling was normal and freely movable. The patient felt no pain in the tumor and she had never had any headache. The growths were removed by operation. It was very difficult to obtain definite history as to the time when this patient had had yaws and as to the time when the growth appeared, but as far as I could make out the yaws were well developed when the swelling was first noticed.

Moderately Developed Cases.—CASE III.—A young man, a Ga native, who had had yaws about seven years ago, felt pain in the nose and got a person to look into it, who said that there were yaw spots on the mucosa, and later a small swelling on each side of that organ was noticed. These small swellings grew slowly to their present size, and the patient said that they were still increasing. He complained of frontal headache and of slight pain in the swellings in wet weather. On inspection two symmetrically placed swellings were seen on each side of the nose, looking somewhat like small eggs. They were oval in shape, with the long axis directed downwards and outwards. The left measured two inches by two inches and the right three inches by two and a half inches. A profile view showed that they were slightly concave on the side towards the orbit. They did not affect the orbital or nasal cavities, nor did they project into the mouth or affect the nasal ducts or the cartilages of the nose. They were attached to the nasal bones, the nasal process of the superior maxilla, and to the superior maxilla itself. They were smooth, but on the left side the tumor rose to a central ridge. The skin over the swellings was quite normal and was freely movable. In order to see clearly, the patient often had to bend his head somewhat. The growths were removed by operation.

CASE IV.—The patient was an Akwapim woman, aged about twenty years. This case was similar to Case III., but the swellings, which had started when the patient (who had suffered from yaws) was seven years of age, were rather more rounded. She would not consent to operation.

An Advanced Case.—CASE V.—A man, a native of Appolonia,

about forty years of age, stated that the swellings began with pain in the nose after yaws, when he was about six years old. They grew steadily and slowly till eight years ago, when they stopped, and they have not increased in size since then. On inspection there were two oval swellings situated on each side of the nose, the left measuring two and a half inches by one inch and the right three-quarters of an inch by half an inch. They projected upwards over the orbit, the long axis in each case being directed downwards and outwards. They did not project into the mouth, the nose, or the orbit, and the nasal duct was free. They were attached to the nasal bones, the nasal process of the superior maxilla, and to the maxilla itself. The skin over the tumor was normal and it was freely movable. The patient complained of headache and found that the swellings interfered with his vision considerably, particularly on the left side. He refused to submit to operation.

An Asymmetrical Case.—CASE VI.—An Ashanti boy, aged six years, from Donkeo Inquanta, had yaws, and while suffering therefrom, just a year previous to his consulting me, the swelling appeared on one side of the nose, and had been growing ever since. There was no sign of any lump on the other side. He was advised to go to Kumassi for operation.

THE TREATMENT.

I have attempted to reduce these swellings by the administration of iodide of potassium, but have not met with any success. The only treatment appears to be the removal by operation. The method I adopt is as follows. The eyes being protected by a pad over each, an incision is made along the long axis of the tumor and the skin is freed on all sides so that its base is exposed. If the swelling is very small in a child it may be necessary to make a cross cut through the skin as well, in order to get sufficient room to work in. The bone being exposed, a portion of the swelling can easily be cut away by bone forceps, because it is very soft. If large, a few nicks with a Hey's saw are found most useful in enabling a large portion of the mass to be removed entire. After as much has been removed as possible with the bone forceps, more may be got away by means of the

gouge or the gouge forceps or the nibbling forceps. I have
experienced difficulty in removing the deeper portions, particularly those close to the orbit. I need hardly say that
in the latter the eye has to be carefully guarded from injury.
After removal of the bone the wound is well washed out
with an antiseptic lotion. The bleeding is slight and is
easily controlled by pressure. The wound is closed by a
continuous suture and it heals up readily.

THE MORBID ANATOMY.

I have never had any chance of examining the growth
post mortem, but the portions which I have removed *en
masse* by operation have enabled me to make some investigations. The periosteum strips off readily, and under this
is a thin shell of compact bone, which appears somewhat
ridged on the side towards the periosteum. The rest of the
tumor consists of cancellous bone. The whole swelling
cuts readily with bone forceps and consists of quite soft
bone. On making microscopical preparations there were
signs of ossification in membrane proceeding under the
periosteum, and the rest appeared like ordinary wide-meshed
cancellous bone. The whole process appeared to be that
of a slow "osteoplastic periostitis."

ÆTIOLOGY.

Two views on the ætiology of this disease have been
brought forward up to the present time, as far as I know—
viz., that the swellings were of a racial character and that
the process was started by the larva of some insect. With
regard to the first I have only to mention that the disease is
found in Ashantis, Grunshis, Fantees, Abantas, the Ga
people, etc., races quite different from one another, to show
that this cannot be entertained. As to the second, I have
never met with evidence which would support the idea that
the disease was started by a larva. On the other hand there
is always the history of yaws and of the tumor starting
during the attack of yaws—*i. e.*, during the period of eruption or soon after. Then, again, the patients complain of

pain in the nose with, in some cases, distinct history of a sore and sometimes discharge preceding the swelling. This might be due to some irritation or ulceration of the nasal mucous membrane by the yaws. I have never had the opportunity of examining any person at this stage of the disease, but in the more developed cases I have examined the nose for marks or signs of old ulceration, but have not found them. If, however, the nasal process of the superior maxilla be examined a few foramina are to be seen, and these are often joined together by a small groove indicating the position of a bygone suture. The foramina are for small bloodvessels, which are said to communicate with those of the mucosa of the nose. The site of these foramina is the situation where henpuye starts, and I venture to bring forward the theory that the causation of this peculiar disease is due to an osteoplastic periostitis brought about by the absorption of the poison of yaws from the nasal mucous membrane through the small vessels (or lymphatics) keeping open the foramina which indicate the suture above mentioned.

THE GEOGRAPHICAL DISTRIBUTION.

I am only aware of cases reported from the Gold and Ivory Coasts of West Africa and the West Indies. I never met with it in Mamprusia, nor have I met any trader coming from Moshi with it, nor have I met with it in Fra Fra, and I can find no one who has seen it in the eastern parts of the colony. But in the folllowing districts it has been noted: Ahanta, Appolonia, Fantee, Accra, Aquapim, Akim, Assin, Sefwhi, Ashanti, Attabubu, Kwahu, Kintampo, Berekum, Gaman, the Neutral Zone, and Wassaw. It is perhaps most common in the Sefwhi, Wassaw, and Appolonia districts which adjoin the French Ivory Coast, where cases are also known.

I look upon henpuye as a localized osteoplastic periostitis in the region of the nasal process of the superior maxilla, generally symmetrical, due to yaws, and found among the natives of West Africa and the negroes of the West Indies.

THE MADDOX ROD OR THE PHOROMETER; WHICH?

IN the last issue of the Journal there appeared an abstract with the above title, and believing the subject to be of much interest at the present time, our readers have been invited to send us their opinions on the matter, as based on the experience obtained in practice. The communications below have been received and are presented in the order of their reception. We shall be glad to hear from any physcians who are interested [ED.].

DEAR DR. DEADY: In reply to your favor requesting my opinion regarding the respective merits of the Maddox rod and the diplopia test, I wish to say that my experience leads me to rely more and more upon the obscuration test, and while I have not followed out the comparison to any great extent, such as is shown by your tables, results obtained by relying upon the rod test in the detection of heterophoria, as well as in determining when the weak muscles have been sufficiently developed, have been such as to warrant my continuance of its use.

E. D. BROOKS.

I have with interest watched the discussions of late, as to the relative value of the Maddox or Stevens tests for heterophoria, as I have for years used them both.

My muscle tests have been made for the last five years at least, with a Risley phorometer, which combines both tests upon one arm and has proven for me a most satisfactory instrument.

I am sorry to say that I have not kept any comparative statistics of my examinations; at the same time they have all left an impression upon my mind, which is this: that I feel more confidence in the results obtained from the use of the Maddox test in the routine tests that I always make of refractive cases. If this test shows any marked degree of heterophoria it has been my habit to retest the patient by the Stevens method, which is usually the same, provided the patient has a sufficient amount of intelligence to give correct answers to the questions put to him. During this test the patient is allowed to sit for some time in front of the prisms, and the eye muscles allowed to relax from that first impulse at muscular effort that follows the placing of the prisms in front of the eyes.

To my mind both tests are good and fairly accurate in the hands of one who is thoroughly familiar with their use and shortcomings, provided your patient is able to answer correctly.

Many times, on re-examining a patient, I have discovered what appeared to be a great change in the muscular conditions, but after repeated examinations I have usually found it was the patient, and not the muscles, that was erratic.

When Dr. Hubbell speaks of $\frac{1}{4}°$ of difference between the Maddox and Stevens tests, he has more confidence than I have in the average judgment of patients that come under our care. Sayer Hasbrouck.

Dear Doctor : Your note asking my opinion of the comparative usefulness of the Maddox rod and the phorometer is at hand.

In the detection of heterophoria I regard the rod as the most convenient and trustworthy instrument used.

The distance at which the test is made and the dissimilarity of the images seen usually eliminate all actual effort to hold the eyes in any particular position other than that in which they stand the most easily. Accordingly the deviation is quickly noted and readily measured.

So satisfactory has this modest little instrument been in my examinations that I now rarely resort to other methods. The amount of deviation sometimes shown between this and other instruments is so slight as to make little or no difference in the measures employed for correction.

It is to be noted that cases not unfrequently occur in which a hyper-sensitive, or, on the contrary, an enervated condition exists, which is not fully indicated by any instrument. An educated judgment will here have to supply conclusions not to be drawn by any hard-and-fast rules.

After the rod and the phorometer came into use and an opportunity was presented to compare the results obtained by each, I made a careful test of eighty pronounced cases of errors of refraction accompanied by heterophoria. Of this number only nine showed a persistent difference of deviation and in none of them a difference greater than 1½°. But this was not always on the one side or the other, as six out of the nine showed a higher degree of deviation by the rod than by the phorometer. Eighty cases may not be enough upon which to base an orthodox conclusion; but my experience with the rod has been so satisfactory that I now seldom use the phorometer at all. It appears quite possible practically to estimate the degree of heterophoria as accurately with the one instrument as with the other; and while it is true that a correction of the error of refraction will commonly correct the deviation, still all cases of optical defect should be tested with the rod or phorometer before the lenses are prescribed.   WM. A. PHILLIPS.

MY DEAR DR. DEADY: Dr. Hubbell limits the discussion "to the comparative value of the diplopia test, by Stevens' phorometer" and the Maddox rod test.

It would be interesting to follow out the idea with other phorometers,—and with the Wilson phorometer my records do not show quite such a marked difference in results,—but I have not taken pains to get comparative results in any considerable number of cases.

Dr. Hubbell says: "In the diplopia test, the dissociation is effected by changing the visual axis of one eye by means of a prism. The displacement of one image cannot be done without associating with it, more or less, an impulse to some form of ocular effort. . . . In the obscuration test (Maddox rod) no such effort is invited, no change of innervation takes place." But in the rod test the light seems nearer to the patient than in the prism test. This may account for much of the difference in results and amount to "an extraneous impulse to muscular contraction."

Dr. Hubbell is entirely justified in his conclusion as made upon experiments with the Maddox rod and the Stevens phorometer. I shall watch cases along similar lines with the Wilson phorometer and report later.

In the mean time the rod and the prism tests may well be taken in each case and let judgment decide as to treatment.

THOS. M. STEWART.

I agree with the writer that the rod test is the more scientific test for heterophoria, and of late years have virtually discarded the prism test, except in special cases. The tables are interesting, but their value would be materially increased if the author would supplement them with tables showing the refraction, and inflammation or its results.

Was it an accident that Stevens' phorometer showed the same amount of right hyperphoria in one-ninth of the cases, and in thirteen of thirty-three cases of left hyperphoria? In which of these cases was there anisometropia and of what kind was it?

What was the refraction of the two cases of exophoria, two of left and one of right hyperphoria by the phorometer; and was the refraction the same in the six cases which were orthophoric by both rod and prism?

Such studies are necessary to a clear understanding of the relative value of these tests.

JOHN L. MOFFAT.

DEAR DR. DEADY : Your letter and inclosed article on " The Maddox Rod or Phorometer ; Which ? " has been received and examined with interest.

I have examined a good many cases in my office by both methods and find variable results, but where there is a radical difference I have found the Maddox rod the more accurate, and from experience I have learned to rely upon it instead of the phorometer, as in prescribing prisms in hyperphoria in connection with glasses for constant use I rely wholly upon the rod test.

J. M. FAWCETT.

DEAR DOCTOR : Concerning the discussion of Maddox Rod vs. Phorometer about which you wrote me—can say that I believe that the Maddox rod is the more reliable test. My reasons on theoretical grounds for so believing are briefly these.

Given a case for examination ; the test which *least disturbs* the muscular co-ordination under investigation must give the best result.   Now I think that when we throw the images into non-corresponding retinal points that we almost certainly cause some tension of certain muscles, because it is putting the eyes in an *unnatural* relation with one another ; and this is done by the phorometer.   The Maddox rod is theoretically free from this objection.

Practically the deviations are more certainly measured, because a patient *knows* when the streak cuts the light ; and you cannot trust their eye alone to tell when the lights are exactly in a line. Have used *both* tests in every case I have examined in my private practice, and I find the Maddox the more reliable test.   It is more to be depended upon.   Edw. Hill Baldwin.

Grant, Dundas.—Case of Emphysema of the Orbital Wall of the Anterior Ethmoidal Cells, Caused by blowing the Nose.—*Jour. Lar., Rhin. and Otol.*, March, 1900.

This case was shown to the British Laryngological, Rhinological and Otological Association.

W. M., twenty-eight years, came under my care yesterday on account of a sudden swelling of his eye which had taken place two hours previously, and which had occurred suddenly as he was blowing his nose without a handkerchief, and which gave him the impression as if something were running out of his eye. The swelling crackled in a manner characteristic of emphysema, and the first suspicion was that he must have had some disease of the orbital wall of the anterior ethmoidal cells, and that on examination there would be found some evidence of ethmoidal disease. None such was to be elicited, and the only history obtainable was that he received several kicks on the nose and back of the ear two months ago. This has probably resulted in a fracture of the orbital wall of certain of these cells.　　　　PALMER.

Lack, Lambert.—Case of Nasal Polypi, with Suppuration and Absence of Maxillary Sinuses.—*Jour. of Lar., Rhin. and Otol.*, April, 1900.

A man, aet. twenty-eight years, complains of nasal obstruction and purulent discharge, with a disagreeable odor in the nose. The polypi having been removed, the pus appeared to flow from under the anterior ends of the middle turbinates. After wiping the discharge away and bending the patient's head forward, it reappeared in large quantity. On transillumination the cheek on both sides appeared quite dark, and the patient had no subjective sensation of light. The diagnosis of antral suppuration was now considered almost certain, and the patient was advised to have both antra punctured from the alveolar margins. This was accordingly attempted under gas, but although the antrum drill was forced in for its full length, no cavity was reached.

Puncture from the inferior meatus was next attempted, and considerable force was used in two different points ; but with no better result. It would seem therefore that the antra must be very small, if not entirely absent.

Discussion.—Mr. Spencer thought it might be one of those convoluted inferior turbinals which form a gutter in which pus collects. The majority considered it suppuration in the ethmoidal region.   PALMER.

Lawson, Arnold.—Cicatrix Horn Growing from the Cornea.—*The Lancet*, February 3, 1900.

The patient was a female child, aged eight years, a hydrocephalic idiot. The history given was that about one year previously a white spot had appeared on the right eye and that the eye began to project. Six months later a growth was first noticed on the right cornea, and this had constantly increased in size. Latterly a white spot had appeared on the left eye. On examination of the eyes there was seen a large conical tuberculated excrescence protruding between the lids of the right eye. It was half an inch in length and its base attached to the cornea covered about four-fifths of its surface. The left cornea exhibited a yellowish infiltration just below the pupil, over which the cornea was bulging ; the anterior chamber was deep, the iris was immobile, the tension was slightly raised, and the eye was quite blind. Both globes were very anæsthetic, and there was considerable muco-purulent discharge from a chronic inflammation of both conjunctival sacs. The growth upon the right eye was accidentally detached a few days after admission into the hospital, and it was then seen to have been attached to the corhea at the apex of a central staphyloma, which was left covered by a fleshy soft core which had formerly been embodied in the center of the growth. The cornea was entirely opaque, and the eye was quite blind. After removal of the right eye a few days later examination of the globe revealed a co-arct retina with evidences of chronic degenerative changes in all the various structures. The anterior chamber was completely abolished, the iris throughout its extent being firmly adherent to the back of the cornea, which was bulging centrally. The apex of the corneal staphyloma had evidently been the site of a large perforation, which was closed by the fleshy granulations which formed the core of the growth. The growth itself measured half an inch from apex to base and one and a half inch around its base.

The interior portion was soft and crumbling, but the external layers were hard and horny and cut with difficulty. A wedge-shaped piece was cut away from the growth and specimens were cut and stained with carmine. The microscope showed that the external layers consisted of several faintly fibrillated strata of a dense, homogeneous nature. The layers occupied about one-quarter of the entire thickness of the walls, the rest being entirely composed of small nucleated cells, those most external being stratified. Adopting Mr. Bland Sutton's classification of human horns, this growth would be an example of a cicatrix horn, the rarest of all varieties of horn, and one which had been usually found in connection with cicatrices of burns and scalds. The probable ætiology in this case was an overgrowth of granulation tissue closing the perforation in the cornea, which, owing to an unhealthy condition of the wound and eye, which was anæsthetic and atrophic, had become exuberant, simulating exactly the condition known as " proud flesh " elsewhere. By a process of accumulation and heaping up, the granulations gradually formed a cap over the cornea, whilst the external layers gradually became stratified and horny from the pressure of fresh growth from the central core and by the action of the air. The nature of the growth was evidence that the corneal epithelium bore no share in its production and discounted the possibility that it might be due to a huge crust of inspissated conjunctival discharges. DEADY.

Lodge, Jr., M. D., Samuel.—A Case of Fatal Sphenoidal Suppuration.—*The Laryngoscope*, March, 1900.

W. S., aet. thirty-one years, admitted to Royal Halifax Infirmary May 15, 1899, complaining of pain in right ear and right side of face of six months' duration. For two months right side face swollen and copious bloody, purulent discharge from right nostril. Nine years ago had syphilis. Insomnia from pain.

On admission : Temperature 100° ; skin over right superior maxilla red and œdematous ; thick purulent discharge from right superior meatus, sequestrum in region of right cribriform plate ; naso-pharynx, chest, and abdomen normal ; urine, sp. gr., 1014 ; trace of albumen. Fundi (of eye) normal.

May 16—No pus found in antrum on exploration and flushing. Patient taking 60 grs. pot. iod: (t. i. d.) and mercurial inunction. Temperature in ear usually higher than that in mouth until just before death. June 8.—Mortuus est.

Post-mortem Examination.—Skull. Base of brain was bathed in thick greenish pus, principally in the neighborhood of the pituitary body, the pus extended back over the pons and medulla. No brain abscess. Ventricles contained more than normal quantity of fluid. Frontal sinuses and cribriform plate of ethmoid and ethmoidal cells normal.

To right of the sella turcica there was some necrosis of the walls of the sphenoidal sinus. Probe readily passed from base of skull through sphenoidal sinus into the nose. Large free opening from said sinus into nose, which sinus was full of muco-pus. Cavernous sinus not thrombosed. Right antrum of Highmore contained about a dram of thick glairy mucus.

PALMER.

Killian, Prof. Gustav.—Case of Acute Perichondritis and Periostitis of the Nasal Septum of Dental Origin.— *Münch. med. Wochen.*, No. 5, 1900.

There have been recorded two cases of perichondritis of the septum due to alveolar periostitis. Suppuration of dental cyst was cause in the following case.

A young man had pain in second left upper incisor ; two days after obstruction of nose supervened, with pain in forehead and high fever. There was a sudden copious discharge of fetid pus from right nostril seven days later. The entire mucosa of the septum was raised from the cartilages, etc. It is considerably swollen over right side of the triangular cartilage, but less so posteriorly. Severe headache in forehead and frontal eminence, and still little fever. The pus was escaping through a small hole into the left nostril. It was freely incised. The triangular cartilage was distintegrated, and the pus had burrowed between the soft tissues and vomer and vertical plate of the ethmoid. The choanæ were constricted by thickening of the septal mucous membrane. The wound healed in a fortnight without sequestrum, while the toothache lasted but two days.

Six months later the patient had recurrence of pain in the same tooth of two months' duration ; it was extracted and pus continued to exude from the socket. A probe. passed 2½ centimeters to the floor of the nose and septum, showed a cavity covered with membrane in the anterior parts of upper jaw, which was a cyst at the root of the tooth. The anterior cyst walls were removed with bone forceps, and the remainder scraped. The cavity gradually healed.

The cyst probably broke through under the septal mucous membrane. In exceedingly few cases of perichondritis does the process extend to the osseous septum. Only once has the author seen record of a case which was as extensive as this. The offensive odor also points to a dental origin.   PALMER.

Hawthorne, C. O.—The Eye Symptoms for Locomotor Ataxia, with a Clinical Record of Thirty Cases. —*Brit. Med. Jour.*, March 3, 1900.

It is now generally recognized that the disease known as locomotor ataxia may include among its clinical manifestations symptoms other than those which depend on pathological changes in the spinal cord. A number of these are associated with the functions of the eyeballs. The Argyll-Robertson pupil is universally admitted as valuable confirmatory evidence of a diagnosis of locomotor ataxia ; ocular paralyses, if less frequent, are certainly not less significant ; and optic nerve atrophy is at least so well known in connection with the disease that its occurrence in any individual case would hardly call for comment.

A further step forward in our knowledge of the clinical possibilities of locomotor ataxia has been the recognition of the fact that ocular disturbances may precede the evidences of any spinal lesion. This advance necessarily means that the occurrence of any one of the ocular events above mentioned must, unless otherwise explained, generate the suspicion that the case may in its later events display the phenomena known to depend upon sclerosis of the posterior columns of the spinal cord.

It is very difficult to collect the evidence necessary to show in what proportion of cases this suspicion is justified by the event. For it is certain that ocular disturbances may long precede the manifestation of spinal symptoms. In the case of optic atrophy the interval may, according to Gowers, extend even to twenty years. Thus it can only be in very exceptional instances that one and the same physician will have the opportunity of observing at least a number of these cases through all the stages of their progress. Yet, if true, it is of manifest importance, for the sake both of exact knowledge and of accurate prognosis, that it should be clearly recognized that an optic-nerve atrophy, an ocular paralysis, or a loss of the pupil light reflex, unless capable of other explanation, belongs in all probability to the order of events incident to locomotor ataxia, and that any one of these may well be the introduction to a more widely-spread manifestation of the disease.

For reasons stated above, the collection of complete histories necessary to afford actual demonstration of the truth of these propositions is difficult ; and all the more so as there is reason to believe that in those cases in which the early stress of the disease falls upon the nervous apparatus of the eyeball the spinal symptoms are apt to be slight in degree as well as delayed in development. This is certainly the case when the ocular disturbance takes the form of optic-nerve atrophy. " In a large number of such cases," says Gowers, " ataxy never comes on, the spinal malady becoming stationary when the nerve suffers."

Of course, in a given case of optic-nerve atrophy without spinal symptoms the question may fairly be raised whether it is right to place such a case in the locomotor ataxia group. All that can be said in reply is (1) that from cases of optic atrophy pure and simple one passes by an unbroken series of steps through cases with more and more distinct evidence of locomotor ataxia to, at the end of the series, optic atrophy in association with characteristic ataxic symptoms, and (2) that, as already stated, a simple case of optic atrophy may remain unchanged for many years, and yet in the end display undoubted evidence of the development of a spinal lesion. But if optic-nerve atrophy may be the primary symptom in the disease, if the ocurrence of spinal symptoms may follow it after an interval of many years, and if again it may remain without at any time any existing ataxia, it is not unreasonable to presume that both the Argyll-Robertson pupil and an ocular paralysis may each have exactly corresponding relations to the development of the spinal evidences of locomotor ataxia. The collection of evidence to support this suggestion is even more difficult than in the case of optic-nerve atrophy. The latter condition must ere long compel the patient to seek medical advice, and thus the opportunity for a complete investigation of the state of his nervous apparatus is afforded at a relatively early date. But an Argyll-Robertson pupil may exist, and presumably exist for years, without any inconvenience to the patient. Such a patient, therefore, will not consult his medical adviser until spinal or other symptoms display themselves, and thus the precedence of the pupillary condition cannot be determined. In the case of an ocular paralysis medical assistance is, no doubt, usually promptly invoked. But such an occurrence is open to a number of ætiological explanations, for example, rheumatism, cold, etc., which it is difficult to exclude with confidence. Hence it is much less precise in its significance than either a double optic atrophy or the Argyll-Robertson pupil. It must be by the collection of observations extending over a long term of years that actual demonstration of the relationship of the ocular disturbances now in question to the occurrence of spinal disease can be established. But while falling short of the merit of actual demonstration, the presentation of the facts displayed by a number of cases which could only be observed over relatively brief periods is not without value. If no one case affords a complete history of all the stages of the disease the picture presented may none the less be fairly complete, provided the cases are sufficiently numerous, and they are seen at different points of development. It is believed that in the present series these conditions are fulfilled. The conclusions they afford, as far as the present purpose is concerned, are : (1) That an optic-nerve atrophy, an ocular paralysis, or an Argyll-Robertson pupil may exist as an isolated symptom for a considerable time, presumably for years ; (2) that any two of these may be associated together, with a correspondingly increased presumption that the diseased process causing them is of the locomotor ataxia order ; (3) that any one of the three, or a combination of two or all of them, may exist in conjunction with a greater or less degree of evidence of spinal disease ; and (4) that occasionally a case which commences with purely ocular symptoms may be seen to develop with comparative rapidity characteristic symptoms of the spinal lesion of locomotor ataxia.

The cases therefore may be held to justify the view that an optic-nerve atrophy, an ocular paralysis, or the Argyll-Robertson pupil (not capable of other explanation) must be regarded as affording a definite basis for suspicion in reference to a possible development of spinal disease. On the other hand, it must be admitted that the prognostic indication, so far as spinal disease is concerned, is not an absolute one, for the ocular defect may exist certainly for many years without any evidence whatever of the involvement of the spinal cord.

The cases here recorded have all been the subject of detailed and in most cases repeated examination, and unless the contrary is stated, it may be taken for granted that the thoracic and abdominal viscera are normal, to physical and other methods of examination. In all cases, too, in which no specific statement is made, it is to be understood that the visual acuity, the visual fields (both for white and colors), and the fundus oculi have been proved to be normal. This last statement of course does not apply to cases in which optic atrophy exists. Particular care has been taken to be accurate in regard to the condition of the pupils and the knee-jerks. In nearly, if not absolutely in every instance where a departure from the normal is chronicled, the record has been confirmed by more than one observer, and in the case of a deficient knee-jerk the conclusion stated has never been formulated until the conditions insisted on by Gowers, Buzzard, and Jendrassik have been fulfilled. With a few exceptions in which only a single observation was possible, the patients have been watched for months, and in some instances for several years. The cases are arranged in series, with a view to show how, from a purely ocular condition, one may pass through gradually accumulating evidence to the same ocular condition in association with the characteristic signs of the spinal lesion of locomotor ataxia.

I.—CASES IN WHICH OPTIC-NERVE ATROPHY IS THE PRIMARY OR DOMINATING CONDITION.

(a) *Optic Atrophy, without Other Evidence of Disease.*

CASE I.—W. T., aged twenty-five. Failure of vision extending over two years, with reduction of visual acuity to the power of counting fingers at three feet. Double optic atrophy; pupils medium, with distinct light response ; knee-jerks distinct and no evidence of spinal disease, and no cerebral symptoms other than one or two attacks of giddiness. Urethritis, but no syphilis.

CASE II.—F. R., aged thirty-eight. Double optic atrophy, with almost complete loss of vision, the defective sight having been observed for at least eighteen months ; pupils dilated and immobile ; no evidence of spinal disease, unless possibly some degree of failure of sexual power ; no cerebral incidents ; no history or evidence of syphilis.

(*b*) *Optic Atrophy, with Other Ocular Evidence Suggestive of Loco-motor Ataxy.*

CASE III.—(By permission of Mr. Ernest Clarke, F. R. C. S.) R. C., aged thirty-nine. Double optic atrophy, reducing right visual acuity to the power to count fingers at four feet, and left to mere perception of light ; right pupil dilated and three times the size of the left ; neither any light response, but free movement on convergence ; entire absence of symptoms and objective signs of spinal disease ; " gleet " twenty years before, no syphilis.

CASE IV.—A. S., aged twenty-five. Double optic atrophy, with observed failure of vision for twelve months. V. A. right-hand movements only ; left, $\frac{6}{18}$ part ; pupils 2.5 mm., no light response, but contract on convergence ; knee-jerks difficult to obtain, but movement, though possibly wanting in promptness, is normal in extent ; no ataxia or other evidence of spinal disease ; mother of three healthy children, no miscarriages.

(*c*) *Optic Atrophy, with Some Evidence of Spinal Disease.*

CASE V.—W. A., aged thirty-seven. Double optic atrophy, with reduction of visual acuteness to " hand movements ; " pupils dilated and immobile ; knee-jerks absent, but no other evidence of spinal disease ; venereal sore when aged twenty ; no recognized secondaries, and father of four healthy children.

CASE VI.—J. G., aged thirty-five. Failure of sight (six months) ; optic atrophy, gradually increasing whilst under observation of twelve months ; pupils not definitely abnormal; knee-jerks absent throughout, but no further appearance of spinal disturbance ; urethritis, but no history of syphilis ; father of two healthy children, wife no miscarriages.

CASE VII.—F. L., aged thirty-nine. Double optic atrophy, reducing visual acuteness to $\frac{6}{24}$, pupils very small, and with

Argyll-Robertson phenomenon ; subsequent to failure of sight (twelve months) has had shooting pains in thighs, and failure in retention power of bladder ; knee-jerks distinct ; no ataxia or sensory defect in lower limbs ; venereal sore twenty years before ; no recognized secondary syphilis ; wife healthy: seven pregnancies, five miscarriages.

(*d*) *Optic Atrophy, with Distinctive Evidence of Spinal Disease.*

Case VIII.—C. H., aged thirty-eight. Failure of sight (two years) from double optic atrophy ; pupils medium, with Argyll-Robertson phenomenon ; moderate double ptosis, but no ocular paralysis ; shooting pains in lower limbs (eight years) ; knee-jerks absent; considerable ataxia and failure of control over bladder ; syphilis at nineteen years.

Case IX.—G. S., aged forty. Pallor of disks and peripheral contraction of visual fields ; four months later loss of knee-jerks and gradual development of ataxia ; pupils normal throughout ; death at the end of twelve months with symptoms of meningitis ; syphilis at twenty-five years.

II.—Cases with Argyll-Robertson Phenomenon.

(*a*) *Argyll-Robertson Phenomenon, without Other Evidence of Disease.*

Case X.—A. L., aged thirty-three, the subject of slight hypermetropic astigmatism. Pupils small, not quite circular, with Argyll-Robertson phenomenon ; no other ocular defect, and no evidence of a spinal lesion. No history of syphilis.

Case XI.—K. S., aged forty-three. Pupils rather small, unequal, quite destitute of light response, though moving freely in convergence ; no other ocular defect except some presbyopia ; no evidence of spinal disease, though left knee-jerk not easily obtained. Unmarried ; syphilis seems highly improbable.

Case XII.—G. G., aged sixty. Pupils small, with distinct Argyll-Robertson phenomenon. Knee-jerks, not easily obtained, but not definitely abnormal, and no other evidence of spinal disease. Patient suffers from defective vision, probably from tobacco poisoning (central scotoma for red) ; no history or evidence of syphilis.

(*b*) *Argyll-Robertson Phenomenon, with Other Ocular Disturbance Suggestive of Locomotor Ataxia.*

Case XIII.—D. T., aged forty-two. Pupils below medium size, destitute of light response, with free movement in convergence ; had for seven days suffered from diplopia, and under observation gradual development of complete paralysis of right external rectus ; no other ocular defect. Knee-jerks distinct, and no suggestion of spinal disease ; chancre of lip and secondary syphilis nine years before.

(*c*) *Argyll-Robertson Pupils, with More or Less Evidence of Spinal Disease.*

CASE XIV.—T. F., aged fifty-five. Right pupil 2mm., left 3 mm., each with Argyll-Robertson phenemenon ; no other ocular defect except presbyopia. Ten years ago had difficulty in passing urine, and since then occasionally voids it involuntarily, and for eighteen years has been liable to seizures of pain in calves, insteps, and heels ; knee-jerks normal, and no objective signs of spinal disease. Venereal sore when aged twenty, but no second-ary symptoms, and father of six healthy children.

CASE XV.—H. W., aged thirty-eight, is the subject of hyper-metropia, 4.5 D. Pupils very small, especially left ; neither moves under light, but distinct contraction during convergence. Admits recent difficulty in descending stairs, saying he " fre-quently misses the bottom step," and has suffered from " sciatica " for two years. No objective evidence of spinal dis-ease, and urinary and sexual functions undisturbed. Admits gonorrhea, but denies syphilis. Wife miscarried eight months after marriage ; no further pregnancies.

CASE XVI.—R. S., aged forty-three. Hypermetropic and presbyopic. Pupils small, unequal, not quite circular, and with definite Argyll-Robertson phenomenon. Knee-jerks cannot be obtained (confirmed on three different dates), but no other sign or symptom of tabes dorsalis, unless " rheumatic pains " in lower limbs for several years. Unmarried ; no history of syphilis. Four years ago had, after " catching cold," to have urine withdrawn by a catheter, but no subsequent disturbance of bladder function.

CASE XVII.—E. W., aged forty-eight. Myosis with Argyll-Robertson phenomenon ; right ptosis and crossed diplopia (one month), without obvious ocular paresis ; absence of right knee-jerk (confirmed on two occasions), and failure in retention power of bladder (six months), but no other evidence of spinal disease; vulvar sores and skin eruption six years before.

III.—Cases in which an Ocular Paralysis is the Earliest
or Dominating Symptom.

(a) Ocular Paralysis, without Other Evidence of Disease.

Case XVIII.—(By permission of Mr. J. T. James, F. R. C. S.)
F. D., aged thirty-seven. Dilated and immobile pupils, without
any other ocular defect. No evidence of spinal disease ; syphilis
nine years ago ; no change while under observation for three
years.

Case XIX.—K. K., aged twenty-eight. Iridoplegia, double,
followed by paralysis of left external rectus, the condition being
under observation for nearly a year, but without the discovery of
any satisfactory explanation. No evidence of spinal disease.
Married, four healthy children, no miscarriage ; during one
pregnancy very free loss of hair (now grown again), but no other
occurrence to suggest syphilis. No family or personal history of
gout or rheumatism.

Case XX.—G. H., aged thirty-three. Dilated and immobile
pupils, with incomplete ptosis and divergence of eyeball on each
side. Present condition of four years' duration, and separated
by an interval of three years from venereal sore and skin eruption.
No other ocular defect ; no evidence of spinal disease, and general health good throughout. No change while under observation for three months.

(b) Ocular Paralysis, with Other Ocular Evidence Suggestive of Locomotor Ataxia.

Case XXI.—E. S., aged forty-three. Diplopia from paralysis
right external rectus, pupils small, each with Argyll-Robertson
phenomenon ; visual left acuity only $\frac{6}{12}$, and small but distinct
central scotoma, with some contraction of the peripheral field ;
knee-jerks distinct, and no ataxia or other evidence of spinal disease. Three early miscarriages, no full-time child. No change
while under observation for nine months, but on two occasions
severe attack of vomiting and abdominal pain, extending over
several days and without recognized cause (? gastric crises).

Case XXII.—A. M., aged fifty-five. Left ptosis and paralysis
of external ocular muscles supplied by third nerve in 1887, the
pupils being normal, followed by incomplete recovery. In 1897
development of identical condition on the right side, and pupils
found to be small and with Argyll-Robertson phenomenon ;

knee-jerks very slight and with great difficulty, but no other evidence of spinal disease. No history of syphilis.

CASE XXIII.—H. F., aged thirty-seven. Right ptosis with diplopia (seven days) and defective inward excursion of right eyeball ; pupils very small, not quite equal, and with Argyll-Robertson phenomenon ; optic disks pale and marked contraction of visual fields, but normal central vision ; knee-jerks scarcely to be obtained, but no other evidence of spinal disease. No history of syphilis. Father of four healthy children. Seen after a month's interval, paralysis of all external right ocular muscles supplied by third nerve, and knee-jerks absent.

(c) Ocular Paralysis, with More or Less Evidence of Spinal Disease.

CASE XXIV.—G. S., aged forty-one. Ptosis and complete ophthalmoplegia externa on left side, with dilated and immobile pupils and some degree of right ptosis, these conditions or some of them having been present for five years. Knee-jerks distinct, and no ataxic phenomenon, but imperfect control over bladder, and failure of sexual power during last six months. No admitted syphilis.

CASE XXV.—J. L., aged forty-two. Diplopia and drooping left upper eyelid for four years. Ptosis left side, and marked defect of ocular movements in each eye ; left pupil dilated and immobile ; right small, contracts during convergence, but no light response ; no other ocular defect. Knee-jerk scarcely obtained on either side ; no ataxia, but attacks of " twitching pains " in lower limbs, and for some time difficulty in starting the flow of urine. Venereal sore in 1882, and subsequent loss of hair, but no other secondary symptoms. Patient watched for twelve months without appreciable change.

CASE XXVI.—L. D., aged forty-four. Crossed diplopia (one month), without obvious ocular paralysis, and pupils small with Argyll-Robertson phenomenon. Knee-jerks absent ; no ataxia to usual test, but has noticed tendency to stagger in the dark ; is troubled with pains in the knees, has difficulty in commencing the act of micturition, and recent marked failure of sexual power ; venereal sore at twenty years, and subsequent sore throat, but no skin eruption or loss of hair. Father of three healthy children.

CASE XXVII.—J. H., aged forty-seven. Double vision of two months' duration ; similar attack three years ago, with complete recovery. Paralysis of right external rectus; pupils, visual acuity, and visual fields normal. Knee-jerks absent, but no other evidence of spinal disease. Patient the subject of albuminuria, and presents physical evidence of an aneurism of the ascending aortic arch. Youngest child has marked evidence of inherited syphilis.

CASE XXVIII.—W. M., aged thirty-five. Paralysis of left third nerve, without iridoplegia or cycloplegia; pupils normal. Knee-jerks absent, but no ataxia or other evidence of spinal disease. Several venereal sores ten years ago, but no recognized secondary syphilis. There is, however, evidence of a former iritis.

CASE XXIX.—M. C., aged fifty-four. Paralysis of left external rectus, with history of two previous attacks of diplopia during last four years; no other ocular defect, unless some imperfect light response in left pupil; knee-jerks absent, and complaint of "sciatica" for two years, but no other evidence of spinal disease. Albuminuria distinct, and physical signs of hypertrophy of left ventricle. No history of syphilis.

CASE XXX.—(By permission of Mr. N. M. MacLehose, M. B.) H. Y., aged thirty. Homonymous diplopia observed over a period of six months without appreciable ocular paralysis; pupils of medium size, with definite Argyll-Robertson phenomenon; knee-jerks absent, and in later months decided ataxia and sensory defects in lower limbs; visual acuity unaffected to ordinary test, but gradual contraction of visual fields, especially on right side; chancre and secondary syphilis four years before.

There are in these series of cases many facts which might reasonably be made the subject of remarks, and several of the cases are certainly of great individual interest. But they are here displayed in the above grouping for the purpose of illustrating the clinical order and sequence in which, as a matter of actual experience, the ocular disturbances of locomotor ataxia may manifest themselves in relation to the spinal evidences of that disease. Of course, in those cases in which there exists only a single ocular symptom unaccompanied by any sign of spinal disease, it may be objected that it has yet to be demonstrated that such cases are of the nature of locomotor ataxia. It is doubtless to be desired that such cases should be under exact observation as long as the opportunity for further developments exists—that is, for the entire life of the patient. But to insist upon such a condition is a mere counsel of perfection. One must make reasonable use of such evidence as the brevity of life and the exigencies of practice permit. And the evidence here set forth affords at least a very strong presumption, to say the least of it, of the truth of the doctrines stated in the earlier paragraphs of this paper. Probably the particular proposition which is most likely to be contested is the one which places the Argyll-Robertson pupil equally with optic-nerve atrophy, and an ocular paralysis, as a possible first event in the eruption of the phenomena of locomotor ataxia. But on turning to the records it will be found that the facts support this suggestion almost as strongly as they support the corresponding suggestion in reference to optic-nerve atrophy and ocular paralysis. Attention in this respect may be particularly given to Case XIII. The man complains of a quite recent diplopia, and he has undoubtedly had syphilis ; the pupils show the Argyll-Robertson phenomenon. It is in the highest degree probable that, had the patient been under observation a week or two earlier, the condition of the pupils would have been the sole existing ocular abnormality. Yet in the light of the development of an ocular paralysis, it can scarcely be doubted that, whether he develop spinal symptoms or not, his nervous system is the site of diseased processes of the locomotor ataxia order. When to these facts there are added, as in Cases XIV. to XVII., illustrations of the various forms and degrees of evidence of spinal disease that may be associated with the Argyll-Robertson pupil, it seems impossible to resist the conclusions that the condition of the pupil so named may be the first evidence of locomotor ataxia ; that it may precede by varying intervals other evidences of the disease ; and that at least very probably, in a certain number of cases, the symptomatology of the disease may be permanently restricted to this one event. In some examples of its spinal form locomotor ataxia is undoubtedly an extremely chronic disease, with few and imperfectly developed symptoms ; and it is thus not unnatural to expect that similar limitations may obtain in the ocular manifestations of the disease. That evidences of grave nervous disease may be limited to the pupil is well seen in Case XVIII., where a syphilitic patient was under observation for three years without the discovery of any abnormality other than paresis of each sphincter iridis. There is certainly no obvious reason why a similar restriction should not

determine the Argyll-Robertson pupil as a purely isolated phenomenon with, it must be added, the same unfortunate possibilities that are undoubtedly attached to the patient whose case
has just been quoted. The conclusions above adopted in reference to the Argyll-Robertson pupil are applicable, *mutatis
mutandis*, to optic-nerve atrophy and to ocular paralysis, as is
abundantly demonstrated in the corresponding series of the
cases recorded in this paper.   DEADY.

Menzies, J. Acworth.—Detachment of Corneal Epithelium (?).—*British Med. Jour.*, March 17, 1900.

The following case seems to be worthy of record because of
the long duration of the symptoms and the immediate relief
ultimately obtained. Mrs. W. consulted me on August 4, 1899,
and gave the following history: Five years previously the right
eye was struck and "cut" by a cricket ball. Since that time
there had been pain exactly as if there was a foreign body under
the lid or embedded in the cornea. There was a pricking feeling
on winking, and the patient could not bear to have the upper lid
touched in its outer half. She could only obtain ease by keeping
the eyes closed and perfectly still, or wide open with the lids
motionless. On examination no foreign body could be seen, and
the lids were normal. In the lower outer quadrant of the cornea
careful observation showed that the epithelium was ruffled and
freely movable over a small area, and in part of the same area
was a tiny circular, slightly opaque, raised patch of the corneal
tissue. Nothing more could be made out. I prescribed a bandage and some boric lotion with cocaine. Two months later, on
October 6, I again saw the patient, who was then in precisely
the same condition as before, and had been so during the two
months' interval. She was in such misery that I decided to
adopt surgical measures at once. Accordingly, after instilling
cocaine, I carefully explored the painful area with a needle,
but could detect no foreign body. I then scraped the part
thoroughly with a sharp spoon, removing the epithelium for some
little distance around, and a fair amount of corneal tissue in the
affected area. The following day there was some smarting, but
the eye could be moved freely under the lid, and there was no
pain on pressure over the previously tender spot. Progress was
uninterrupted. The epithelium grew over the denuded surface,

and no opacity resulted. The eye now is perfectly right and the vision is normal.

I should have put the difficulty I had in making a diagnosis down to my having overlooked some detail, had it not been that the patient was for a considerable time under treatment at an eye hospital. The explanation I am inclined to adopt, for want of a better, is this, that the original blow caused the anterior elastic lamina with the epithelium to become detached. The nutrition of the epithelium might thus be kept up, and every movement which pressed upon the surface would bring the detached membrane down on the corneal nerve filaments. But it must be confessed it is not easy to understand how this condition could remain stationary for five years. DEADY.

Hines, M. D., Oliver S.—Iodide of Stanmum in Tuberculosis.—*The Amer. Hom.*, March 15, 1900.

The author thinks iodide of stannum often preferable to stannum in tuberculosis. He uses it when the patient has a clear complexion and long eyelashes and where the progress of the disease is rapid. He reports a case for which the 2x trituration was given, in which there was "a marked tubercular affection of the chest, increased vocal fremitus, an abundance of thick yellow and sweetish sputum, sweat at night, and rapid emaciation." The result was encouraging. PALMER.

Kyle, M. D., D. Braddon.—Initial Forms of Tubercular Laryngitis.—*Inter. Med. Mag.*, March, 1900.

The enumeration and exact description of these prodromal symptoms are so important that we copy them in full.

The following, which is a translation of an article by Monsarrat of Paris (*Rev. Hebdom. Laryngol., d'Otol., et de Rhinol.*, No. 43, October 28, 1899), covers the ground so thoroughly that it is worthy of repetition:

"Laryngeal phthisis completely developed presents multiple and varied symptoms, some more characteristic than others. In one patient are found symptoms functionally grave, out of proportion to the lesions relatively benign. In another, physical signs take first place; there may be an ulceration completely obliterating one cord, or considerable œdema of the arytenoids and vestibule, which closes the opening of the glottis. Having reached the period when tuberculosis is easily recognized, the various patients are able to date their laryngitis from diverse pathologic beginnings. This one will present solely the history of a cough, the other a raucous voice, in another pain will take precedence. In mentioning these various modes of commencement we insist on the connection which may exist between each of them and the localization at the beginning of tuberculosis, on one or the other parts of that complex organ known as the larynx. Let us divide the symptoms into the functional and the laryngoscopic. The connection or antithesis between them will be noticed.

" An initial symptom, quite frequent in tubercular laryngitis, is, without a doubt, cough. This symptom, common to all maladies of the respiratory tract, would have no diagnostic value, except that it is characteristic. On it alone the diagnosis of laryngeal phthisis could never be based. At the beginning, cough puts us on our guard, especially when it is causeless; that is to say, when auscultation of the chest fails to reveal anything abnormal. This cough is always persistent, sometimes violent, hawking, and provoking.

" The physical signs of the chest do not correspond to the tenacity of the cough; it is therefore possible for the larynx to be accused. As regards this cough, the 'hemming' so often described, and which draws attention most often to a possible rhinopharyngitis, may cause us to think at the beginning of tuberculosis, but only after examination of the rhinopharynx has established its integrity. There is a cough, well known at the beginning of tubercular laryngitis, a little dry cough, commencing insidiously, often at the moment when the patient is about to speak, which the individual himself does not notice, but to which his friends attach an importance too often justified by the outcome. The cough may be hacking, followed or not by expectoration, and often accompanied by vomiting. It is certainly right to consider it as a symptom of the beginning of the disease.

" The speaking voice is often altered, dysphonia appears, and the patient who is attacked presents little alteration in his larynx; no ulceration, the cords accurately approximate, and they are very slightly congested; the laryngeal image does not reveal anything by which this profound alteration in the voice can be explained. There is no cough. There will come a time in the disease, however, which will cause us to see that this, too, is an initial form, and oblige us to give a prognosis exceedingly guarded.

"The voice may be eunuchoid. Castex has noted it among the tuberculous. The raucosity of the voice should also recall the statistics which demonstrate the fact that a fifth of the cases of this condition are tubercular. But these three symptoms, dysphonia, raucosity, eunuchoid voice, are also found in other maladies of the larynx; conditions, however, easily diagnosticated by the laryngoscope. If nothing justifies these affections of the voice, one should think of tuberculosis. It is these initial forms, apparently paradoxical, but analogous to that, which we are going to mention under the subject of pulmonary lesion not sufficient to provoke cough in the beginning if the larynx has not been initially affected. The forms that are recognized in the mirror are evidently very numerous. We will mention some: Congestion of the cords, monocorditis, recurrent laryngitis, and a nodular form at the free border of the vocal cords. We do not take into consideration any variety of ulceration, no matter how insignificant, as for the most part the velvety aspect of the cords leads us to think at once of laryngeal phthisis. But this has not appeared at the beginning, and we are only considering initial forms. The symptoms which we are attempting to describe are those suggestive of tuberculosis, and we only say that tuberculosis of the larynx may begin by a nodule, by a congestion, by a monocorditis, etc.

"Congestion of the vocal cords, whose ætiology is difficult to explain, often coincides with slight dysphonia, with cough. This congestion, fugacious, if not tuberculous, disappears with rest, if it is not aggravated by a chronic rhinopharyngitis. In the majority of cases the patient returns. Despite a treatment, properly instituted, the congestion persists; it extends on the cords; it may remain there, or it may reach over the ventricular bands to the arytenoidal apophyses; this is a form of commencing laryngeal phthisis, especially if, after a period of calm, there is found in a patient a new congestion. It is recurrent laryngitis, another form of initial tuberculosis more grave than the first. Against laryngitis of this form treatment is of no avail.

"Another variety of initial tuberculosis is monocorditis. The patient becomes suddenly aphonic; laryngoscopic examination

shows a cord perfectly red, congestion of which is evident, not
only by the color, but by its altered volume. Contrast with the
sound cord is often striking. Movements of the affected cord
may be observed, but it is generally paretic. Acute monocorditis
should cause us to think that it is an initial form of tuberculosis.
This monocorditis often corresponds to the side of the lungs
which is afterward or at that time attacked by the bacillus. Certain authors admit that this relation is absolutely constant, and
their statistics allow no exception to the rule. On the other
hand, Bayle's theory, setting forth the direct penetration of the
tubercular infection, becomes less often justified. It is the
lymphatic route which most often produces bacillary infection.

"Tubercular laryngitis may often begin by a nodule situated
on the border of the vocal cords. It is important not to confound
it with singers' nodules, these latter being more conical and more
rounded. The tuberculous nodule may grow slowly, not ulcerate
for a long time; interfering so little with the speaking voice that
the patient often refuses any intervention. But the day comes
when we see this nodule desquamate, and we may observe the
evolution of the tuberculous ulceration which displaces it. We
make no mention of the other forms of commencement characterized by a congestion of the entire organ, by œdema of the epiglottis, by a lividity quite characteristic which invades the entire
endolaryngeal mucosa, forms most usual for the tubercular
involvement of the larynx. A form especially noticeable is that
which begins with a sensation of a lump in the throat. It is true
that this variety is not observed except in the nervous; it is not,
however, to be compared to the globus hystericus. Tuberculous
patients, in whom the tuberculous process in the larynx begins
with a sensation of a lump in the throat, may be in very good
health, but this particular impression is often the first symptom
which they observe in a laryngitis, which finally becomes tuberculous. At the moment when the patient complains of this
symptom it may happen that laryngoscopic examination fails to
detect any lesion. It is useless to add that this form is especially
met with in the female. It most nearly resembles that form that
begins with a dysphagia that persists to the end; but at the beginning of tubercular laryngitis this dysphagia alone is noted without
any other symptoms." So it can be seen that laryngeal phthisis
may begin by a variety of symptoms, some common, the others

rare. It is needless to insist upon the importance of an early diagnosis. PALMER.

Ball, James Moores.—On Removal of the Cervical Sympathetic in Glaucoma and Optic-Nerve Atrophy.— *Jour. A. M. A.,* June 2, 1900.

I propose to consider the surgery of the cervical portion of the great sympathetic nerve in certain ocular diseases. European oculists and surgeons have performed sympathectomy for glaucoma and exophthalmic goiter. I have gone further, and in one instance removed the superior cervical ganglion for simple atrophy of the optic nerve. I have performed sympathectomy four times up to July 20, 1899. First the cases will be reported; then the conclusions will be drawn.

CASE I.—EXCISION OF SYMPATHETIC FOR GLAUCOMA
ABSOLUTUM.

Mrs. B. S., aged thirty-six, has had pain in and around the right eye for two months, and examination showed vision in this eye reduced to light perception; tension + 3, and the pupil widely dilated. The anterior chamber was shallow, the cornea cloudy and slightly anæsthetic, the media slightly cloudy, still allowing the fundus to be seen. The episcleral vessels were enlarged. Circumcorneal injection was present and the optic nerve cupped. A diagnosis of chronic irritative glaucoma was made. The left eye presents immature cataract, and vision in this eye is 20/70.

Knowing of the flattering results obtained by Jonnesco and others, by excision of the superior cervical ganglion in absolute glaucoma, I explained the operation to the patient, and obtained permission to operate. On May 15, 1899, the patient was anæsthetized, chloroform being employed. An incision four inches in length was made on the right side downward from the mastoid process, extending along the posterior border of the sterno-cleido-mastoid muscle. The external jugular vein was cut and tied. The sterno-cleido-mastoid was then separated from the trapezius muscle, and the spinal accessory nerve was cut. A deep dissection was then made, exposing the carotid sheath. This was opened to enable us to locate the pneumogastric nerve beyond question. The carotid, internal jugular vein, and pneumogastric nerve were then pulled forward, enabling us to see the rectus capitis anticus major muscle, on which the superior cervical ganglion rests. Tearing through the fascia, the ganglion was found and stripped. The ganglion was then cut high up with curved scissors and all its branches severed. About one inch of the trunk of the sympathetic below the ganglion was removed. The wound was closed with interrupted sutures and the neck placed in a plaster cast. The time required for operation was fifteen minutes, and immediately after it was noticed that the right eye was suffused with tears, the right conjunctiva much injected, and the right nostril moist. The intra-ocular tension was + 2. The patient slept well all night, without medicine, being free from pain for the first time in over two months. Tension had steadily decreased to + 1.

On May 16, slight ptosis was noticed on the right side. This symptom is yet present. On May 19 the circumcorneal injection was much less; the conjunctival hyperæmia and lachrymation were still present, while the ptosis was slightly increased and tension was + 1.

At the present date—July 23, 1899—this patient has no pain. The retinal arteries are increased in size. Tension is + 1. Vision has increased from light perception to ability to count fingers at three feet. The conjunctival injection which followed the operation has disappeared; the optic nerve has a color more approaching the normal. The ptosis is less.

This was the first sympathectomy made in America for glaucoma.

CASE II.—DOUBLE SYMPATHECTOMY FOR GLAUCOMA SIMPLEX.

Miss M. E., a German, aged forty-three, was sent to me on June 14, 1899. For two years sight had been failing, until at this time vision was as follows: R. E. = 0; L. E = light perception. Tension was + 3. Both optic nerves showed marked cupping of the disk; the vessels were pushed to the nasal side. She stated that she had never had pain in the eyes, and had not consulted an ophthalmic surgeon.

I advised her to submit to an excision of the left superior cervical ganglion; she consented, and on June 15 the operation was performed by myself, assisted by Dr. E. C. Renaud, at St. Joseph's Sanatorium, in the presence of Drs. J. C. Murphy, A. R. Kieffer, and S. A. Grantham. The operation was difficult, owing to the abnormal position of the vagus nerve. This was outside of and external to the carotid sheath, and was much smaller than normal; it was not larger in diameter than the head of a pin. It was identified by irritating it and watching the effect on the heart. The superior cervical ganglion was removed and one-half inch of the trunk of the sympathetic below. Shortly after the operation there were lachrymation, ocular congestion, and contraction of the pupil on the corresponding side. On the second day she counted fingers at 2½, and on the third at 3½ feet. Slight ptosis was present.

She left the hospital on the eighth day. At this time she counted fingers at four feet. There was only slight, if any, reduction of tension during the eight days she was in the hospital. In counting fingers she saw with the nasal side of the retina—temporal field. I did not see her again until June 30, and she was then counting fingers at five feet. Tension on that day was normal. She had light perception in the right eye.

On July 16 I excised the right superior cervical ganglion without difficulty, and on July 7 she counted fingers at seven feet with the left eye, and could see the hand at four inches with the right. I examined her on July 20, when vision remained the same, the tension of the right eye was + 1, and of the left + 2. She was well pleased to have the small amount of vision she possessed.

CASE III.—SYMPATHECTOMY FOR OPTIC-NERVE ATROPHY.

T. J., aged forty-six, an inmate of the St. Louis City Hospital, a laborer, was admitted on account of blindness. There was no history of syphilis, rheumatism, nor any systemic disease. The patient was of limited mentality. No history of his family could be obtained. He claimed to have had good health all his life, with the exception of an attack of malarial fever several years ago. The patient had been a moderate drinker of alcoholic beverages. In appearance he was robust, and he complained only of loss of vision which, in the left eye, had been failing for eleven months, in the right for seventeen weeks, according to his statement. Until seventeen weeks before this he could see enough with the right eye to get around. Since then vision had steadily declined until he had light perception only—and this only apparent when light was concentrated on the eye by the ophthalmoscopic mirror. Vision of the left eye = o.

The pupils were widely dilated. The ophthalmoscope showed, in the right eye, a white disk, particularly on the temporal side ; the arteries slightly reduced in caliber, veins normal. There was shallow, atrophic cupping of the nerve head. The retina and choroid were normal, the vitreous and lens clear. The left eye showed a disk of a dead white color throughout the whole area, arteries very small, atrophic excavation pronounced, veins reduced in caliber, and choroid normal. The macula was not visible in this eye, owing to the much-reduced blood-supply. The vitreous and lens were clear. Vision was as follows : R. E. = perception of concentrated light. L. E. = o.

Diagnosis.—R. E. = optic-nerve atrophy. L. E. = complete atrophy of optic nerve and retina.

Treatment : Resection of the right superior cervical ganglion of the sympathetic was done. The operation was followed by conjunctival congestion, lachrymation and contraction of the pupil, slight ptosis and hypotonia.

No appreciable change in the patient's vision followed, and ophthalmoscopic examination made two weeks after operation showed no change in the appearance of the fundus, except that a cilioretinal artery in the upper part of the disk had doubled in caliber.

So far as I know, Case III. is the first instance in the history of medicine of an excision of the superior cervical ganglion, or of any part of the sympathetic system, for the relief of optic-nerve atrophy. Although the operation was not of benefit in this particular instance, yet I am not willing to concede that it will prove valueless in cases of non-inflammatory atrophy in which vision is not entirely lost. In truth, I expect it to prove beneficial in such cases, sufficiently often to justify the procedure.

I was led to make this experimental operation for several reasons : 1. The use of glonoin is often followed by an improvement in vision in cases of simple atrophy of the optic nerve. 2. Glonoin enlarges the retinal vessels, as has been proved by ophthalmoscopic examination. 3. There is no question that in glaucoma simplex—a disease in which there is an atrophy of the optic nerve—improvement in vision follows sympathectomy. 4. Excision of the cervical sympathetic is followed by an increase in the blood-supply of the orbital contents.

PATHOLOGIC CHANGES IN THE EXCISED GANGLIA.

The microscopic examination of three of the excised ganglia was made by my friend, Dr. Carl Fisch, of St. Louis. The specimens were those from Cases I., II., and III. Of the two ganglia removed from Case II. only the first one—the left—was examined.

Transverse and longitudinal sections of the three specimens were studied microscopically, by means of a great number of different staining methods. Owing to the method by which the ganglia had been preserved—weak formalin solution—the employment of the Golgi—Marchi—and the more delicate Nissl stains was rendered impossible. In general it may be said that the pathologic changes found were the same in the three cases, although a little less pronounced in No. 2 than in 1 and 3.

Most striking of all was a very marked hyperplasia of the connective tissue, which in some places resulted in dividing up the ganglion into small groups of nervous elements separated by broad bands of fibrous elements. The walls of the vascular structures showed decided sclerosis ; the connective-tissue sheaths of the ganglionic cells were much increased in thickness. In Case I. small foci of round-cell infiltration were seen in this hyperplastic growth, of an inflammatory character. No plasma nor mast cells could be demonstrated.

The ganglionic cells were markedly pigmented. Together with a number of cells normal to all appearance there were great numbers showing different stages of degeneration. As a rule the nucleus, besides having lost part of its peculiar staining property, had assumed the parietal position ; the nucleus was reduced in size or even missing in a large percentage of the cells. While in some cells the chromatic elements were well preserved, in others the process of chromatorhexis and chromatolysis could be followed up through all of its stages. Only comparatively few cells were seen showing the normal dendriform processes ; very often the processes were short, ending bluntly, or they had even disappeared altogether. The general peripheral network of processes was much reduced in volume and compressed by the pressure of the connective-tissue formation. Only very few medullated fibers were seen. Unfortunately it was impossible to study their structure with the Marchi method.

The general pathologic aspect was that of a decided sclerosis, originating in inflammatory processes going on in, and starting out from, the walls of the vascular structures. The changes of the nervous elements were most likely not idiopathic, but due to pressure and inhibited nutrition.

The plates accompanying this paper have been made from drawings of sections of superior cervical ganglia.

TECHNIQUE OF THE OPERATION.

The ordinary precautions for surgical cleanliness are to be observed, and general anæsthesia employed. The incision should be made along the posterior border of the sterno-cleido-mastoid muscle, starting at the mastoid process and running downward to within an inch of the clavicle. The sternomastoid is separated from the adjacent muscles, the spinal accessory nerve cut, and the carotid sheath reached. This dissection is made with the fingers. The carotid sheath should always be opened in order to locate the pneumogastric nerve. I consider this very important because : 1. The nerve is sometimes outside the sheath, as happened in my second case, in which the pneumo-gastric was much atrophied and was external to the sheath. 2. Differentiation of the cervical sympathetic from the vagus is sometimes difficult. Often, in operating on the cadaver, I have found both nerves inclosed in the same fascia. It is needless to say that excision of the vagus instead of the sympathetic would not only defeat the object of the operation, but would add a serious complication. Differentiation of these nerves after open-ing the carotid sheath is not usually difficult, for in working upward the operator comes upon the ganglionic expansion of the sympathetic. The ganglion is seized with forceps and stripped. Its branches are cut first, then the cord passing below is severed, and lastly the ganglion is cut above, as high as possible. It is best to use curved scissors and to have the finger under the ganglion while traction is made, thus cutting on the finger and avoiding injury to the underlying structures.

If the middle ganglion is to be removed, it will be best to excise it first and then work upward. If the entire chain of the sympathetic is to be removed, as is done for epilepsy, and as is now advised in exophthalmic goiter by Jonnesco, the operation is one of great difficulty, owing to the location of the inferior ganglion. This is situated near the neck of the first rib. One of my friends, who is a skillful surgeon, in removing this ganglion ruptured the vertebral artery near its origin and was obliged to tie the subclavian to check the hemorrhage. After the latter has ceased the wound is closed with superficial sutures. The hemorrhage in removal of the superior ganglion is usually trifling, only a few small vessels being cut. The external jugular vein was cut in my first case, but not in the others. The patient leaves the hospital on the eighth or ninth day.

Jonnesco's method, according to his latest communication on the subject, is different. He always employs the premastoid route where only the superior ganglion is to be removed, reserving the postmastoid for the excision of the entire chain. The carotid sheath is split, the internal jugular vein and sternomastoid drawn outward by a retractor; a second retractor draws the vagus and internal carotid inward. In the space made the superior ganglion is found. The deep vertebral fascia is opened, all the branches of the ganglion isolated and cut by blunt, curved scissors; when this has been done the ganglion is attached only by nerve strands above, a strong pull is made, and the ganglion gives way. The excision is then completed by cutting the inferior strands. In closing the wound, he uses both deep and superficial sutures.

He mentions a transient dysphagia and pain in the craniomandibular joint as occurring after this operation.

EFFECTS OF EXCISION OF SUPERIOR CERVICAL GANGLION.

The effects of removal of this ganglion are immediate and remote : The immediate are relief of pain, lachrymation and conjunctival injection, together with a discharge from the corresponding nostril, unilateral sweating, and contraction of the pupil. Often there is an immediate reduction in intra-ocular tension. These effects are noted within five minutes after the excision.

The remote effects are ptosis, which appears on the third or fourth day, improvement of vision, and in some instances a tardy contraction of the pupil and a tardy reduction of the intra-ocular tension. To these there must also be added a slight sinking of the eyeball into the orbit, and a feeling of heaviness in the head. What I have just written applies particularly to cases of glaucoma.

In exophthalmic goiter, after the excision of the ganglia, the exophthalmus and tachycardia are said to improve almost immediately and a reduction of the goiter soon follows.

Although Jonnesco speaks of the immediate reduction of the intra-ocular tension, yet this does not always occur. In my second case, at the end of eight days the tension was + 2. On the sixteenth day the tension was normal. In my first case reduction of the tension was immediate. The relief from pain in the first case was immediate and lasting. This patient had not been free from pain for two months previously. The slight ptosis following sympathectomy is to be attributed to paralysis of Müller's muscle. Sinking of the eyeball is no doubt due to paralysis of the unstriped peribulbar fibers found in Tenon's capsule. Contraction of the pupil is usually an immediate result ; it may, however, appear tardily. Thus in my first case the pupil was unchanged until the fourth day after the operation ; and it did not become at any time as markedly contracted as in the other two patients. In the third case—that of optic-nerve atrophy—the pupil was markedly contracted within five minutes after the excision.

The lachrymation, conjunctival injection, and nasal moisture are transient symptoms which are usually absent after the first day.

In this connection it is interesting to note that Mr. Jonathan Hutchinson, as early as 1866, recognized many of the ocular symptoms of paralysis of the cervical sympathetic, and wrote a paper thereon.

HOW DOES EXCISION OF THE CERVICAL SYMPATHETIC REDUCE INTRA-OCULAR TENSION ?

This is a question difficult to answer—difficult for the reason that we are not sufficiently acquainted with the physiology of the production of aqueous humor under normal surroundings. Panas and Duvigneaud have assumed rightfully that " If the nervous mechanism of intra-ocular secretion or, to speak without hypothesis, the action of the nervous system on intra-ocular tension can be known, the pathology of glaucoma will be cleared up, iridectomy will be explained, and perhaps a new and scientific basis for the treatment of glaucoma will be established." Many observers have sought to solve the problem. Donders attributed the hypertension to a neuro-secretory cause and believed the trigeminus to be the agent of excessive secretion. He held that section of the trigeminus should relieve intra-ocular tension, while section of the cervical sympathetic could have no particular influence.

His views were overthrown by experiments made by Wegner in 1866, on rabbits. By means of manometers placed in the anterior chamber, he sought to record variations in the intra-ocular tension. He proved to his own satisfaction that the trigeminus takes no part, while section of the cervical sympathetic produces hypotonia, and irritation of its upper end, and causes hypertonia. He held that section of the cervical sympathetic enlarges the blood vessels of the eye ; the blood then flows under reduced pressure, and intra-ocular secretion is lessened. Almost identical results were obtained by Adamück—1866-68— who experimented on cats.

Von Hippel and Gruenhagen believed that the cervical sympathetic contains vasoconstrictor fibers for the eye. Their experiments were made on cats and dogs. They found that irritation of the upper end of the cervical sympathetic causes in the cat hypertonia, while its extirpation increases intra-ocular tension. While, according to Wegner, the hypertonic action proceeds from the enlargement of vessels caused by cutting the cervical sympathetic, and the contraction of the blood vessels caused by the irritation of the nerve causes a hypertonic action, the contrary view is held by Adamück, Von Hippel, and Gruenhagen.

However this may be, there is no doubt that the trigeminus plays no great part in the production of ocular tension. Furthermore, the inefficiency of Bedal's operation—stretching the nasal nerve—is explained by the fact that it is the cervical sympathetic, and not the trigeminus, which influences intra-ocular tension.

Jonnesco believes that the ocular sympathetic fibers from the brain and spinal cord pass through the superior cervical ganglion; permanent or intermittent irritation of these is accompanied by dilatation of the pupil, narrowing of the small intra-ocular arteries, contraction of the peribulbar muscular fibers, and probably an increased action of the elements which produce the aqueous humor. "As a matter of fact," says Jonnesco, "any increase of the blood pressure will produce a permanent or intermittent narrowing of the arteries and cause the extravasation

and increase in aqueous humor; then it is probable, although
not definitely settled, that a permanent or intermittent irritation
of the excito-secretory fibers is followed by an increase in the
secretion of aqueous humor; the permanent or intermittent
dilatation of the pupil pushes the iris into the iris-angle, closes
the canals of the filtration zone, and hinders or prolongs the
exit of aqueous humor from the eye; the permanent or intermittent contraction of the unstriped peribulbar muscular fibers
closes the efferent veins of the eyeball, and hinders the venous
circulation of the eye—hence the dilatation of the intra-ocular
veins."

He holds that excision of the superior cervical ganglion
destroys all vasoconstrictor fibers of the eye. The arteries relax,
the blood pressure is lowered, and extravasation is reduced.
This operation destroys the excito-secretory fibers, thus limiting
the amount of aqueous produced. The fibers which dilate the
iris are destroyed, hence the contraction of the pupil reopens
the iris-angle and removes the obstacle to the outflow of aqueous.
The nerve-fibers supplying the unstriped muscular apparatus
contained in Tenon's capsule are destroyed, hence the pressure
on the efferent veins is removed and ocular circulation is re-
established.

Jonnesco believes that the starting-point of the nervous
derangement producing glaucoma is central: "When one removes the ganglion the point of origin of the influence will not
be removed, but the communication between this center and the
eyeball is destroyed."

Regardless of the differing views of physiologists concerning
the mechanism of the reduction of ocular tension, based on
experiments made on the lower animals, there can be no difference of opinion concerning the effect of excision of the superior
cervical ganglion in the human subject. The operations made
by Jonnesco and others on the Continent, and by myself in
America, prove that removal of the superior cervical ganglion
causes a marked reduction of intra-ocular tension in glaucomatous cases. That the same effect occurs in eyes with normal
tension is evident from my third operation—that done for
optic-nerve atrophy.

EXTENT OF SYMPATHECTOMY IN DIFFERENT DISEASES.

Up to the present time excision of the cervical sympathetic

has been performed for the following diseases : epilepsy, exoph-thalmic goiter, glaucoma, and optic-nerve atrophy. The ques-tion naturally arises : How extensive an operation is necessary in these affections ? This I will attempt to answer :

In epilepsy it is necessary to excise the entire cervical chain on both sides for the reason that, according to Jonnesco's theory, it is necessary to convert a state of cerebral anæmia—which he assumes is the condition in epilepsy—into one of cerebral hyperæmia. Since the carotid plexus is formed by branches from the superior ganglion, and the vertebral plexus arises from branches which have their origin in the inferior cervical ganglion, it is evident that the entire cervical sympathetic must be removed.

In exophthalmic goiter, although Jonnesco in his first opera-tion excised only the superior and middle ganglia, he now believes it necessary to remove the inferior as well, for this reason : from the superior ganglion the ocular fibers arise ; from the inferior the vasodilator, cardiac-accelerator, and, prob-ably, the secretory nerves of the thyroid gland. If eye, thyroid, and cardiac symptoms are to be relieved the entire chain must be excised.

In glaucoma removal of the superior ganglion alone is neces-sary. All of the sympathetic fibers of the eye, with the excep-tion of those which pass directly from the cerebrum by way of the trigeminus, are connected with the superior ganglion.

In optic-nerve atrophy, if it should be proved that non-inflammatory atrophy of the optic nerve can be improved by sympathectomy, removal of the superior ganglion alone will be necessary, for reasons already given.

If the glaucoma is unilateral, it is necessary to remove only the corresponding ganglion.

HISTORY OF SYMPATHECTOMY.

In 1889 Alexander of Edinburgh resected the superior ganglion on both sides. In 1892 Jacksh resected the vertebral plexus and cut the cord connecting the middle and inferior ganglion. The third operator was Kummel, who excised the superior ganglion on one side only. In 1893 Bojdanik made a bilateral resection of the middle ganglion. In 1896 Jaboulay made a bilateral section of the sympathetic cord, above and below the middle ganglion. These operations were all made for epilepsy.

In regard to exophthalmic goiter, Jaboulay made a simple section of the sympathetic early in 1896. In September of the same year Jonnesco excised the superior and middle ganglia.

Jonnesco was the first, in 1896, to do a bilateral resection of all three cervical ganglia, though it is claimed by a Polish surgeon, Baracz, that he proposed the same in 1893. To Professor Jonnesco furthermore belongs the credit of having first excised the superior ganglion for glaucoma in September, 1897.

Ball of St. Louis was the first to remove the superior cervical ganglion for optic-nerve atrophy. The date of this operation was June 24, 1899.

Terrier, Guillemain, and Malherbe, in their "Chirurgie du Cou," 1898, were among the first to give the surgery of the sympathetic a place in a text-book.

Among those who have operated on the cervical sympathetic for the relief either of glaucoma or exophthalmic goiter, or both, are Abadie, Réclus, Gerard-Marchant, Chauffand and Quénu, Jeunet, Bled, Ball, Renaud, and Bartlett.

Panas is opposed to sympathectomy in glaucoma. He reports seeing a patient in whom, three months after the operation, vision was still declining.

François-Frank, at a meeting of the Paris Academy of Medicine, held May 22, 1899, spoke of the effect of sympathectomy on the circulation of the thyroid gland, brain, and eyes, and on the heart. He believes that the operation can easily produce good results.

Doyon has described the trophic changes produced in the rabbit by excision of the cervical sympathetic.

CONCLUSIONS.

From a study of the cases of sympathectomy made by Jonnesco and others, and from the observation of my own cases, I offer these conclusions:

1. Excision of the superior cervical ganglion is a most valuable procedure in glaucoma.

2. It is of more value in glaucoma simplex than in inflammatory glaucoma.

3. In inflammatory glaucoma, on which iridectomy has been done without benefit, excision of the superior cervical ganglion should certainly be tried.

4. In cases of absolute glaucoma with pain, sympathectomy is to be tried before resorting to any operation on the eyeball.

5. In cases of simple optic-nerve atrophy, sympathectomy may possibly be beneficial if done before vision is entirely lost.

6. In cases of exophthalmic goiter, which do not improve under hygienic medicinal and electric treatment, excision of the cervical sympathetic on both sides is to be advised.

7. In unilateral glaucoma excision of the sympathetic ganglion is to be done only on the corresponding side.

8. In the hands of a careful operator, excision of the superior and middle ganglia is a safe operation, but removal of the inferior ganglion can be done safely only by the most skillful surgeons.

9. The postmastoid route is to be preferred in excision of any part, or all of the cervical sympathetic.

10. The fact that glaucoma is improved by sympathectomy and the finding of pathologic changes in the excised ganglia suggest the conclusion that this affection is due either to a permanent irritation of the cervical sympathetic, or to an irritation located elsewhere and transmitted by means of the cervical sympathetic.

I wish to extend my thanks to Drs. E. C. Renaud and Willard Bartlett for valuable assistance in the preparation of this paper ; to Dr. Carl Fisch for the pathologic report.   DEADY.

Heath, M. D., Charles.—A Case of Sinuses in the Vault of the Naso-pharynx.—*The Jour. of Lar., Rhin. and Otol.*, May, 1900.

Case shown at the Lar. Soc. of London :

A woman, æt. thirty-one years, had suffered several years with discomfort in nose, throat, and mouth, with dyspepsia. Mucosa of nares and pharynx markedly atrophied. Atrophied condition made post-rhinoscopy easy. " The eustachian eminences were seen to be enormous, filling the fossæ of Rosenmüller, and reaching nearly to the pharyngeal roof. Just behind the upper edges of the choanæ, on each side, there appeared a transverse elliptical opening, which was about half an inch long and a fifth of an inch across at the widest part on the left side, and slightly less in each dimension on the right ; a probe apparently extends about a quarter of an inch into the cavity." In the discussion following some thought them to be small recesses formed by cicatricial tissues, other formed by peculiar distribution of adenoid tissue, and still genuine sinuses.   PALMER.

Roughton, B. S. (Lond.), F. R. C. S., Edmund W.— The Diagnosis and Treatment of Chronic Purulent Nasal Discharges.— *The Jour., of Lar., Rhin. and Otol.,* May, 1900.

We ascertain by interrogation, (*a*) if the discharge is purulent or muco-purulent ; (*b*) whether it is unilateral or bilateral ; (*c*) whether it is continuous, intermittent, or influenced by change of posture ; (*d*) if there is offensive smell perceived by the patient or by others ; (*e*) pain is not usually complained of unless there is obstruction to drainage, and consequently retention of pus under pressure.   Unilateral discharge suggests a foreign body in a child or sinus involvement in an adult.   If it is intermittent or influenced by position probably originates in a sinus.   Subjective fetor suggests sinusitis ; while objective fetor, ozena ; and combined subjective and objective is the rule in syphilitic necrosis.   Location of pain is of very little, if any, use in diagnosis.

Rhinoscopy.—Attention directed to (*a*) situation of the pus ; (*b*) polypi ; (*c*) atrophy of the mucous membrane ; (*d*) crusts ; (*e*) ulcerations ; (*f*) adenoids ; (*g*) nasal obstruction ; (*h*) foreign bodies.   Under (*a*) beside usual cleansing of nasal cavities and re-examination to ascertain situation, he recommends " tamponading," *i. e.,* by blocking up first one part, then another, with pledgets of wool, and noticing whence the discharge reappears. (*e*) Ulceration may be syphilitic, simple, tubercular, or lupoid in origin.   " It must not be forgotten that a perforation " of the septum " may be entirely the work of a misused finger-nail." (*g*) The normal mucoid discharge damned up by nasal obstruction frequently becomes purulent.

Special methods of diagnosis as follows are mentioned : transillumination ; examination of upper teeth ; catheterization of the ostium, maxillares, naso-frontal canal, and outlet of the sphenoidal sinuses ; external examination of antrum and frontal sinuses ; exploratory puncture of the antrum through the inferior meatus, alveolar process, or canine fossa.   Diagnosis of ethmoiditis is principally by exclusion.

Treatment of the accessory sinuses may be summed up under the following indications : (*a*) removal of the cause ; (*b*) evacuation and drainage of pus; (*c*) antiseptic irrigation; (*d*) removal of morbid material, when present.   PALMER.

Williamson, R. T.—**Remarks on the Diagnosis and Prognosis in One Hundred Cases of Double Optic Neuritis with Headache.**—*Lancet*, May 12, 1900.

The detection of optic neuritis is of the greatest importance in the diagnosis of cerebral affections. Nevertheless, in certain cases of double optic neuritis with headache considerable caution is necessary before coming to a conclusion as to the exact nature of the disease. Though these two symptoms are present in the majority of cases of brain tumor and are so frequently due to this cause they are also met with in other diseases. In some cases of granular kidney, for example, the patient comes under treatment for headache and failure of vision; and ophthalmoscopic examination may reveal intense optic neuritis like that of cerebral tumor (neuritic form of albuminuric retinitis). At first the symptoms appear to indicate cerebral tumor, but a careful examination of the urine and cardio-vascular system will clearly reveal the cause. Limited space does not permit an enumeration of all the causes of double optic neuritis with headache. The results of the examination of one hundred cases presenting these two symptoms reveal, however, several points of interest. Most of these cases have been seen by us conjointly; some were seen separately, whilst others (in Groups I. to VIII.) were examined by one of us (R. T. W.) whilst holding the post of medical registrar at the Manchester Royal Infirmary. For permission to include the latter amongst our cases we are indebted to the medical board of that hospital.

With respect to the diagnosis and termination these one hundred cases may be grouped as follows:

I. Brain tumor, verified by necropsy, 27.

II. Cases terminating fatally; probably, majority due to brain tumor; but no necropsy obtained, 27.

III. General symptoms of brain tumor; but necropsy revealed distention of the ventricles of the brain with fluid; no tumor (serous meningitis of ventricles), 2.

IV. Cerebral abscess (fatal), 3.

V. Tuberculous meningitis (fatal), 2.

VI. Chronic interstitial nephritis ; neuritic form of albuminuric retinitis (fatal), 3.

VII. Toxic conditions and blood diseases :

Chronic lead poisoning, 3.

Ulcerative endocarditis, (fatal), 1.

Purpura hemorrhagica (fatal), 1.

Henoch's purpura (fatal), 1.

Chlorosis with cerebral symptoms (recovery), 3.

VIII. Headache and double optic neuritis (without localizing symptoms) ; probably syphilitic (recovery, with blindness, 2 ; with impaired vision, 4), 6.

IX. Headache and double optic neuritis (without localizing symptoms) ; no evidence of syphilis ; duration six and two and a quarter years, respectively. Termination still uncertain, 2.

X. Headache and double optic neuritis (without localizing symptoms) ; no evidence of syphilis ; recovery with blindness, 8 ; with impaired vision, 3 ; with good vision, 8, 19.

The following are brief abstracts of the notes of the cases in Group X. which have come under our observation and which we have followed for a considerable period of time. The number of years during which each case has been followed is given in parentheses after the brief note.

1. A boy, aged ten years. Double optic neuritis, headache, and vomiting ; slight internal strabismus of the left eye. Recovery with normal vision. (Seven years.)

2. A young woman, aged seventeen years. Headache, vomiting, and double optic neuritis. Recovery, but with impaired vision in one eye and blindness in the other. (Five and a half years.)

3. A young woman, aged eighteen years. Double optic neuritis, headache, and vomiting ; several epileptic fits. Recovery, with useful vision in one eye ; vision in the other is very defective. (Seven years.)

4. A young woman, aged eighteen years. Double optic neuritis, headache, and vomiting. Recovery, but complete blindness followed. (Four years.)

5. A young woman, aged nineteen years. Double optic neuritis, headache, and vomiting. Recovery with good vision. (Three years.)

6. A man, aged twenty years. Double optic neuritis, head-

ache, and vomiting. Recovery, but complete blindness followed. (Two and a half years.)

7. A girl, aged ten years. Double optic neuritis, headache, and vomiting ; knee-jerks were absent. Recovery, but complete blindness followed. (Three years.)

8. A boy at the age of thirteen years had double optic neuritis and headache ; recovery ensued. At the age of fifteen years he had a return of headache and double optic neuritis ; also vomiting. At a later date there was partial anæsthesia in the distribution of the right fifth cranial nerve ; the right cornea was opaque ; there was complete blindness in both eyes. Partial anæsthesia of the face and blindness remained, but otherwise the patient recovered and felt quite well nine months after the second attack.

9. A girl, aged sixteen years. Double optic neuritis, headache, vomiting ; slight internal strabismus of the right eye. Recovery with normal vision. (Four and a half years.)

10. A boy, aged ten years. Double optic neuritis, headache, and vomiting. The head had increased in size. Recovery, but with complete blindness. (Three years.)

11. A woman, aged nineteen years. Double optic neuritis, headache, and vomiting. Recovery with normal vision. (Three years.)

12. A boy, aged fifteen years. Double optic neuritis, headache, and vomiting. Recovery. (Two and a half years.)

13. A woman, aged twenty-one years. Double optic neuritis, much swelling of the disks, headache, and vomiting. Complete recovery with normal vision. (Four and three-quarter years.)

14. A girl, aged fifteen years. Double optic neuritis, headache, and vomiting. Recovery with good vision. (Five and a quarter years.)

15. A boy, aged twelve years. Double optic neuritis, headache, and vomiting ; slight internal strabismus of the right eye. Recovery with good vision. (Four years.)

16. A man, aged forty years. Double optic neuritis, headache, and vomiting. Recovery, but with complete blindness. (Eighteen months.)

17. A youth, aged seventeen years. Double optic neuritis, headache, and vomiting. Recovery, but with total blindness. (Five years.)

18. A woman, aged twenty-two years. Double optic neuritis, headache, and vomiting. Recovery, but with total blindness. (Two and three-quarter years.)

19. A girl, aged fourteen years. Double optic neuritis, headache, and vomiting; internal strabismus (left) for fourteen days. Recovery, with normal vision. (Two years.)

The following are brief notes of the cases in Group IX.:

20. A girl, aged twelve years. Headache, vomiting, and double optic neuritis in December, 1893. Recovery in twelve months, but vision was much impaired. She remained well with the exception of occasional headache until December, 1899. Then the severe headache returned. She became ataxic and optic neuritis reappeared. In April, 1900, the headache was much less and the patient felt much better, but she was completely blind. (Six and a half years.)

21. A young woman, aged seventeen years. Headache, vomiting, and double optic neuritis. Vision was impaired. Vomiting ceased; the headache continued for over two years, but recently disappeared after lumbar puncture. (Two and a quarter years.)

In all cases of double optic neuritis a systematic and careful examination of the patients should be made. The urine and cardio-vascular system should be examined for signs of chronic interstitial nephritis; the gums should be examined for the lead line and other indications of lead poisoning should be sought for; the question of chlorosis or other "blood disease" should be considered; and the ears should be examined for signs of otitis. But when all these conditions have been excluded and when the symptoms are apparently due to a cerebral affection, there is one group of cases in which localizing brain symptoms are absent and in which the chief indications of disease are headache, double optic neuritis, and often vomiting. In most of these cases syphilis can be also excluded. A diagnosis of brain tumor is given, and the growth is thought to be situated in some region in which the localizing symptoms are at first indefinite—cerebellum, temporo-sphenoidal lobe, or prefrontal region. Such a diagnosis often proves to be correct. Localizing symptoms may develop later and a necropsy may show the accuracy of the opinion expressed. But sometimes, to the surprise of the medical man, a fatal termination does not occur;

the symptoms sometimes disappear and the patient recovers, though very often impairment or loss of vision remains. The patient may continue in good health for years or for a lifetime afterwards. Most medical men who have paid much attention to cerebral diseases will have met with a case or cases of this kind. The chief object of our article is to call attention to this class of cases and to indicate the frequency of their occurrence. Nineteen out of one hundred cases of double optic neuritis with headache in the table just given could (after careful examination) be placed in this group (X.).

What is the cause of the symptoms in this group of cases? Possibly in some cases the symptoms are caused by a non-malignant tumor (or tuberculous mass) which ceases to extend and becomes quiescent and encapsuled. One of us has recorded a case in which symptoms of cerebral tumor (including Jacksonian epilepsy and hemiplegia) gradually subsided and temporary recovery ensued; but three years later symptoms of cerebellar tumor developed and death occurred. The necropsy revealed a recent large tuberculous mass in the cerebellum and an old capsuled tuberculous mass just beneath the motor cortex in the right cerebral hemisphere. The latter had evidently been the cause of the early cerebral symptoms from which the patient had recovered. An instructive case has been recorded by Dr. T. K. Monro of Glasgow. The patient, at the age of sixteen years, suffered from severe headache with failure of vision which passed on to complete blindness. For thirty-three years he was an inmate of a blind asylum, ophthalmoscopic examination showing double optic atrophy. He died at the age of sixty-three years, from cancer of the stomach, and the post-mortem examination also revealed a large myxomatous tumor in the left half of the cerebellum. In all probability the early cerebral symptoms had been associated with optic neuritis which had passed on to optic atrophy and the cause had been the myxoma in the cerebellum which had remained quiescent for forty-six years.

In some cases of double optic neuritis with headache and general cerebral symptoms, when recovery occurs the cause is probably distention of the ventricles of the brain with fluid—serous meningitis of the ventricles (Quincke). This condition was present at the necropsy, and no tumor growth could be found in two out of the one hundred cases tabulated. It is probable that a number of the cases in which a diagnosis of cerebral tumor has been made, but in which recovery has occurred, have been due to this condition—serous meningitis of the ventricles. Probably the two cases in Group IX. and possibly some of the cases in Group II., in which death did not occur for several years after the onset of symptoms, were of this nature. Other cases which recover may be due to a basal meningitis.

The table given above is instructive both as regards the diagnosis and prognosis in cases of double optic neuritis with headache. It shows the necessity for careful examination before giving either a diagnosis or prognosis, and the clinical group of cases No. X. ought always to be borne in mind whenever the diagnosis is obscure and localizing symptoms are absent.

There are two other points to which we would draw attention. In ten out of the one hundred cases the patient recovered completely from the headache and general cerebral symptoms and regained perfect health, but the optic neuritis was followed by atrophy and complete blindness. In the face of this terrible termination we cannot help thinking that simple trephining of the skull and the removal of bone, without any interference with the brain, as suggested and practiced by Mr. Victor Horsley for the relief of optic neuritis and pressure symptoms, is a method of treatment worthy of more frequent trial when vision is failing markedly. Dr. James Taylor has published cases which appear to show that this method of treatment may be of service in checking the optic neuritis and failure of vision. In the class of cases in Group X. if there should be a suspicion that the symptoms may be due to serous meningitis of the ventricles, lumbar puncture appears to be worthy of trial, since several cerebral cases are now on record in which this treatment appears to have been of great service, and in which the cause of the cerebral symptoms was probably that just mentioned.   DEADY.

Murrell, W.—A Case of Double Optic Neuritis from Serous Effusion (Quincke's Disease).—*Lancet*, April 28, 1900.

A schoolboy, aged seven years, was admitted into Westminster Hospital on January 28, 1900, the only history obtainable being that on the previous morning he had been brought home in a "fit," which lasted the greater part of the day. On admission he was perfectly sensible and talked freely, but on being put to bed he passed into a condition of semi-consciousness which lasted for many days. He took no notice when spoken to, and remained absolutely mute. The face and upper extremities exhibited choreiform movements of a slow and coarse type. These movements were apparently purposive in character, and at times he endeavored to clutch at objects within his reach. Sometimes the arms were widely extended, and then slowly flexed, as if performing the act of embracing. Sometimes the movements conveyed the idea that he was feebly endeavoring to strike those around him. There was no paralysis of the face or of the muscles of the limbs. The movements were, as a rule, bilateral, although sometimes the facial movements were unilateral, but not always on the same side. There was no rigidity of the muscles, retraction of the head, or opisthotonos. There was nothing to indicate that the patient suffered from headache, although at times the brows were contracted and the face wore a worried and anxious appearance. The bowels were open twice a day and urine and fæces were passed in bed. The motions were normal in character. The patient was unable to swallow, and had to be fed by the nasal tube. There was no nystagmus, the pupils were normal in size and contracted well to light. There was well-marked double optic neuritis. The temperature was 99.8° F., and the pulse was 108. There was no tenderness or swelling of the joints, and there was no rash on the skin. No tache cérébrale could be obtained. There was a little cough, but there was no expectoration. The breath and heart-sounds were normal. The urine was acid, had a specific gravity of 1018, and contained neither albumen nor sugar. The spleen was not enlarged. The patient showed no signs of anæmia, but the blood was not examined. There was no wasting of the muscles, and the knee-jerks were present, although somewhat sluggish. The tongue was clean, and presented no sign of having been bitten. The patient would not protrude it voluntarily, and it had to be examined with the spatula.

The condition of the patient remained practically unchanged for twelve days. The highest temperature recorded was on the second day, when it reached 100°; on the following day it was 99.8°, and from that time onward it was normal. The double optic neuritis continued, and the disks were observed to be getting paler. On February 13 (the seventeenth day of the illness) the patient was much more sensible, and recognized his mother, putting his arms round her neck. He was still unable to talk, although apparently he endeavored to do so, from time to time uttering a few unintelligible words. On being asked if he would like an orange he nodded his head, and he showed some signs of interest in a watch which was shown to him. The incontinence of urine and fæces continued, but food was taken with less diffi- culty. The movements gradually subsided. On the 17th the patient could say his own name, but beyond that could utter only inarticulate sounds, and failed to recognize letters or words, either written or printed. On the 20th he was able to speak plainly, although incoherently. He endeavored to get out of bed, and during the night was so noisy that he had to be removed from the ward. Urine and fæces were still passed under him. On the 22d he was quieter, and for the first time indicated that he wanted the bed-pan. The optic neuritis was less marked. On March 1 the patient was able to get up, and seemed to be quite well. On the 8th the following note was furnished by Mr. G. Hartridge, who had frequently examined his eyes during the course of his illness: "Pupils five millimeters each. React well to light, to convergence, accommodation, and consensually. Right vision $\frac{6}{8}$, left vision $\frac{6}{8}$. Right disk getting white; not much swelling of the disk; edges clearing. Retinal vessels, specially veins, very full and tortuous. Left disk pale (less so than right), dim; edges blurred." The only medical treatment adopted was the administration for a few days of 15 minims of liquor arsenicalis three times a day. DEADY.

Stephenson, Sydney.—Concussion of the Retina.—
Brit. Med. Jour., January, 1900.

Several years have elapsed since Dr. R. Berlin described a series of cases in which he had observed a peculiar retinal change after the eye had been struck with a blunt object, as, for example, a stick or a stone. Under those circumstances he noticed a cloudiness of portions of the retina, not involving the retinal blood vessels. The milky appearance reached its height in twenty-four to thirty-six hours, and disappeared in two or three days. Berlin pointed out that the rapidity with which the cloudiness developed, and the length of time that it persisted, stood in direct relationship with the severity of the original injury. This curious condition, which Berlin called *commotio retinæ*, was associated with some reduction of sight, episcleral congestion, and a difficulty in getting the pupil to dilate when atropine was dropped into the eye. Small retinal hemorrhages were sometimes present. Berlin explained the ophthalmoscopic picture by supposing that a rupture of the choroid was followed by bleeding and œdema of the retina. This theory has recently been opposed by Denig. That observer, as the result of experiments upon rabbits, believes that the blow upon the eyeball causes the vitreous to impinge upon the retina, to tear the internal limiting membrane, and to force the vitreous into the nerve-fiber layer. The alternate elevations and depressions thus brought about in the nerve-fiber layer of the retina are, according to Denig, the cause of the ophthalmoscopic appearances.

Since the publication of Berlin's original paper few cases of *commotio retinæ* have been recorded. Indeed, the retinal changes are of so fleeting a nature that an opportunity for observing them must occur comparatively seldom. This fact leads me to place upon record brief notes of a somewhat interesting case:

E. S., aged eleven years. First seen on July 25, 1899.

History.—At 6.45 P. M., on July 24, the patient was struck in the right eye with a cricket ball, made of cork and covered with rag cloth.

Present State.—Right eye: Small abrasion of the skin of the lower lid, with a surrounding area of redness. Some general conjunctival congestion, with a definite ecchymosis in the ocular conjunctiva, opposite the lower-outer quadrant of the cornea. Tension *minus* 1. The pupil distinctly sluggish and a trifle larger than the other one. Anterior chamber deep. A narrow line of blood clot lay at the bottom of the anterior chamber. V. $\frac{6}{9}$ (ii. letters). Pupil dilates imperfectly to a mydriatic. With the mirror alone some parts of the fundus oculi were seen to be unduly white. When examined more closely with the ophthalmoscope there was found a wide but defective zone of whitish fundus, situated peripherally upward, inward, and outward. No such appearances could be made out in the lower part of the fundus. The retinal vessels, which lay anterior to the affected areas, showed no changes. In most places it was possible to get beyond the whitish patches so as to see the edges of the latter. These margins were irregular, and showed white, tongue-like projections running into normal fundus. Some small islands of cloudiness lay, however, beyond the area of general haziness.

Around the yellow-spot region was a white radiating appearance, but no definite white mass was present in that place. Left eye: No fundus changes. V. $\frac{5}{6}$ (iv. letters). Tension normal.

Treatment.—Vaseline to abrasion of skin of lid; atropine drops (2 grs. to the ounce—to each eye twice a day); rest in bed.

Progress.—July 26. R. V. $\frac{5}{12}$; tension still rather low. The blood clot present in anterior chamber and also on anterior capsule of lens renders it difficult to see the fundus clearly; but no white patches can be made out in the fundus.

July 27. A little blood is still present in the lower part of the anterior chamber. The parts of the retina that were milky have resumed almost their natural appearance, and the changes above mentioned are now represented merely by a faint, whitish, ill-defined stippling of the areas in question. Around the yellow spot is a system of fine radiating lines, which extend for some distance into the surrounding fundus. This is doubtless due to œdema of the retina.

July 28. R. V. $\frac{5}{6}$ (i letter); tension still slightly *minus*. Ecchymosis present in ocular conjunctiva, but the blood has disappeared from the anterior chamber. Pupil not so wide as that of the left eye, although atropine is being used to both. Faint cloudiness lower third of the cornea, made up of almost transparent dots, as may be seen with a $+$ 20 lens in certain positions of the eye. Fundus changes have disappeared; faint radiating lines, however, may still be seen around the yellow-spot region.

July 29. R. V. $\frac{5}{6}$ (ii letter) T—I. Pupil now as large as that of the other eye. Yellow-spot region still surrounded by a wide band of fine, closely set, radiating gray lines. It may be noted that the corresponding region of the left (unaffected) eye is encircled by an ordinary oval reflex.

August 1. R. V. $\frac{5}{6}$; (Tn.). A small ecchymosis still present in the ocular conjunctiva on the outer side of the cornea. No blood in anterior chamber; no corneal cloudiness. Radiating appearance still present around yellow spot of fundus.

August 9. R. V. $\frac{5}{6}$, L. V. $\frac{5}{9}$; (Tn.).

August 12. Vision unaltered. Radiating lines still present around yellow-spot region of affected eye.

September 5. The right pupil rather larger than its fellow, but no break in the continuity of the edge of the iris can be discovered to account for this. The action, both to light and to accommodation, of the pupils is equal. The radiating lines formerly present around the yellow spot of the right eye have been replaced by an ordinary oval reflex, like that present in the other fundus. Tn.; R. V. $\frac{5}{6}$ (i letter), L. V. $\frac{5}{6}$ (i letter); No 1 Jaeger read easily.

September 7. Under atropine. R. V. $= \frac{5}{18} + 1.5$ D. Sph. $= \frac{5}{6}$. L. V. $= \frac{5}{12} + 1.0$ D. Sph. $= \frac{5}{6}$. DEADY.

BOOK REVIEW.

DISEASES OF THE NOSE, THROAT, AND EAR. Part I. Diseases of the Nose and Throat. By S. H. VEHSLAGE, M. D., Assistant Surgeon to the New York Ophthalmic Hospital (Throat Department). Part II. Diseases of the Ear. By G. DE WAYNE HALLETT, M. D., Assistant Surgeon to the New York Ophthalmic Hospital. New York: Boericke & Runyon Co., 1900. Price, cloth, $3.00.

We are glad to receive this volume, for which we have been looking for quite a while; because it fills a vacancy in our homeopathic literature which has long needed filling.

It will be found a clearly and concisely written volume, very instructive and advantageous to the student and busy practitioner; it is not intended to be exhaustive enough for the specialist in these branches.

Among the many commendable points, we would call attention to thorough consideration of the subject of Diphtheria, and we are glad to say that the treatment of this disease is sufficiently broad to include antitoxin,—let it be rational, allopathic, or whatever we may denominate it. While, on the other hand, we regret not to see the appreciable doses of iodide of potash more highly recommended as antidotal to the syphilitic poison, when manifest in these localities.

The manner in which the general, topical, or mechanical and hygienic portion of the treatment is handled is to be strongly approved. The homeopathic indications are well written. Like almost all books by homeopathic authors, it shows the peculiar bent of the homeopathic physician's mind is upon the therapeutics or cure of the patient rather than upon the fine development of the pathology, aetiology, etc., of the disease.

The publishers have done well in the binding, selection of type, and leading,—making it easy to read, but we are sorry to notice a number of small typographical errors have crept in, to mar it for a somewhat critical eye.

BOOKS RECEIVED.

The following books have been received and will be reviewed in the next issue of the journal.

Sajous' "Annual and Analytical Cyclopædia of Practical Medicine." Vol. V., "Methyl-Blue to Rabies." The F. A. Davis Co.

"Diseases of the Eye," Nettleship ; Sixth American from the Sixth English edition. Lea Bros. & Co.

"Injuries to the Eye in their Medico-Legal Aspect." By S. Baudry, M. D. The F. A. Davis Co.

VOL. XII.   OCTOBER, 1900.   PART 4.

THE JOURNAL OF OPHTHALMOLOGY, OTOLOGY AND LARYNGOLOGY.

EDITOR,
CHARLES DEADY, M. D.

ASSOCIATE EDITOR,
A. W. PALMER, M. D.

EDITORIAL.

EARLY in the year 1888 the late Dr. Geo. S. Norton laid before me his project of establishing the first homeopathic journal devoted to the interests of practitioners following the special lines of Eye, Ear, and Throat work, and asked me to become one of the associate editors. I was enthusiastically in favor of the plan, and much of that year was spent in making the necessary preparations for the initial issue, which appeared in January, 1889.

We had able and abundant support from our professional friends and the JOURNAL was a success from the start, its columns being filled by articles from the pens of the best men in the departments covered. Two years later occurred the untimely death of the editor in chief, and I was confronted with the necessity of attempting to fill the position he had honored by his talent, knowledge, and experience—a responsibility which had not entered into my calculations, but which I accepted and the requirements of which I have endeavored to fulfill to the best of my ability.

For nearly ten years I have given all the time that could be spared from a life crowded with official and professional work to the support of the inheritance from my lamented friend, and I have been content so to do while my mind was at ease and only labor was involved. For the past two or three years, however, serious and protracted illnesses in my family have so distracted my mind that literary work has at times been almost impossible, and the constant supervision necessary has been burdensome in the extreme.

For this reason I have decided to sever my connection with the editorial department of the JOURNAL with the present issue and to take my place in the ranks of its contributors and supporters, to whom I have been indebted for so many kindnesses in the past, which I here desire to acknowledge, and for which I wish to express my sincerest gratitude.

With the issue of January, 1901, the chief editorship will be assumed by my personal friend, Dr. John L. Moffat of Brooklyn, N. Y., who will need no recommendation to those who know him. Intellectually one of the best men who ever received the degree of the New York Ophthalmic Hospital, which was conferred on him in 1881, his broad culture, indefatigable industry, and the experience derived from the preparation of the Transactions of the Homeopathic Medical Society of the State of New York, during the thirteen years which he so ably served as its secretary, peculiarly fit him for the position which he has accepted at my urgent request.

Under his management the JOURNAL will become a bi-monthly, new departments will be added, the editorial staff will be increased, and in some other respects the administration of the publication will be upon new lines.

I most earnestly bespeak for him the cordial support of the profession, and feel the most absolute confidence that he will deserve and requite it in the fullest measure.

CHARLES DEADY.

EXPERIMENTS ON ANÆSTHESIA OF THE SEMI-CIRCULAR CANALS OF THE EAR.[1]

BY PROFESSOR G. GAGLIO OF MESSINA[2].

MOTOR disturbances consequent upon lesions of the semicircular canals of the ear form the basis of the opinions and hypotheses which have been put forward as to the function of these organs. One cannot refrain from admiring the ingenious arguments and occasionally frivolous views which illustrate this chapter of physiology, although the authors, far from being agreed, have arrived at so many and diverse conclusions.

And the disagreement starts on their first question, which is fundamental: Are the disorders following the destruction of the semicircular canals due to the abeyance or to the paralysis of an organ, or are they better attributed to reflex phenomena, occasioned by stimulation (experimental irritation) of the organ?

The former opinion has been supported by Flourens, who first demonstrated the characteristic motor disorders provoked by section of the semicircular canals, and concluded that they were due to loss of a controlling function of movements.

"The action of the semicircular canals and the opposite fibers of the brain," says Flourens,[3] "is much more an action which controls, a force which rules, rather than one which excites and determines.

---

[1] *Journal of Laryngology, Rhinology, and Otology*, London.

[2] Translated by Macleod Yearsley, F. R. C. S., Surgeon to the Royal Ear Hospital.

[3] "Recherches exp. sur les propriétés et les fonctions du système nerveux" (Paris, 1842, p. 497).

" As long as the semicircular canals or the opposite fibers of the brain are intact, the movements are moderated or controlled ; on the contrary, as soon as the semicircular canals or the opposite fibers of the brain are wounded, the movements break out violently.

" There is, then, in the semicircular canals and in the opposite fibers of the brain a force which controls and moderates movements."

The hypothesis of Goltz, who regards the semicircular canals as furnishing all sensations of position and equilibrium of the head ; that of Mach and Breuer, according to which they give us the sensation of movements of the head ; the hypothesis of Cyon, who sees in the semicircular canals the peripheral organ of space, by means of which we acquire knowledge of the direction of our head and our movements ; the hypothesis of Ewald, who sees in them a source of stimulations maintaining muscular tone, ought to be considered as resting upon the fundamental idea that the motor disorders which are observed following their lesion are due to a function being placed in abeyance.

Others have denied that the semicircular canals have any direct action on movement, and have supposed that the motor disorders observed following their injury are due to reflex acts, as shown by experimental irritation and operative traumatism. Autenrieth, Thomaszewicz, McBride, Preyer, Schäfer, Lussana, Vulpian, etc., share this view, and consider the disorders consequent upon the lesion as the effect of abnormal excitation of sensory vertigo.

Löwenberg (1862)[1] arrived at the following conclusions :

1. The disorders of locomotion produced by a lesion of the semicircular canals are due to stimulation, and not to a paralysis.

2. The stimulation of these canals produces convulsive movements by reflex action, without any participation of the will.

3. The transmission of this reflex stimulant occurs in the optic lobes.

[1] " Ueber die nach Durchschneidung der Bogengänge," etc. (*Archiv f. Augen- u. Ohrenheilkunde,* vol. iii.)

Laborde has supported the opinion of Löwenberg, that the absence of co-ordination following the lesion of the semicircular canals results from stimulation of a reflex kind.

Fano and Masini[1] have regarded the disorderly movements determined by the destruction of the semicircular canals as dependent on abnormal sensations, and, having seen them persist even after the ablation of the optic lobes, they have admitted, like Wlassak, that the central seat of the disorders consecutive to these lesions should be sought in the bulbo-spinal portions.

Clinically, as one knows, Charcot considered the phenomena of loss of equilibrium and motor impulse, consecutive to these lesions, as being provoked by cerebellar reflexes.

Finally, others—as Stefani—have admitted a double mode of action—that is to say, that the phenomena following lesions of the semicircular canals should be attributed to an absence of knowledge of the position of the head, and to movements which give rise, by reflex paths, to irritation of the canals.

These different methods of considering the effects of section of the semicircular canals—that is to say, as proving the absence of a function, or as being of an irritative nature —depend partly on theoretical conceptions of their function, partly on the fact that the experimental stimulation of these organs is likewise followed by characteristic movements of the head and eyes.

Flourens, in his memoir on the semicircular canals, which is a model of research in experimental physiology, pointed out that pigeons give signs of keen pain when the semicircular canals are cut, and that the pain and oscillatory movements of the head are similarly elicited by pricking inside of the canals with the point of a needle. But with the pricking of the interior of the canal the movements of the head are feeble, and speedily disappear ; they reappear, however, on renewing the pricking.

Breuer and Stefani found that pulling of the membranous

[1] "Intorno agli effetti della lesioni postate sull' organo dell' udito " (*Lo Sperimentale*, 1893, vol. xlvii. fasc. v.)

canal causes violent twisting of the head. Increase of pressure in the canals acts as a stimulus and provokes transient motor reactions in the animal, as Ewald clearly proved; but, on the other hand, as Cyon first demonstrated, the lymph can be withdrawn from the canals without the animal showing any motor disorder.

Endeavors to excite the semicircular canals by means of chemical substances have given little or no results; nevertheless, Landois reports that, by directly painting them with a solution of common salt, he caused pendulum-like movements of the head, which persisted a little, and now and then ceased completely.

All experimenters have observed that electrical stimulations of the canals induce violent twisting movements of the head, but they have interpreted these results differently.

Cyon, in a recent work,[1] declares that he could never attach any weight to results obtained by investigators by electrical stimulation of the canals, since, on the one hand, it is impossible to stimulate the isolated canals with electric currents, and, on the other hand, it is difficult to exactly observe disorders of movement in animals fixed in restraining apparatus; and, finally, if one wishes to practice electric stimulation on animals unrestrained, it is extremely difficult to stimulate the precise spot. To justify this warning, it is sufficient to remember the very opposite conclusions at which authors have arrived with *stimulations of the labyrinth.*

As is obvious, the same argument has been made use of concerning the semicircular canals as that which has been brought forward regarding experimental lesions of the nervous system in general, with the design of establishing a distinction between the phenomena of absence of function and the irritative acts which accompany them. The discussion which concerns the semicircular canals has been long, and rich in ingenious arguments, although it has not reached agreement amongst experimenters. On the con-

[1] "Bogengänge und Raumsinn" (*Archiv f. Anat. u. Physiol.*, 1897, B. i.-ii. pp. 52, 53).

trary, it has separated them into two opposing camps—those who consider the effects of lesions of the canals as acts due to absence of function, and those who look upon them as acts of traumatic or functional irritation.

In all these experimental researches to distinguish the consequences of stimulation from those of insufficiency of function of the injured canals there exists a weak spot; that is, they fail to estimate the action of cocaine applied directly to the canals. With the local application of cocaine we must pay attention to (1) the temporary disappearance of sensibility to pain in the canals, and, in consequence, the abolition of reflexes set up by pain ; (2) the temporary suppression of the specific activity of the nerve endings of the canals. By means of cocaine we can hope to separate the irritative acts, which are temporarily suppressed, from acts due to loss of function, shown up by anæsthesia of the nerve terminals of the injured semicircular canals.

The result of many experiments is that cocaine not only suppresses sensibility to pain, but also is capable of completely abolishing the special sense and functional activity of the nerve elements. When applied to the tongue and to the olfactory mucosa, it abolishes respectively the sense of taste and of smell. Oddi and Belmondo, by painting the posterior roots of the spinal nerves with cocaine, were able to produce effects identical with those of section of the root ; Ugolino Mosso, by applying a ten per cent. solution of cocaine to the phrenic nerve, made the diaphragm stop contracting ; François Frank, by injecting cocaine into the sheath of the vagus nerves of a dog, obtained effects identical with those following section of these nerves; Aducco, by painting the cerebral psycho-motor centers with cocaine solution, rendered them unexcitable.

The nerve into which cocaine is injected and the nerve center to which it is applied present the same temporary effects as if the nerve had been cut or the center removed.

We can, then, depend upon cocaine, applied directly to the semicircular canals, to abolish the pain which follows their injury, and to abolish the sensations which, following the opinion of a great number of physiologists, pass from the canals to the nerve centers, and which are the source of the sense of equilibrium (Goltz), or the movements of the head (Mach, Breuer), or the muscular tone (Ewald).

Experiment has shown that cocaine, applied to the cut semicircular canals, allows the motor disorders which were manifested after their injury to persist.

I have made numerous experiments on pigeons by cutting either the horizontal, the inferior vertical, or the superior vertical canal, sometimes on one side, sometimes the homonymous canals of the two sides, and by applying afterward to the injured canal two or three per cent.— sometimes nearly five per cent.—solutions of hydro-chloride of cocaine, either by forceps or by small pledgets of wool impregnated with the solution and kept in place. After the section of the canals and the succeeding application of cocaine, I have never observed any essential difference in the motor disorders following section only; sometimes, alone, one can easily demonstrate an increased intensity of disorders of movement.

If the horizontal canal on one side be cut, in spite of the immediate application of the cocaine solution, fleeting oscillations of the head are manifested in the horizontal plane, from right to left and left to right, with paresis of the limb on the side of the injured canal and circus movements in walking.

Section of the horizontal canal on both sides determines the maximum of intensity of the head oscillations; these are maintained persistently, and cocaine does not exercise any calming influence.

If the inferior or posterior vertical canal be cut on both sides and, immediately after, the cocaine solution be applied, violent oscillations of the head appear, backward and forward, forward and backward, following the vertical plane, with a tendency for the animal to hold the head bent on the back and to turn over backwards.

If the superior or anterior vertical canal be cut on both

sides and the cocaine applied immediately, intense oscillations of the head are likewise seen to appear, backward and forward, forward and backward, in the vertical plane, with a tendency for the animal to turn a forward somersault.

Finally, if several canals be cut, both right and left, the complex and disorderly movements which are manifested do not disappear at all, in spite of the local application of cocaine.

Not only in no case, after the application of cocaine, has a sedative action on the disorders of movements following the different lesions of the semicircular canals been observed, but sometimes one can easily demonstrate an augmentation in the characteristic movements described.

This last observation suggested a series of experiments to find out the action of cocaine instilled directly into the uninjured semicircular canals; that is to say, to see what are the consequences of anæsthesia of the canals.

The experiment has shown that the effects of anæsthesia of the semicircular canals obtained by the application of cocaine are equivalent to those which the section or destruction causes.

To carry out these researches, I laid bare the bony semicircular canals of a pigeon; then, having made sure of the homonymous canals on both sides, I scratched, with the point of a very fine scalpel, a spot of the bony covering of the canals, until I saw the lymph therein. Through this tiny orifice I introduced a very fine hypodermic syringe needle fitted to a rubber tube, and, by sucking with the mouth, I removed several drops of lymph, or I soaked the lymph up by means of a little roll of filter-paper.

All these preliminary operations, if done with care, only cause slight and fleeting oscillatory movements of the head, which becomes perfectly still in a few minutes.

Having thus removed a portion of the lymph, I introduced, using the same syringe, a few drops of cocaine solution through the original opening made into the canal. Almost immediately oscillatory movements of the head were manifested, which acquired a maximum intensity when cocaine was injected into the homonymous canal of the other side. These movements were as impetuous and as disorderly as if the canals had been cut or destroyed.

They were evidently determined by the anæsthetic action of the cocaine, and not by an excess of pressure from the injected fluid.

For comparison, following the same method as that employed in using cocaine, I injected a physiological solution of chloride of sodium. When this was done with care, I found that no motor reaction was excited in the animal, or mere fugitive oscillatory movements of the head induced.

It is, then, to the specific action of the cocaine, to the anæsthesia it produces in the terminal nerve organ of the semicircular canals with which it comes in contact, that the tumultuous movements of the animal should be attributed, analogous to those excited by section of the canals.

These disorders of movement last from half an hour to an hour, according to the duration of the anæsthetic action of the cocaine.

Occasionally, following the injection of a two per cent. solution of hydrochloride of cocaine into two homonymous canals—for example, the horizontal canals, previously robbed of their lymph—I have observed disorders of movements just as if these canals had been carefully divided ; that is to say, the animal showed strong oscillations of the head, from right to left and left to right, in the horizontal plane, and circus movements. These disorders passed off in from half an hour to an hour, after which the animal entirely resettled itself.

The disorder which disappeared last is that which I have constantly seen to be one of the first to show itself after the slighter lesions of the canals—that is, the inability of the animals to fly. Sometimes an animal which has sustained a slight injury to one canal, especially if limited to one side, cannot be distinguished by its movements from a normal animal, but if thrown into the air it will tumble clumsily to the ground, beating its body on the earth.

Very often disorders of movement observed following the injection of cocaine into homonymous canals were of a very complex nature, and equivalent to those induced by injury of several canals; that is to say, the animal manifested oscillations of the head, sometimes lateral, sometimes up and down, down and up; sometimes it turned the head in a vertiginous manner, sometimes it tended to hold it curved on the back, sometimes it bent and rolled it, resting the occiput on the ground, the beak upward.

This last position, characteristic of a lesion of the semicircular canals, and particularly of the anterior canals, which all experimenters have described, probably represents a movement of compensation by which the animal, finding a *point d'appui* on the ground, tries not to fall forward and to restrain the violence of the movements its head makes.

Amidst all the various inco-ordinate movements, I have nearly always noted, following the instillation of cocaine, attempts at vomiting, or effectual and repeated vomiting, which have also been observed, but less frequently, following section of the canals.

Evidently the cocaine injected into a canal ought to spread itself easily to the other canals, and consequently give multiple results, as if several canals had been destroyed at the same time. Between the horizontal and posterior canals there exists at the point where they cross an aperture of communication; and truly, following the injection of cocaine into one of these two canals, one ordinarily observes the combined phenomena of the lesions of both canals; the animal rolls its head, folded on the back; it tends to turn over backward or to make complete somersaults backward, one after another. When the fluid is placed in the canal with a certain pressure, it should be able to spread itself across the vestibule to the ampulla of the anterior canal.

Solutions of cocaine hydrochloride, two to three per cent., instilled into the canals previously partly deprived of their lymph, give a more limited action than solutions of five per cent., which, besides easily giving rise to complex motor disorders, sometimes cause death by poisoning.

The experiments which, in anæsthetizing the nerve-terminal apparatus of the semicircular canals by means of cocaine, induced motor disorders identical with those which are observed to follow section or destruction of the canals, clearly show that the disorders of movement are phenomena due to absence of function, and not the consequence of sensory and traumatic stimulations.

The paralyzing action of cocaine directly applied to nerve tissue is so precise and so general that one cannot think it, in this case, due to any irritant action of cocaine otherwise than to one which it would be absurd to exclude.

One finds the experiments that I have made in applying irritating substances directly to the cut canals in accordance with the anæsthetic action of cocaine. If the characteristic oscillations of the head were a consequence of irritation of the different canals operated upon, we ought to see the disorders increased when we apply with fine forceps, after section, solutions of irritant substances directly to the injured nerve elements.

I have tried various substances in this manner, solutions of sodium chloride, dilute acetic acid, tincture of iodine, solutions of metallic salts—corrosive sublimate, perchloride of iron, alum—essence of mustard, croton oil, etc., and I have never clearly seen the contact of these bodies followed by acute reactions of movement.

Landois, by painting the semicircular canals with a solution of sodium chloride, obtained pendulum oscillations of the head, and these continued a short time. But already other experimenters,[1] finding out the uncertainty and insufficiency of the results obtained from the direct application of irritants to the canals, have been obliged to abandon this method of research.

A grave inconvenience in the direct application of irritants consists in the fact that in making these substances act energetically, they disorganize the very delicate nerve

[1] Ewald, " Physiologische Untersuchungen über das Endorgan des Nervus octavus," Weisbaden, 1892, p. 253.

elements, so that their final effect is equivalent to that of a destruction of the canals.

It is to this mode of action that I attribute the oscillatory movements of the eyeballs and the head, described by Högyes[1] as following injections of hydrochloric acid, of strong nitric acid, and of perchloride of iron, which were made to reach the labyrinth by way of the tympanic cavity.

All my experiments agree in showing, in the plainest way, that the characteristic motor disorders following section of the canals are due to the suppression of a function, and not to a reflex action caused by sensory and traumatic stimuli. This is indeed a fact which was perfectly patent to the first experimenters, when they recognized that the forms of movement presented by animals following lesion of a given canal were precise and constant, and that the motor disorders, which were established immediately after the section, had a long duration, persisting sometimes the whole life of the animal. All this accorded badly with the theory of a reflex action, started by irritation, which should present together most complex and inconstant phenomena, destined to lessen and disappear in course of time.

In the present state of our knowledge it is difficult to establish what is the function of the semicircular canals. In basing it on known experiments, one has all the arguments put forward, all the hypotheses that can be made or expressed on the question ; I ought, therefore, to end my work here, and not venture into discussions but little profitable, convinced as I am that further experiments alone will put in evidence the true function of the semicircular canals. Nevertheless, having operated upon the canals of a large number of animals—not only of pigeons and birds, but also of dogs and rabbits—after having made a great number of experiments which I have not even mentioned in this paper, and having thoroughly read with a deep interest the works on the question, I have

[1] " Ueber die wahren Ursachen der Schwindelerscheinungen bei der Drucksteigerung in der Paukenhöhle" (*Pflüger's Archiv*, 26).

grown to feel that I ought to explain my investigation, and I shall do so briefly and without pretending to refute other opinions.

I do not believe that the head possesses in the semi-circular canals a special organ for the sense of equilibrium, which, in truth, appears unnecessary, for the general conditions of sensibility which determine the sense of equilibrium in other parts of the body ought to suffice. Goltz based his hypothesis on the displacements and changes of pressure of the endolymph in the canals, which would serve to more or less excite the ampullary nerve endings. But it has been shown, and I have seen it also in several experiments, that in certain experimental conditions all the lymph may be poured out without causing any disorder of equilibrium (Cyon).

And "the peripheral organ of the sense of space," which, following Cyon, is represented by the semicircular canals, seems to me neither useful nor well demonstrated. We explore space with all our senses, and it is the sum of the impressions which they bring to our nerve centers which gives us the consciousness of relation to space, of the position of equilibrium, and of the movement of our bodies.

Never in my experiments have I been able to detect in animals under investigation a want of concordance in actual space and space perceived by them. I have seen, on the contrary, pigeons, whose canals had been operated upon by different methods, find and peck at grain, and strike just the spot where they find the grain on the ground, but without the power to hold it in the beak and swallow it; I have seen such pigeons keep their equilibrium well on the edge of a table or on a staff, and keep it properly, without slipping or preparing to fly, just as if they possessed consciousness of their position in space, of their weakness, and the defect in them of necessary co-ordinated movements.

Among these motor disorders, this inability to fly is the first to show itself and the last to disappear in pigeons which have been subjected to injury of a canal, even limited to one side only. When one takes a strong pigeon in one's hand to operate, and it struggles vigorously, one is surprised to see that when a semicircular canal is cut it only puts forth a feeble resistance, and that if it is thrown into the air it cannot sustain itself, and falls awkwardly to the earth. If a canal is wounded on a single side, the pigeon shows no other trouble than this incapacity for flying, with which is associated an abnormal gait, in the sense that in walking the pigeon strikes his feet hard upon the ground, as if making a great effort to move ; if the horizontal canal of one side be injured, these troubles may be accompanied by a tendency to circus movements, as if the muscles of one part of the body were stronger than those of the other part.

These observations show that lesions limited to the semicircular canals determine general motor disorders, and a weakness more or less general.

The laryngeal muscles also suffer. After limited injuries of the canals, I have noted that pigeons, immediately following the operation, coo in a hoarse tone, which continues for several days. After extensive operations they become completely mute.

Let us now consider the characteristic pendulum oscillatations which the head makes after injuries of the canals on both sides. The experiments in which the application of cocaine reproduces these disorders show that the oscillations are determined, not by a stimulation, but by a failure of function. It appears to me that they can be equally well explained by a failure of function of muscle groups.

As is well known, each semicircular canal exercises its influence over the two parts of the body, right and left; that is why the section of the canal of one side causes transient disorders, the failure of function being compensated for by the function of the opposite homonymous canal. On the contrary, the loss of homonymous canals on both sides results in permanent disorders.

These disorders consist essentially in oscillatory movements of the head, right to left and left to right (horizontal canal), down and up and up and down (vertical canal).

If the semicircular canals were so connected with ascertained muscular groups that injury of the horizontal canal brought about functional modifications in the lateral muscles of the neck, abductors and adductors, and that injury of the vertical canals brought about modifications in the extensor and flexor muscles of the head, we could explain these curious movements, which follow so constantly injury of the canals, and which have surprised all experimenters. And this functional modification ought to be of a nature to determine in antagonistic muscles rapid contractions and succeeding relaxations, consequently jerking movements and oscillations.

The physiological contraction of a muscle proceeds from a summation of elementary ones; they last a certain time, and may be compared to tetanus of the muscle; but in the muscular groups ascertained under the influence of the semicircular canals such a functional depression can be produced that the fusion of divers elementary contractions is wanting, so that the muscle does not rest contracted during a certain time, but accomplishes movements by bounds.

This is precisely what happens after lesions of the semicircular canals. I have proved it in a most conclusive manner in pigeons several weeks after operation, when they tried to peck grain from the ground; they rapidly dipped the head, struck the grain with the beak, but were evidently unable to seize it; they were obliged to leave it, to stoop again, and try afresh to carry out an impossible act. It was sufficient to gently bend the head forward, and keep it so with the hand, for them to catch the grain in the beak and swallow it.

All experimenters have succeeded in proving that the tumultuous movements of the head shown by pigeons under operation on the semicircular canals are apparently violent, but in reality a light pressure of the hand upon the head suffices to stop these movements, without the hand feeling any resistance.

The pigeon in this condition greatly resembles an animal deprived of its cerebellum. A great number of investigators, commencing with Flourens, have already remarked in several experiments a certain analogy between animals whose semicircular canals and those whose cerebella have respectively been the seat of operation. I will cite for example the dogs whose cerebella Professor Luciani has ablated, and which I have had occasion to study for a number of years at the Physiological Institute of Florence. These animals had an undecided gait, the head oscillated in a lateral direction and up and down, and these oscillations became so intense, when seeking to take ·food, that they were often unable to do so. It was sufficient then to hold the neck firmly with the hand to enable them to retain and eat food.

Luciani[1] has described, as a result of the removal of the cerebellum, functional modifications in the muscles, and particularly a want of contractile force (*asthenia*), a lack of tonicity of the muscles in a state of rest (*atony*), and a want of fusion in the elementary contractions of the muscle, which make up the physiological contraction—a lack which has, for consequence, tremors, the staggering and rhythmic oscillations (*astasia*).

We are in a position to admit that something analogous results in fixed muscular groups after section of the semicircular canals—but it would be very difficult to make a detailed examination of the functional modifications of muscles—and that certain phenomena are capable of different explanations; nevertheless, among the disorders which pigeons show after section of the canals want of energy is specially remarkable in contraction, and want of fusion in the elementary contractions which make up the physiological contraction.

Luciani admits that the cerebellum gives force and tonicity to the muscles, of which part is a lingering influence, which continues traveling along the efferent tracks to the nerve centers, and renders the functional control of the muscles possible.

[1] Luciani, *Il cervelleto*, Firenze, successori Le Monnier, 1891.

We are able to admit the same thing for the semicircular canals—that is to say, to think that an influence partly endures normally, which, passing to the nerve centers, expends itself on the muscles, and according to which canal is injured, particularly in fixed muscular groups.

It is the duty of Science to dispel the singular and curious elements of phenomena by reducing facts, which at first sight appear very different, to general rules ; but in bringing together, without effort of reasoning, what is observed to follow section or removal of the semicircular canals, and what takes place after removal of the cerebellum, the function of the semicircular canals appears less strange and less astonishing.

And there is no lack of other examples of this continued influence, easily excited, which is transmitted from a sense organ by way of the nerve centers to nerves and muscles. Cyon has already demonstrated that, following section of the posterior spinal nerve roots, the excitability of the anterior roots diminishes, and Belmondo and Oddi[1] have confirmed this fact by showing that, even in anæsthetizing the posterior spinal roots by means of cocaine; there is a diminution of excitability in the corresponding anterior spinal root.

From the intervertebral ganglion passes, then, in the posterior root, an exciting influence, slow and continued, which is reflected along the cells of the spinal marrow to the anterior roots.

In the auditory labyrinth the cochlea has of itself a reflex influence on the muscles, but to a much less degree than the semicircular canals. It has been proved that if pigeons deprived of both cochleæ keep a normal gait they lose the faculty for flying—that is to say, the necessary force for maintaining themselves in the air by moving the wings. We must admit that, equally for the cochlea, a slow action continues, which, by way of the nerve centers, is carried to motor nerves and muscles.

[1] Belmondo and Oddi, '' Intorno all' influenza delle radici spinale posteriori sull' eccitabilita delle anteriori '' (*Revista sperim. di Freniatria*, 1890 ; *Arch. it. de Biol.*, t. xv. p. 17).

It is interesting to observe, on this subject, that the motor disorders which follow removal of the semicircular canals are lessened if the cochlea be afterward also removed;[1] the animals no longer exhibit oscillations of the head or twistings of the neck; they have a fairly regular gait, but they have altogether lost the capacity for flying. This experiment has been differently interpreted. Following our method, the explanation of these facts is that motor disorders are very evident when different muscular groups are affected in their function by injury of one or other semicircular canal, but when the whole labyrinth is destroyed, all the muscles are equally deprived of their tone and their energy of contraction.

The discussion, which, up to now, we have for greater clearness limited principally to the oscillatory movements of the head, applies equally to the movements of oscillation of the eyeball—nystagmus—which are also an invariable act, determined by injury of the semicircular canals. Nystagmus consecutive to section of these canals has also been noted in pigeons: but it is especially in mammals that it has been studied most. In mammals oscillatory movements of the head following destruction of the canals are weak, whilst, on the contrary, those of the eyeballs are very pronounced.

In the pigeons whose semicircular canals I injected with cocaine, I have seen that head oscillations were equally accompanied by nystagmus.

After destruction of the membranous labyrinth in dogs, nystagmus is very strongly induced in the eye corresponding to the injured side, and I have found that cocaine, locally applied immediately after the destruction, increased the oscillations of the eyeball. In a dog, in which I destroyed the whole auditory labyrinth on both sides, the movements of nystagmus in both eyes were strong and continuous, and the head showed feeble oscillatory movements from right to left and from left to right; having afterward instilled into the two destroyed labyrinths a three per cent. solution of cocaine, I saw lateral movements

[1] Fano and Masini, *l. c.*, pp. 11, 22.

of the head appear very markedly, and the nystagmus in both eyes was strongly augmented.

These experiments confirm the fundamental idea of this investigation, namely, that the disorders of motion which animals exhibit after the destruction of the semicircular canals are phenomena of functional insufficiency.

Nystagmatic movements of the eyeballs are equally observed following excitation as following destruction of the semicircular canals and other parts of the membranous labyrinth. They have been minutely studied, principally in order to explain by visual vertigo the motor disorders following injury of the canals, since, under these circumstances, there is cessation of movements associated with the eyes, which compensate the movements of the head and body, and allow the visual image to always fall on identical points of both retinæ.

The object of this work is not to criticise the opinions put forward on the question, but to insist upon the conclusion that the nystagmatic movements of the eyeballs, which are observed to follow destruction of the labyrinth, are phenomena not of excitation, but of paralysis—that is to say, of loss of function of an organ which normally, by a reflex path, influences the function of the muscles of the eyes. In other words, we admit that the semicircular canals and other parts of the membranous labyrinth originate. normally a wave of excitation, slow and continuous, which, carried to the nerve centers and following them, extends to the nerves and muscles of the eyes.

These nystagmatic movements, in fact, are very enduring, and cannot be explained by the persistence of an irritant cause; further, the action of cocaine applied locally is especially instructive; it never allays the nystagmus which follows the destruction of the labyrinth; on the contrary, it manifestly augments, perhaps completes, the paralysis induced by the destruction of the organ.

A notable fact is that, amid all the muscles of the body, it is those which accomplish the most agile movements which especially suffer in their function after these lesions.

It is so in birds: the first faculty to be lost after the slightest injuries of the canals and other parts of the membranous labyrinth is that of flight, *i. e.*, the function of the very agile wing muscles. Pigeons, which have a very mobile head, show markedly, after injuries of the canals, the strongest oscillations of the head.

J. R. Ewald, in comparing different birds, after having cut all their horizontal canals on both sides in the same way, found that disorders of movement are most pronounced in swallows, very slight in geese, and he puts the functional lesion of the muscles in direct connection with the greatest precision of the work which they carry out.[1] Indeed, it seems to me, the functional lesion of a muscle has a direct connection with the greatest agility of the movement accomplished by the muscle; flight, in fact, is not a work of precision, but of force and agility, and when the labyrinth is injured, it is that which is the first to suffer.

In mammals the organs most mobile are the eyes, and it is precisely the eye muscles which suffer longest in their function when the auditory labyrinth is destroyed in these animals.

Occupied in logically demonstrating the conviction which I possess touching the cause of these motor disorders determined in animals by the destruction and anæsthesia of the semicircular canals and other parts of the labyrinth, I have mentioned none of the authors who have more or less recognized this labyrinthine influence on muscle function. The disorders of the function of the muscles in animals under experiment are so marked that many observers should have recognized them, and all the restraint of theories has failed to keep the observer from the truth.

Bornhardt[2] has expressed the opinion that the muscular sense is affected by injury of the semicircular canals.

---

[1] *Pflüger's Arch.*, vol. xli. p. 463.

[2] Bornhardt, "Zur Frage über die Function der Bogengänge des Ohrlabyrinths" (*Centralb. med. Wissensch.*, 1875); *Ibid.*, "Exp. Beiträge zur Physiologie der Bogengänge des Ohrlabyrinths" (*Pflüger's Arch.*, vol. xii. p. 471).

Högyes[1] has upheld that the labyrinth exercises by a reflex path an influence over the ocular muscles, and he has shown in detail that the left vestibular branch carries nervous reflexes for the muscles that move the left eye up and out, and which turn the vertical meridian inward, while for the right eye it acts on the muscles which move it down and in, and which turn the vertical meridian outward; the right vestibular branch in its turn carries nerve stimuli for the muscles which move the right eye up and out, and which turn the vertical meridian inward, while for the left eye it acts on those moving it down and in, and turning the vertical meridian outward.

Ewald considered the motor disturbances produced by destruction of the semicircular canals and other portions of the labyrinth as phenomena of functional insufficiency, and he admits that from the whole auditory labyrinth sensory stimuli pass out continually, which go through the nerve centers to the striped muscles, keeping them functionally normal; he has christened this function of the labyrinth by an expression already made use of by Högyes, that of *labyrinthine tonus.*

Ewald has put his doctrine in agreement with that of Goltz, by admitting that the labyrinthine tonus is influenced by movements of the head, and that it gives us the sense of the direction and force of these movements, practically representing a sense organ for equilibrium.

Wlassak has observed that after unilateral extirpation of the labyrinth in the frog, it set up a predominance of action of the flexor and adductor muscles of one part of the body, and of extensors and abductors of the other part.

Other authors, also, who attribute other functions to the semicircular canals, have allowed them a secondary influence over muscle innervation.

Cyon[2] connects the motor disorders following destruction of the canals to the following causes:

---

[1] Högyes, " Ueber die wahren Ursachen der Schwindelerscheinungen bei der Drucksleigerung in der Paukenhöhle " (*Pflüger's Arch.*, vol. xxvi.).

[2] *Archiv für Anat. und Physiol.*, 1897, p. 78.

1. To a visual vertigo, due to loss of co-ordination between actual and ideal space.

2. To false representations, which react upon the position of our body in space.

3. To disturbances in the distribution and graduation of muscular innervation.

He finds it very natural that the same organ to which, according to him, we owe the knowledge of space, and which helps us to a high degree in the proper orientation of our bodies, should rule this force of innervation, which ought to be equally distributed to various muscles to bring about normal movements.

In the explanation of these ideas, Cyon points out less of the modifications in the muscles than of the functional alterations in the nerve centers, and, theoretically considering with these centers those which preside over the choice of fibers along which the impulses should pass, and those which regulate the force of innervation to be distributed to nerve fibers and to muscles, he argues that these second centers are those which suffer more from extirpation of the semicircular canals.

Amid such an eclecticism of explanations the idea of a special organ for the sense of space grows dim and vanishes, and that which, for Cyon, is fundamental becomes extremely problematical.

But what many experimenters have been obliged to admit, in evolving different theories, is that these are modifications of muscular innervation pre-eminently. These modifications, which, without the least doubt, are of reflex origin, are explained in the simplest way by the loss of influence of sensory impulses, which normally the semicircular canals carry to the nerve centers that distribute the innervating force to the different muscle groups.

By turning to experiment one endeavors to discover which are these nerve centers.

The cerebral centers and the cerebellum can be ablated in pigeons without any of the effects of injury to the semicircular canals fundamentally disappearing, although in the first case they become lessened and in the second increased. Therefore the mesencephalon and, particularly in birds, the optic lobes have to be considered as the seat of reflexes. Therefore tentative experiments in ablation of the optic lobes have been made, with the conclusion that this mutilation as well allows the motor disturbances of the section of the canals to remain fundamentally, and that consequently it is in the bulb that the seat of reflexes must be sought (Wlassak, Fano).

But the gravity of this operation, the complication of irritations that show themselves, throw doubts on the results of similar experiments. One must, therefore, very reasonably conclude that it is on several nerve centers that the semicircular canals distribute their influence.

Certainly one fact of which the importance impresses is to see animals whose semicircular canals have been operated upon suffer the most severe mutilations of the nerve centers, and yet show, as long as they breathe, the characteristic motor disturbances.

I remember pigeons which showed the classical oscillations of the head after section of the canals, and to whose wounded canals I applied concentrated solutions of cocaine. Sometimes these pigeons showed serious symptoms of cocaine poisoning, which ended in a cessation of respiration. The heart still beat, and therefore I practiced artificial respiration. At the end of several minutes of this procedure I saw natural respiration reappear, and with the movements of spontaneous respiration also reappeared the head oscillations, although the animal lay in a state of grave collapse.

In this condition of serious depression of the nerve centers the oscillations, which were among the last phenomena to disappear when the life of the animal was extinguished, were among the first to show themselves when the first necessary functions of life were revived.

This demonstrates that the nerve centers functionally injured by the destruction of the semicircular canals are included among those which are the most fundamental to life.

THE PROGRESS IN LARYNGOLOGY AND RHINOLOGY DURING THE LAST HALF CENTURY.

BY FRED D. LEWIS, M. D., BUFFALO, N. Y.

IN reviewing the literature of this, one of the youngest specialties, for the past fifty years, I find that the progress has been from practically nothing to its present high standard. As a specialty it was non-existent at the time of the organization of this Society. To be sure, some work was being done in the nose and throat by the family physician or surgeon, but it was of a very crude nature. The armamentarium of the most progressive men of that time consisted of a nasal dilator, forceps, scissors, tongue depressor, and tonsillotome. The requirements of the progressive man of to-day are legion. In fact the advance made in the past fifty years in laryngeal and rhinological practice has been far greater than during the whole previous history of the practice of medicine. The reason of this rapid advance is easily to be found. With the introduction of the laryngoscope, a light was thrown on the normal and morbid actions of the pharynx and larynx, and permitted a study of living parts that previously could be examined only after death.

To whom, and at what time, can we give the credit of this truly great discovery? The old saying that, " There is nothing new under the sun," might seem to apply to this discovery when one searches the writings of the fifties and early sixties, and notes the attempt to deprive Professor Czermak of the credit due him. It might be well to quote here from the *Lancet*, vol. I, 1863, from an article written

by Professor Czermak on the " Practical Use of the Laryngoscope," in which he claims the credit of the discovery by
quoting from a work by Dr. Locher as follows:

" That we do not consider him as an inventor, in the
real and beautiful sense of the word, who first conceives and
carries out a new idea, and then lays it aside, without even
a presentiment of its importance, but him, on the contrary,
who first discovers the practical application of the idea
(even when it has originated elsewhere), and helps toward
its public recognition."

The laryngoscope, as described by Liston and Garcia,
was practically identical with the one now in use, but was
square instead of round, with the shank attached to one
of its corners. From the report of the New Sydenham
Society of London for 1861, we find this method of its use
described as follows:

" The method which I have employed is very simple:
it consists in placing a little mirror, fixed in a long handle
suitably bent, in the throat of the person experimented on,
against the soft palate and the uvula. The party ought
to turn himself toward the sun, so that the luminous rays
falling in the little mirror may be reflected in the larynx."

Signor Garcia perfected the laryngoscope in 1854 and
presented a paper before the Royal Society of London in
1855. The merit of Garcia's discovery was not appreciated
in England, but becoming known to Türck of Vienna, it
was shortly afterward communicated to Professor Czermak.
The inconvenience of depending on the sun for illumination, its uncertainty of being unclouded when wanted, and
the many conditions that would prevent its use when perhaps most needed, were recognized by Czermak, who substituted an artificial light, first by holding a lighted candle
with a reflector before the eyes, by means of a handle held
between his teeth. Later he employed the mirror of an
ophthalmoscope and then the mirror now commonly in
use, holding it in position, either by the aid of the hand
which holds the stem, by a support held in the mouth, by
the head band, or by an arrangement similar to a pair of
spectacles.

That Czermak was at that time given the credit of bringing the laryngoscope into general use may be further proven
by quoting from the *British and Foreign Medical and
Chirurgical Review* of 1864 :

" We should not be doing justice to the subject if we did
not associate very prominently with the whole subject of
the laryngoscope the name of Professor Czermak of
Prague: .

" The historical sketch which we formerly gave to the
invention of the laryngoscope, has now to receive the back-
ground of some important additions. In an interesting
communication which Mr. Windsor recently furnished to
this journal, it is shown that, as early as 1807, Bozzini
employed an arrangement of mirrors for illuminating internal cavities and spaces in the living animal body. In
the work which he published at that time, it does not
appear that he specially recommended this simple apparatus
for inspecting the larynx, but he advised its employment
for examining the posterior nares. In 1829 Dr. Benjamin
Babington exhibited some mirrors at the Hunterian
Society, closely resembling those now in common use,
with which he said it was possible to inspect the larynx.
In 1838 M. Brumès showed a mirror, about the size of a
two-franc piece, to the members of the Medical Society of
Lyons, and described it as being very useful for examining
the larynx and posterior nares. In 1840 Liston, in a third
addition to his ' Practical Surgery,' made that reference to a
mode of examining the larynx which led Professor Czermak, in his first pamphlet, to speak of the Liston-Garcia
laryngoscope. In 1844 Dr. Warden succeeded more than
once in inspecting a diseased larynx, and in 1846 Avery
invented his laryngological speculum. We have already
pointed out the merits and shown the defects of Avery's
instrument, and we have little to add with reference to
Garcia, Türck, and Czermak. Research or accident may
perhaps show that the idea of examining the larynx by
means of reflected light was of even earlier origin than we
have here indicated ; but to Professor Czermak will always

be due the great merit of having so simplified and improved the instrument that it can be applied with comparative facility to the relief of suffering humanity. From 1807 to 1857 the invention, if such it may be called, was of no use to anyone; but when, in the latter year, the clumsy dentists' mirror passed into the dexterous hands of Dr. Czermak, a transformation was soon effected, and with the laryngoscope a new key was obtained to the portals of life."

The introduction of the laryngoscope was followed, as a natural consequence, by better diagnosis, a more accurate knowledge of the physiological and pathological conditions, the determination of the mechanical action of the vocal cords in phonation, the presence or absence of diseased conditions or abnormal growths, the necessity for many new and delicate instruments, the more accurate application of caustics, liquids, powders, sprays, or vapors to affected parts, and of course a greater percentage of recoveries.

In fact I believe the discovery of the laryngoscope was one of the greatest blessings to humanity of the last century.

As we became more familiar with the parts to be treated, and recognized what good might be accomplished by operative measures, and knew that such operations would be difficult or impossible under general anæsthesia, and that they would be extremely painful to the patient without an anæsthesia of some kind, cocaine was given to us.

The introduction of cocaine to the profession as a local anæsthetic is due to Dr. Koller, who first called attention to its usefulness in eye surgery in 1884. Previous, however, to cocaine, as early as 1860, bromide of potassium was reported as a local anæsthesia for the larynx.

One of the great advances also in this department, it seems to me, is the recognition of the far-reaching reflexes that may result from improper respiration, or pressure within the nasal cavities. Also positive deformities may be the result of impaired breathing, as may be seen in the neglected adenoid cases with their rat mouths, high, arched palates, high shoulders, and pigeon breasts; with impaired hearing and expression of stupidity stamped on their countenances.

There have also been many discoveries in general medicine, that have been of great value to the laryngologist in the treatment of his patients, such as the recognition of bacterial causation of disease, the determining of the nature of bacilli or morbid growths by the aid of the microscope, the necessity of absolute cleanliness, and the employment of antiseptic measures in all operations, the preparation and use of new drugs, etc., etc., but this is hardly the bureau in which they should receive more than mention.

In regard to the instruments that have been devised from time to time, that work along these lines may be more thoroughly, accurately, and scientifically performed, to enumerate them would be wearisome and consume time that can be more profitably spent. One need only visit a well-equipped instrument house, exclude from their stock the five instruments mentioned earlier in my remarks, and the rest will show to what an extent, and of what great value, has been the advance in this direction.

188 Franklin Street.

CASE OF NASAL GRANULOMA, PROBABLY TUBERCULOUS.

REPORTED BY MR. JOHN CUMMING, F. R. C. S. E.

(Under care of Dr. Hunter Mackenzie in the Edinburgh Eye, Ear, and Throat Infirmary.)

MISS A. came complaining of complete obstruction of, and occasional severe bleeding from, the right nostril of about one year's duration. On examination the nostril was found completely blocked with what seemed to be a reddish-brown polypus, which, on probing, was found to be freely movable and very vascular. On attempting its removal in the usual way by the snare it was seen to be very friable, and with a marked tendency to hemorrhage. A pair of dressing forceps pointed with cotton wool was accordingly introduced, and the whole growth was easily detached and pushed into the posterior nares, from which it was removed by the mouth. This was followed by very severe hemorrhage, necessitating plugging of the nostril. The polypus was about two inches long, and had been attached along the ridge of the middle turbinate body. It was of a reddish-brown color, interspersed with white streaks. Microscopically it was found to be a " granuloma with giant cells, probably tuberculous." The area from which it sprang was treated with the electro-cautery, and six months subsequently there was no indication of any tendency to recurrence. It may be added that the patient had enlarged glands on both sides of the neck, some of which had been excised about a couple of years previously. There were no indications of pulmonary phthisis. The middle turbinate body remained raw and inflamed for a longer period than after the removal of an ordinary mucous polypus, but no ulceration or necrosis of bone occurred.

REMARKS BY DR. MACKENZIE.

This case presents certain important features :

1. *Its Hemorrhagic Character.*—It illustrates the diagnostic value to be attached to hemorrhage as a concomitant of polypus of the nose. A polypus which bleeds freely on removal—more especially if there is a history of occasional troublesome spontaneous hemorrhages, and even if to the naked eye it presents the appearances of an ordinary mucous growth—may be safely regarded as malignant, or, as this case tends to show, tuberculous. The only exception to this is in the case of what is known as bleeding polypus of the nasal septum (angioma), which is more generally found in women, and can be readily differentiated from other varieties of polypus by its extremely vascular appearance and by its microscopical characters. The hemorrhagic tendency of these malignant or tuberculous polypi gives them a reddish-brown color, as in the present case.

2. *Seat of the Polypus.*—It is most unusual for tuberculous polypi to spring from the middle turbinate area, that is, from the same locality as the benign. Chiari,[1] in fact, states that one of the diagnostic marks of a tuberculous polypus is its proclivity to be localized to the anterior portion of the septum, where it is particularly prone to recur and be followed by septal perforation and ulceration. In the case now recorded none of these peculiarities was present.

3. *Relation to Pulmonary Phthisis.*—It appears that a tuberculous polypus of the nose may occur as a primary growth, that is, without evidence of the existence of similar disease in other regions of viscera, especially of the lungs, as in the present instance. This has previously been noticed. Thus Wroblewski[2] reports the case of a recurrent tumor of the nasal septum about the size of a hazel nut, which was removed and, on microscopical examination, found to be tuberculous. It occurred five times, and during a period of six years over which these recurrences extended, examination of the lungs and sputum gave negative results. It was believed at first to be an ordinary polypus (although located on the septum), and on removal bled freely. Tuberculous ulceration of the septum ultimately ensued. In the present instance the enlarged glands in the neck tend to give a somewhat unfavorable shade to the prognosis. An endeavor will be made to have the patient inspected from time to time, and the ultimate result will form the subject of another report.

[1] *Archiv für Laryngologie und Rhinologie*, 1893, 1–2.
[2] *Internat. Centralblatt für Laryngologie*, vol. x. p. 17.

NOTES ON CHRONIC SUPPURATION OF THE MIDDLE EAR.

BY A. MIDGLEY CASH, M. D., TORQUAY.

OF all cases of ear disease commonly met with in general practice those of *chronic purulent inflammation of the middle ear* are apt to give most trouble. They are difficult to cure, offensive to deal with, and anxious on account of the complications to which they are liable, and as to the results to which they tend. They require long patience on the part of the patient and of the doctor, and thus they often come to be deemed incurable. Also they require regular attention, and cannot always—as, for instance, in the out-patient department of a hospital or dispensary— receive the care and time which are necessary if cure is to be attained or even improvement brought about. This arises largely from the fact that the local treatment is important as well as constitutional, and neither can by any means be dispensed with. Even with both methods carefully carried out chronic purulent inflammation of the middle ear is frequently sufficiently rebellious. Still, good results are to be attained, and it is well worth the trouble and time given, for the individual with this disease is in a chronic state of danger. This is well known and recognized by all life insurance companies.

Septic thrombosis, cerebral abscess, and pyæmia are all very possible terminations to septic aural catarrh, and may be brought about with startling and unexpected suddenness. The association of this class of cases with *tuberculosis* is a point to be carefully noted. The difficulty of cure is thus increased, as the system is thereby disposed to low-grade, lingering, inflammatory processes. Again, a purulent otitis, however it has been caused, may be the means of introducing the tubercle bacillus into the system, the general thus following the special disease ; in either case a vigorous effort should be made to combat the ear trouble. Good results have been obtained thus, even in constitutions already thoroughly tubercular. The special internal remedies most frequently required are : sulphur, hepar sulphur, calcarea, silicea, mercury, and nitric acid ; these generally are useful, and many others are also required, according to individual symptoms.

In commencing the treatment of a case of middle-ear purulent suppuration and otorrhœa I have usually found a suitable remedy in one of the above medicines, given two or three times a day in doses of two or three grains or drops, as the case may be. The local treatment consists in first thoroughly cleansing the ear, removing the semi-fluid pus which oozes from the meatus, and the caked crusts and *débris* which lie deeper in the ear, often beyond the perforated tympanum. I use a syringe with a long fine nozzle, having a caliber about the size of a fine crow quill. This in a good light can be introduced some distance down the external meatus of the ear, and can thus be brought to bear on special points much better than a coarse, thick nozzle which fills up the passages. A warm sanitas lotion, or one of carbolic acid 'or listerine, does well. A saline solution of one dram of salt to a pint of warm water, or an alkaline one, as bicarbonate of soda, or boric acid, two to five per cent. in strength, may be used. Having gently syringed out the *débris* and pus, the interior of the ear should be carefully dried by pledgets of absorbent cotton wool. In some cases it is well to use the air douche to assist in the removal of discharge. The cavity being thoroughly dry I generally insufflate two or three grains of finely powdered boracic acid by means of the powder blower, and lastly put lightly into the external meatus a dossil of wool ; this should not be packed firmly in so as to confine the discharge, and it should be frequently changed.

If, as frequently happens, polypi and granulations co-exist, these must be removed ; should the polypus have a of it, as Blake's. If, however, the polypi are small, sessile, or more of the nature of granulations, these may be removed by fine forceps with cup-shaped cutting blades. I have found it in some cases convenient to use a fine stick of lunar caustic, mounted on a No. 2 or No. 3 flexible catheter stem; this can be manipulated with considerable exactness at any curve or angle, and can be introduced down a vulcanite speculum and touch exactly the spot desired. A few applications of the caustic will wither up the polypoid tissue; this process has the advantage of being bloodless, and so more can be done at one time, whereas, when a growth is snared, the ear commonly fills up with blood, which interferes with further manipulations for that sitting. When it is possible to get a thoroughly good illumination of the polypus, also if the polypus is vascular and the patient steady, I have sometimes used the galvano-cautery to shrivel up the growth. A fine-pointed platinum cautery must be passed down a vulcanite speculum and pressed lightly against the surface of the polypus; the current is then turned on for a second and then shut off, and the cautery carefully withdrawn. The destructive power of the electro-cautery is intense and its application in the ear requires the greatest care. The polypus rapidly shrivels up under it and dies; local anæsthesia is required. I have generally used a tampon of fine absorbent cotton wool, saturated in a solution of five per cent. cocaine, and five per cent. beta eucaine, making a ten per cent. solution. This is equally effective in its anæsthetic properties to cocaine alone, though possibly requiring a slightly longer time to act, and it is less likely to have any unpleasant toxic effects. These aural polypi are often extremely sensitive, and even with carefully attempted anæsthesia it is not unusual for the patient to experience sharp pain at the moment of avulsion or cauterizing; a pain which may be felt at the spot or sometimes acutely in the throat, conveyed there probably by the tympanic branch of the glosso-pharyngeal nerve. When operative interference is not indicated, polypoid granulations may be shriveled up more slowly by instillation into the ear of rectified spirits of wine, or of the biniodide of mercury solution 1–3000 in

S. V. R. A serious result of suppurative middle-ear dis-
easè is illustrated by a dispensary case under my care at
present. Here, as a sequence, is a chronic reflected otor-
rhea, inflammation has extended along the canal of the
facial nerve, and permanent facial paralysis, along with
almost complete deafness, has been caused.

I.—Case of fifteen years' standing ; chronic purulent otitis
media, deafness, aural polypus, perforated tympanum, and otorrhœa. Miss le M., aged thirty-five ; she was under treatment for a
year ; the result of the treatment—restoration of the tympanum,
considerable improvement in hearing, cessation of aural discharge,
removal of polypus. She took internally aurum met., hep. sulph.,
thuja, calc. carb., and phosphorus, during this time. The local
treatment was first boracic acid and calendula as lotion, and also
as powder blown into the ear, and for a time instillations of the
biniodide of mercury solution. I removed the polypus by touching it carefully several times with the fine platinum point of the
electro-cautery, under which it shriveled and disappeared. The
discharge was extremely fetid and seemed to indicate the presence of dead bone, but the whole thing healed up and all fetid
discharge was gone within a year of commencing treatment ; this
had to be partly by correspondence, as she was a visitor and I
was only able to see her at occasional intervals. When I was
last able to examine the ear, which was two years after treatment had been begun, I found the tympanum restored and presenting its natural anatomical appearance, only showing somewhat dry and parchment-like. Her hearing varied, but on the
whole she reported it as keeping fairly good.

II.—S. L., twenty-two, a clerk, comes of a tuberculous family ;
his mother and two brothers died of phthisis, and a sister is at
the present time under treatment for chronic tubercular phthisis.
Has had chronic otorrhœa from a child and used to suffer from
earache, some degree of deafness, at times much increased.
Watch distance of right ear at present is $\frac{8}{60}$, the right tympanum
is largely ulcerated and its anatomical landmarks obliterated.
A large red polypus was growing from the roof and internal
meatus at tympanic border. A particularly foul-smelling, yellow
discharge, often bloody, exudes from the ear and stains his
pillow in the morning. Liable to severe attacks of headache.
The *local treatment* consisted in syringing out the ear at inter-

of absorbent cotton wool, and insufflating with boracic-acid powder. The polypus was touched with solid nitrate of silver, under which it gradually sloughed off in layers and was syringed out with the *débris*. The internal remedies chiefly used were nitric acid, calc. c., hep. s., thuja, kali mur., merc. sol., and silic. The discharge lessened in violence, and the deafness sensibly improved, which he was able to judge of well by the fact that he could now hear through the office telephone clearly the sounds which formerly he could barely distinguish. At the present time, treatment having extended just over two and a half years, his condition is as follows :

Hearing, right ear, w. d. $\frac{18}{60}$. For general purposes he hears well. The polypus is gone. The tympanum is apparently healed, and shows nearly normal, the hammer handle and short process clearly marked in position. There is a slight discharge for which he has to syringe with sanitas lotion twice a day ; the condition is much improved. There is a gain in watch hearing of ten inches and practically the deafness is cured. Still he has a strong tendency to the tubercular dyscrasia which threatens him through the ear, and he will for a time need to be kept under observation.

III.—Scarlet fever in infancy, destruction of tympanum, chronic middle-ear suppuration, aural polypus with fetid otorrhœa, enlarged tonsils, deafness. B. T., aged seventeen, a pale, stout, flabby girl liable to severe headaches, suffering from some degree of anæmia. After eight months' treatment the present condition is :

Cure of polypus, discharge nearly entirely ceased ; hearing distance of watch $\frac{3}{60}$ cm., hears spoken words very fairly, tonsils much reduced and not now abnormally large, tympanum cicatrizing and presenting a healthy, clean appearance. The polypus I removed with the wire snare and cutting forceps, and cauterized the stump with solid nitrate of silver.

The tonsils were reduced by the galvano-cautery; a fine platinum point being made to puncture their substance wherever most prominent, under which process they rapidly shrank and subsided to normal dimensions. Irrigations of phenyl lotion were used to cleanse the ear, and rectified spirits of wine dropped occasionally.

Insufflations of boracic acid were also used ; plaques of hypertrophic mucous membrane on the fauces needed occasional touching with the electro-cautery point, and by the help of gargles the throat was got into a healthy condition ; baryt. carb., merc. sol., hep. s., and calc. phosph. were the medicines used. Here we had a condition of suppurative middle-ear otitis conjoined with so-called throat deafness, preceded by scarlet fever in infancy.

The girl was of a strumous constitution, and the medicines given appeared to have a salutary effect in improving her general health as well as upon the otitis. To this last the throat treatment also probably contributed.

The tonsils fell back into place, exuberant throat granulations were destroyed and the girl's cold-catching propensity was thereby checked.

IV.—Little girl two years old, of strumous temperament, suffering from chronic middle-ear catarrh with otorrhœa and frequent attacks of high temperature. After going on several weeks in this way the friends sent hurriedly for me. The discharge had ceased some days before, a tender red swelling had formed over the mastoid process and was pointing as for abscess. The ear was everted and forced outward by the swelling, the child was white and looked very ill. I cut down through inflamed tissues into the mastoid process and let out a quantity of matter; the symptoms promptly subsided, the deformity disappeared, and the otorrhœa did not return.

In a day or two the child was as usual; a month later, on some threatening of similar trouble, caust. and sulph. 30 were given and all the symptoms passed away. Here we had a condition of things which is very likely to happen in purulent inflammation of the middle ear; the inflammation finds its way backward into the mastoid cells. Œdema and pus formation occur, and at this stage, if a free incision is made down to the bone and tension relieved, further mischief may be prevented ; if no relief is afforded general extension into the mastoid cells ensues, and septic thrombosis of the sinuses of the brain, with all its attendant dangers, may easily supervene. It seems more than one can fairly expect, that medicine internally could avert such a state of things when threatening. In the case just related I find I had it noted at the time that it was to be observed when deep-seated trouble was brewing, that aconite and bell., given alternately, would seem to check it, and would throw the force of the inflammation outward, where it could be more easily dealt with. Later on calc. carb., caustic, and sulph. were all found useful in this

PREVALENT ERRORS REGARDING THE DIAGNOSIS AND TREATMENT OF "EYE-STRAIN" FROM VARIOUS CAUSES.[1]

BY AMBROSE L. RANNEY, A. M., M. D., NEW YORK.

THAT the eyes often create more or less serious *physical ills* (as well as many symptoms referable only to the eyes) is acknowledged to-day by all oculists.

The marvelous numerical growth of reputable opticians in all large cities within the past decade is proof in itself that the general public, as well as the medical profession, is keenly alive to-day to this important factor in inducing and perpetuating ill-health.

There are many department stores, moreover, in large cities that have lately added an " optical department " to their equipment in order to supply a demand that can no longer be ignored.

Strange as it may seem to cultivated and intelligent medical men, the purchase of glasses by the wealthy as well as the poorer classes is commonly made to-day without advice from any oculist. More harm is thus done to the eyes and general health of the community than can be computed.

In some of the larger cities of America certain manufacturers of lenses for the trade have had for years in active operation so-called " optical schools " under their management. From these so-called " schools " uneducated men (engaged chiefly in the selling of jewelry in small towns) are turned out (with diplomas) as " refractionists," to sell

[1] *New York Medical Journal.*

and prescribe glasses to their customers, after only a few days or weeks of instruction from their so-called "professors," who are too often incompetent themselves.

The entire country is being flooded to-day with such "refractionists." They often announce their calling with a conspicuous public sign; and exhibit their framed diplomas to the credulous lay public, as a guarantee of their attainments.

Signs that read as follows: "Free eye-testing done here," "Eye-testing parlors," and other words of similar import, are to be seen in this city on every prominent business thoroughfare; in spite of laws that are strictly enforced in this State against irregular medical practitioners and bogus "diploma mills" of a medical character.

That untold harm is being done by these men cannot be doubted. The evil is sure to continue and grow until the medical profession and the general public at large are made to realize the truth and importance of the following statements.

1. The proper selection of glasses is most important from the standpoint of future health. Serious harm to the eyes (and general health as well) may follow the bad refractive work done by inexperienced people.

2. No glasses should ever be bought without a prescription being first obtained from an oculist; not a so-called "refractionist," but one who is a medical graduate in good standing.

3. No glasses (even when prescribed by a competent oculist) should ever be used until the correct grinding of the glass and its setting are verified by the oculist who prescribed them.

Serious mistakes are too often made in filling a prescription for glasses, even by opticians of repute. Glasses have by mistake been given to one patient that were ground for another, in my own experience; they have frequently been interchanged by accident, after being properly ground, and were thus put over the wrong eye; they sometimes get reversed in putting them into the frame, thus placing the wrong side of one or both glasses next to the eye ; and many other similar or worse blunders are being constantly made by careless or stupid workmen.

Such mistakes on the part of opticians frequently reflect great and unjust discredit later upon the oculist who prescribed the glasses ; may do serious harm to the patient who wears them ; and lead in many ways to disturbing annoyances that could easily have been avoided.

4. Glasses may be properly prescribed and ground and yet be so improperly set in the frames as to be worse than useless.

Almost every day some patient appears in my office with glasses that do not fit the face ; causing one or both lenses to set too high or too low, or more often too wide for the eyes or too narrow.

Oftentimes extreme decentering of lenses subjects the patient to constant torture ; because they act not only as a refractive correction, but also as prisms that disturb the proper action of the ocular muscles.

In such cases the oculist is very apt to be blamed for the suffering caused. He frequently loses not only the confidence, but also all further patronage, of valuable friends from such mistakes made by others ; simply because he failed to personally inspect the fit of the frames given by some incompetent or careless optician.

Women naturally prefer, as a rule, to wear nose-glasses in preference to spectacle frames. It should be remembered, however, that the slightest bending of the nose-clips of such frames may produce a malposition of one or both of the lenses ; and even placing the frame upon the nose in an improper manner may also seriously modify the effect of the glasses. In patients where a high degree of astigmatism exists, it is always best to educate the patient as to the vital importance of watching the eyeglasses constantly to see if they set properly before each eye. It is almost a part of life's routine for an intelligent woman (wearing nose-glasses constantly) to have the nose-clips frequently readjusted by skillful opticians. They get so easily out of adjustment as to constitute to men a source of great annoyance, as a rule. Spectacle frames are therefore worn by most active men during business hours in preference to nose-glasses.

Some years ago a male patient, to whom I had given strong cylindrical glasses in a spectacle frame for constant use, married a year or two afterward and went West to live. After wearing his spectacles constantly for three years, he was persuaded by his wife to change to nose-glasses and discard his spectacles. One morning after putting his nose-glasses on he suddenly found himself unable to read print with or without his glasses. In great alarm he traveled over one thousand miles to see me. I found one nose-clip very badly bent. On readjusting it, the proper axes of his cylinders were restored and his vision immediately became normal. He returned home wearing spectacles, after having learned a simple, but expensive lesson.

5. No tests made with a view of finally deciding in regard to suspected errors of adjustment of the eye-muscles are of any value until the refraction of each eye is first separately and accurately measured, and, if deemed important, corrected by proper lenses.

I lay the greatest possible stress here regarding this axiom. There seems to be, among the profession at large, and even among certain oculists to-day, a most unaccountable misapprehension regarding the views upon this point of those who are prominent in the investigation and correction of " heterophoria." [1]

For years I have printed this axiom time and time again in italics. Never for the past fifteen years has the history of an eye-case been entered upon my records without as thorough and complete an examination for refractive errors as it is possible to make. Not one case in fifty that have been intrusted to my care has escaped the use of a mydriatic, whenever its employment could possibly have modified the refraction.

Furthermore, the effect of wearing glasses for refractive

[1] A term that covers all forms of maladjustment of the eye-muscles, where actual cross-eye does not exist.

errors upon any apparent maladjustment of the eye-muscles is frequently noted by me for weeks or months (in cases that seem to justify it) before even prismatic glasses are ordered.

6. There is no rational basis for an extreme statement that has been too frequently published by certain oculists (evidently with a limited experience in the investigation of heterophoria), viz., "that errors of adjustment of the eye-muscles are invariably due to errors of refraction."

It is full time that this prevalent error be publicly stamped as absurd, unproved, and a fallacious basis for creditable work!

In my late work, entitled "Eye-strain in Health and Disease,"[1] I have personally published a sufficient number of cases to convince any judicial mind of the accuracy of the foregoing comment. Furthermore, there is not a prominent investigator in this special line of eye-work (who uses modern instruments and modern methods) that cannot indorse it from his own experience.

I have personally reported at least one hundred cases *whose eyes had no refractive error even under atropine,* and yet in whom serious nervous afflictions had existed for many years from eye-strain (embracing epilepsy, headache, neuralgia, sleeplessness, nervous prostration, etc.). They were absolutely restored to health by graduated tenotomies performed upon some eye-muscle, after other methods of treatment and judicious medication had failed to afford relief. Because marvelous results in sufferers from various nervous and eye diseases are often obtained by the correction of refractive errors alone through the instrumentality of spherical or cylindrical glasses, no basis exists for argument that the eye-muscles may not also be solely at fault in other cases and require prismatic lenses or surgical relief.

I believe that the time has passed when any oculist of education and repute can with safety to his reputation make assertions before ophthalmological societies that have

[1] F. A. Davis Company, Philadelphia, 1897.

heretofore been made too recklessly in print and elsewhere regarding the non-existence of maladjustments of the eye-muscles (except in squint cases) and their supposed effects upon the general health. Many of the audience would surely to-day turn such statements to ridicule by overwhelming experience to the contrary.

I have called special attention to the six preceding suggestions, because there yet seems to be a general mis-impression regarding the importance of refractive work in the treatment of heterophoria among the younger oculists, fostered, I fear, by a few of the older men who have heretofore violently opposed all scientific investigation of maladjustments of the ocular muscles by modern instruments and modern methods.

Not long since, while conversing with an attending surgeon to one of the largest eye hospitals of this city, he remarked to me : " Why do you not take refractive conditions into more serious consideration than you do, before deciding positively in regard to maladjustments of the eye-muscles?" I naturally was astonished!

I asked him in reply where he got such an absurdly erroneous impression (which he assured me was more common than I perhaps supposed), and I immediately referred him to my published writings on that subject.

A criticism that can more justly be made in return by me regarding the work done in most of the eye hospitals and dispensaries, as well as in the private offices of many oculists, is this : That investigation of the eyes is too apt to be regarded as final whenever refractive conditions have been estimated by Javal's instrument or by retinoscopy, and the fundus examined by the ophthalmoscope.

The excuses that are offered for cursory refractive work in public institutions, by those of the staffs who have discussed it with me, are that sufficient time cannot always be given to each patient and that the poorer classes cannot be tested under the influence of a mydriatic without depriving them of their earnings for a time.

They argue that retinoscopy and the use of Javal's

ophthalmometer are all that is practically required in those cases where the greatest precision is not sought for or demanded. A few are still inclined to pin their faith on their personal ability to estimate refraction accurately by means of the ophthalmoscope—a time-saving device, but one of extremely uncertain value as a means of estimating refractive errors with precision. All admit that the use of a mydriatic would unquestionably make confirmation of previous tests for refraction positive and final; but they state that it is unfortunately impracticable to test each refractive case (in public institutions) with dilated pupils and a relaxed accommodation.

But what too commonly happens after the refraction of dispensary patients has hastily, and often crudely, been passed upon and prescribed for?

This special class of sufferers naturally buy their glasses where they can get them for the lowest price. As a rule, they get poorly-fitted frames; and, in consequence, de-centered lenses. It is seldom, if ever, that the glasses prescribed at dispensaries are carefully verified and the fit of the frame passed upon by the oculist who wrote the formula. Seldom are these poor sufferers impressed with the importance of keeping the frames in order; to have them straightened when bent by wear or accident; to return and have the glasses verified whenever one becomes broken or slips out of the frame; to test their own vision at home from time to time (with a test card given them for that purpose); to report if any change in vision is noticed; and to be faithful in wearing all astig-matic or hypermetropic lenses not occasionally, but con-stantly.

Is it any surprise to thinking men that investigations made upon dispensary patients for " heterophoria " are generally deemed as unworthy of serious consideration by those who are particularly interested and are scientific workers in this field of science? Even the refractive work in public institutions is done hastily and crudely; and most of the cases are apt to be lost sight of after the first tests are made. How is it possible under such conditions to keep daily records of the eye-tests of any patient for weeks under the influence of prisms of varying degrees? How can any modifications of muscular tests (after an accurate refractive correction has been tried) be carefully noted, when the cases are seldom seen at regular intervals, and not always then by the same oculist?

Where is there a public or eleemosynary institution that can show to-day for inspection, or publish for the general information of the profession, complete and full records of the eye-tests of fifty consecutive cases of any nervous disease or of asthenopia?

I take the liberty of quoting in this connection the following paragraphs from a recent contribution of mine (*Buffalo Medical and Surgical Journal*, March, 1900) relative to the eye-treatment of headache, neuralgia, and nervous prostration:

" None are so blind as those who won't see! There are many in the medical profession, to-day as in the past, who stick to antiquated methods; who unfortunately regard all innovations as either nonsensical or useless; who scoff at all facts which conflict with their pet theories and methods; who refuse to even try what they have groundless prejudices against; who talk learnedly in societies and elsewhere about the results of investigations by themselves or others that can never have been made intelligently, if at all; and who write as fluently of, as they talk derogatorily to, an important field in medicine that they have little, if any, technical knowledge of, no sympathy with, no experience in, and whose results (in such hands) must of necessity have been unsatisfactory.

" Everyone who has worked intelligently and faithfully for years in the scientific study of the eye-muscles knows to day that the opinion of anyone on their anomalies must be of little value—no matter how great the reputation of the man—if he has neither the 'phorometer' nor 'tropometer' as a part of his office equipment, nor any records of the power of each individual muscle and the arcs-of-rotation of each eye upward, downward, inward, and outward.

" There is indisputable proof to-day that ' crossed ' eye toward the nose or temple—chiefly the former—may in some cases be made parallel with its fellow by simply lowering or raising one or both eyes. Such cases were not understood five years ago. They tend to-day to explain why many operations for ' squint ' have, in the past, caused bad overcorrections or yielded negative results. It is known to-day that the muscle at fault in ' cross-eye ' is not always the muscle that to the casual observer appears to restrict the natural movements of the eye. The cutting of the wrong muscle may sometimes give the operator who follows antiquated methods of research before operation—and the patient as well—subsequent food for reflection and a vast amount of regret.

" The sad results, viewed from the standpoint of suffering humanity, that are entailed by indifference and prejudice in men of scientific reputation cannot be estimated.

" By giving expression to others of their opinion concerning what they have not properly and patiently investigated themselves or will not see, thousands of sufferers are doomed to a life of misery."

How can the refractive work done in public institutions (presumably more or less imperfect, for reasons previously given) be of value in determining the effect of the glasses prescribed upon the ocular muscles? I have personally encountered in the rooms of such institutions large, fat, round-faced adults wearing glasses in frames that would fit a child, and hatchet-faced men and women with spectacle-frames on that would fit a giant; yet I have seen such decentered lenses passed upon by the oculists in charge without one word of comment or of disapproval.

CONCLUSIONS.

The following axioms relate to the modern methods of diagnosis and treatment of " eye-strain " and are vital to the best results:

1. All errors of refraction (manifest and latent) should first be very accurately determined, and as far as possible corrected for both distant and near points.

2. A mydriatic should be employed before suspected latent refractive errors are finally decided upon. Exceptions to this rule of procedure are rare.

3. The ophthalmometer of Javal should first be employed to detect and measure corneal astigmatism. Subsequently cylindrical trial lenses should be employed to verify the instrument of Javal or to detect astigmatism of the lens.

4. Neither retinoscopy, trial lenses, nor the ophthalmoscope are positive and trustworthy in estimating " latent " refractive errors. The former is probably the best of the three in skillful hands ; but serious errors may be made, even by a competent retinoscopist.

5. A marked difference in the refraction of the two eyes should be corrected by proper lenses *at all times and for all points.* This is vital to good work on eye-muscles as a preliminary step.

6. Cylindrical glasses should preferably, but not necessarily, be set in spectacle frames, in order to lessen the danger of alteration in the axis of the cylinder.

7. No glass prescribed should ever be worn by a patient until they have been inspected and verified by the oculist who prescribed them.

8. The frames selected by the patient or optician should always be inspected by the oculist with care to guard against decentered lenses. Each pupil should accurately correspond to the center of the corresponding lens. In children, the frames may have to be changed from time to time, on account of the growth of the head and face.

9. Patients should be personally instructed by the oculist to observe any decentering of their own lenses, that often occurs from bending of the frames or nose-clips ; also to personally test the vision of each eye separately from time to time (by means of a test card), to see if the refractive correction remains perfect.

Such education of the laity unquestionably takes much

time and trouble; but it pays in the end by giving the
patient valuable information that may prevent relapses of
some previous nervous- or eye-disturbances.

10. Patients should also be cautioned by oculists to
always have their lenses verified whenever they fall out of
the frames and are replaced, or whenever a lens gets broken
and a new one is made.

The stupid blunders that are not infrequently made by
jewelers and opticians are more apt in this way to be
detected early; and the oculist (who is most apt to be held
accountable for the distress caused by others' blunders)
may hold the patronage of his patients longer by timely
words of caution.

11. All tests made to determine either the power of individual muscles of the orbit or the presence or absence of
equilibrium of the ocular muscles, are of no positive value
until all errors of refraction are determined and properly
corrected by lenses.

12. The first "muscular tests" made upon any patient
by the oculist should be recorded as revealing only the
"manifest" muscular errors (in contradistinction to
"latent" muscular errors); and these tests should invariably be made with the proper lenses placed before the eyes
of the patient to correct refractive errors, if any exist.

13. The "manifest" muscular errors (revealed at the
first examination) should never be regarded as possessing
much clinical importance, except as possible pointers
toward some special type of heterophoria and a guide to
the oculist in searching for "latent" heterophoria.

Nothing indicates so clearly the inexperience of the
absolute tyro in the investigation of "eye-strain" as to
hear and read the statements of oculists (often men of distinction in other lines of ophthalmology) that they "found
only one degree of some anomaly," that "this defect was
too insignificant to be considered seriously," and other
similar opinions formed after only one interview with a
patient suffering from some form of "latent heterophoria."
Such expressions make experienced men wonder and
laugh!

14. The most positive and uniform standard of power in any of the ocular muscles (when studying some puzzling case of suspected heterophoria) is *the normal power of abduction.*

Whenever the abduction falls below 8°, latent esophoria may safely be suspected ; whenever it exceeds 8°, exophoria is apt to be present—although genuine exophoria is less common than most oculists seem to suppose.

Too much stress cannot be laid upon this point, whenever an oculist is called upon to interpret the records of muscular tests in any individual case.

15. A marked difference in the *power of sursumduction* on the two eyes is always to be regarded as a suspicious sign of hyperphoria.

16. It is usually wise to follow up suspected latent hyperphoria with vertical prisms, prior to any investigation of apparent anomalies of the internal or external muscles, whenever hypo-esophoria or hypo-exophoria seem to exist.

Manifest or latent anomalies of the vertical muscles in the orbit should be investigated first, as a rule, and rectified before co-existing anomalies of the lateral muscles are treated. There are exceptions to this rule of procedure, but it is a wise one to follow in most cases.

17. Whenever the refraction of a patient requires the constant wearing of glasses to correct it, the investigation of heterophoria by the wearing of prisms is most easily made through the aid of lorgnette frames that can be attached to spectacled frames by means of small hooks.

I keep a large assortment of such frames as a part of my office equipment, with different bridges and interpupillary distances, so as to fit almost any form of spectacle frame. My office stock of prisms is so made as to be interchangeable and to fit all of my office frames.

18. Operative procedures upon the eye-muscles should never be too hastily performed. It is vitally important, to insure the best results in any case, that the effects of accurate refractive correction (and possibly of prisms also) be noted for a time ; and that repeated muscular tests be

made in any case of heterophoria before any surgical steps
for its radical correction be advised or undertaken.

It usually takes time, patience, experience, modern instruments, and much good common sense to successfully
solve a complex eye-problem and to rectify an eye-condi-
tion that may be causing eye-disturbances, eye-disease, or
nervous derangements.

[We republish this article, first, because it considers a
subject which is exceedingly important and which cannot
be too widely discussed, and second, in order to say that
there is at least one public institution to which its, in many
cases, well-deserved strictures do not apply.

In the New York Ophthalmic Hospital cases of refraction are subjected to a mydriatic, the ophthalmometric
test, to retinoscopy, and to test lenses. The glasses prescribed are examined by the surgeon when brought back
by the patient, the fitting of frames is carefully looked
after, and patients are warned of the necessity of wearing
them properly, and of having them straightened when bent
out of shape by use.

In fact, most of the recommendations contained in the
paper, and all of the important ones, are conscientiously
carried out as a matter of routine in the hospital clinics.
Further, the smallest degrees of astigmatism are carefully
corrected where there are asthenopic symptoms present.—
ED.]

Potter, M. D., E. F.—Persistent Adenoids in a Woman Aged Forty-seven.—*Jour. of Lar., Rhin. and Otol.,* June, 1900.

A clinical report of a case which we note only on account of the rare occurrence of this condition at such an age. Upon reference to literature, the oldest persons in whom hypertrophied adenoids have been found are one reported by Luc, at fifty-four years, and one by Solis-Cohen, at seventy. PALMER.

Thompson, M. D., St. Clair (London).—**The Bacteriology of the Normal Nose.**—*Jour. Lar., Rhin. and Otol.,* August, 1900.

Until 1895 it was taken for granted that the normal nares were teeming with bacteria. Within the last five years this opinion has entirely changed. The cause of this freedom of the nose proper (that portion posterior to the vestibule) is probably threefold, to wit—(a) the motion of the ciliated epithelium, (b) inhibitory action of the mucus, and (c) the phagocytosis of the leucocytes. The author draws the following conclusions: " Considering the large quantity of dust-laden and germ-carrying air which passes hourly into the nasal fossæ, they are remarkably free from micro-organisms. Certain authors have always been able to find some organisms in the healthy nose, though always in small numbers ; others have found none in a majority of cases. This difference is probably due to the fact that the latter observers simply lifted loopfuls of mucus from one spot, while the former generally swept out the nose with pledgets of sterilized cotton wool.

" All researches have confirmed the observation that the vestibules of the nose swarm with organisms. Previous observers have demonstrated the action of the ciliated epithelium in sweeping out intruding matters from the nose, and the effect of the trickling of mucus in cleansing the mucous surfaces. Some (Wurtz, Lermoyes, Praget) claim decided bactericidal power for nasal mucus.

" Others (Thomson and Hewlett) have not been able to do more than prove that the mucus has an inhibitory effect on the development of micro-organisms, while some again have only formed the conclusion that mucus is not a favorable medium for their development. Phagocytosis shares in the work of removal, and for a study of this side of the question the thesis of Dr. Viollet is interesting and instructive." PALMER.

Brailey, M. D., M. A., W. A.—Ocular Headaches.— *Brit. Med. Jour.*, August 11, 1900.

The subject is ocular headaches, that is headaches in association with refractive and muscular ocular errors. While the great majority of headaches are, of course, independent of the eyes, it is a matter of general acceptance that ocular errors produce headache, though by no means in all cases. Are there any errors especially effective in the causation of headaches, or in producing any particular form of headache ?

Muscular errors are by far the most important, though, of course, these must be ultimately of nervous origin. Other influences than muscles are glare and sudden irregularities in the distribution of light, such as flickering.

Muscular ocular movements are :

Intrinsic { pupillary { accommodative
Extrinsic { of recti { and obliqui muscles

Pupillary movements are unimportant except as slightly influencing glare.

Accommodative movements are bound up with the great majority of ocular headaches.

It is a general law that the larger the ocular error the less the effect produced on the head, the reason being that a great defect of accommodative power leads to its abandonment, the patient seeing as best he can without it. So also uncorrected presbyopia is rare as a cause of headache except just at its commencement. It may cause strain and burning, but not headache.

A highly hypermetropic patient will read close with poor vision, but no aching, as also will patients with high hypermetropic astigmatism. Similarly great inequality of refraction gives comparatively little trouble, the worse eye being abandoned to disuse, and muscular action being regulated by the better one.

High degrees of myopia and myopic astigmatism produce little effect, distant objects hardly being seen, while near vision can be remedied largely by adjusting the distance. But low degrees of hypermetropia and hypermetropic astigmatism are often causes, especially when they lead to an excess of effort both in amount and duration beyond what is needed, as with weak muscles or hypersensitive nervous supply; this spasm of accommodation continuing in distant vision, and even under retinoscopy in the dark.

But both spasm and headache are more produced by moderate inequality of refraction, especially if astigmatic, and most of all by astigmatism with asymmetry of the axes. The ciliary muscle appears to act unequally on the two sides in correcting this, or a muscle even in different parts of its circuit in remedying astigmatism or asymmetry of axes. Evidence of this is seen when atropine reveals astigmatism on one side or both, increases its amount, or alters the axis of the correcting lens in amount less than 90°.

So astigmatism, often unequal-sided, may become manifest when presbyopia begins, and refractive defects reveal themselves to retinoscopic examination in eyes blind with fundus changes, such as optic atrophy, in proportion beyond that observed in average seeing eyes. The above refractive errors cause aching in the eyes, often passing presently or the following morning into the brows, immediate aching in the brows, temples back of the head, and occasionally also headache of the type of migraine. Treatment by appropriate glasses is of extreme value.

Errors of the extrinsic muscles produce headache, but less than of the accommodative muscles, though more migraine, more giddiness, and more general distress. Here also the rule holds: the larger the amount of error the less the disturbance; the explanation being that in considerable degrees of strabismus the image falls on the peripheral and so less acutely seeing retina.

But another potent factor in headaches is the tendency to binocular vision, and so we have another rule ; the stronger the tendency to binocular vision the more headache produced by an error of the recti and obliqui muscles.

Binocular vision varies much in its strength in different subjects. Possibly there are natural differences related to the centers as much as to the muscles, for I have seen such indisposition run through families. But binocular vision appears to be generally made rather than born. Babies often squint irregularly till, after a few weeks of life, they get their yellow spots gradually to accord. I have met cases where, instead of bringing them into harmony, the child has developed another retinal point to work with the opposite yellow spot in an eye congenitally squinting, though with fair concomitant movement. Rectification of such apparent squint by tenotomy will produce diplopia.

Other cases are common where the two eyes remain quite independent; for example, where there is congenital want of power of both external recti from central defect. Diplopia is absent, and the child sees to his left with the right eye, and *vice versâ*.

Binocular vision is not strongly established by the early age at which ordinary concomitant squint arises; so diplopia, though present, gives no trouble, and, indeed, is little noticed even in the comparatively rare cases where each eye has normal refraction and vision.

But take the case of a paralytic strabismus—for example, of the superior oblique—suddenly arising in an adult. Here we have much disturbance, and the same with cases where, when the two eyes have been used for different purposes—that is, one for near and the other for far vision—we suddenly attempt by lenses and prisms to unite the images, the results being distress, giddiness, migraine, and other headache. But extrinsic muscles may, like the ciliary, have large latent defects, and I suspect that many obscure cases of headache have their solution here. I quote the case of Mrs. X., aged sixty, neurotic. A surgeon practicing many years ago in London gave, for some ocular distress when she was aged forty, glasses for constant wear, each eye + 1.25 D. sph., 1° prism base in, and in response to her gradually increasing trouble, altered them through eighteen changes extending over twenty years to + 1 D. sph., 6° prism base in each eye for constant distant wear, and + 4.5 D. sph., 7°

prism base in for near work. Then I came in, and finding to ordinary tests no more than the average error of lateral muscles, tried to take away the prisms, but to no purpose. She declared that they " supported her " and " held her up." Consequently I made a closer examination, and found a difference of vertical level, which has increased in the six subsequent years ; so now she is " supported," satisfactorily on the whole, by, for distance, right eye : +1 D. cyl., 115°, 4° prism base in ; left eye :+0.75 D. sph., +0.72 D. cyl., 115°, 4° prism base down.

My belief is that this vertical error was always the essential one, and that its existence weakened the power of the internal recti so much that she was able to wear the huge prisms that she had. Without the glasses she feels an intolerable strain, and cannot bear to look.

One more case of Miss W., aged thirty-eight, a doctor's daughter, with occasional distress. I found low hypermetropic astigmatism and insufficiency of the internal recti. Through several changes she has come to the constant wear of right eye : + 0.25 D. cyl.. 150°, 3° prism base in, left eye the same, with, in addition, 1 ? vertical prism. With these she gets on fairly ; without them she cannot bear to look.

These, I think, are real latent errors ; doubtless very conducive to quackery, and so to be touched cautiously, especially as regards operation.

I cite also a case of great power of adjustment, though with distress, but no diplopia ever. Mrs. M., a doctor's wife, suffering much from migraine, quite unrelieved by spherical lenses. The images at 6 meters show half a meter difference of vertical level. She has now worn for two years, with great benefit to her head, her full refractive correction : Each eye —1.5 D. sph., —0.25 D. cyl., 165°, 3° vertical prism in opposite directions.

I myself have a latent difference of vertical level, though I am happily entirely free from headache, but not quite free from migraine.

Besides individual tendencies other influences alter the disturbing effect of ocular errors.

   1. Age ; they being most potent between ten and forty-five.

   2. Sex ; women being the greater sufferers.

   3. Nationality. My experience does not extend much beyond

English and citizens of the United States, the latter of whom are eminently affected by them, so that a series of doctors and operators has arisen to take charge of that special subsection of practice. Doubtless there are other influences, such as occupation and temporary states of the nervous system.   DEADY.

Ingersoll, A. M., M. D., J. M.—Primary Epithelioma of the Tonsil.—*The Lar.*, June, 1900.

Only 120 authentic cases of epithelioma of the tonsil having been reported, each additional one is of interest.

"M. G., a well-developed, muscular Irishman, æt. forty-two years, family and personal history negative. Within thirteen weeks of first examination he had noticed a slightly painful enlargement of the right tonsil ; this had already been amputated twice with tonsillotome. No disease existed elsewhere. Pain in tonsil steadily increasing.

"The tonsil was covered by a fairly firm, irregular, fungoid mass, projecting out about two cm. beyond the anterior pillar.

"The whole surface presented an uneven, cauliflower-like appearance, covered by a muco-purulent secretion. The mass extended upward on to the soft palate, involving both the anterior and posterior pillars ; it also followed the anterior pillar downward and extended on to the tongue ; posteriorly the growth extended along the posterior pillar downward to its attachment to the pharyngeal wall, but the wall itself was not involved. The surrounding tissue was inflamed and infiltrated. The lymphatic glands at the angle of the jaw, on the right side, were involved.

"From the macroscopic appearance of the tumor the diagnosis of a malignant growth was made and a piece was removed and submitted to Dr. Perkins for microsopical examination : he reported it to be typical epithelioma. The patient refused operation, and died a few weeks later under the treatment of a 'cancer specialist.'"   PALMER.

Wishart, M. D., D. J. Gibb.—Removal of Septal Spurs : A Note upon the Use of the Carmalt-Jones Spokeshave.—*The Lar.*, July, 1900.

This instrument is useful in removal of ecchondroses or exostosis in shape of (*a*) a horn or (*b*) a shelf. Not applicable to

those which are sessile in shape, or those associated with deflections.

After the usual preparations for the operation the spokeshave
is introduced into the nares with the bevel of the cutting edge
always turned toward the septum, passing it gently back over the
spur until it drops into the slot, and then pressing the blade as
closely as possible up to the septum ; by this means engaging the
whole of the spur. The blade must be drawn through with one
sweep. The spur usually remains attached to septum by shred
of membrane, which needs clipping with scissors.

The advantages claimed for this method are (1) the absence
of bleeding until the operation is accomplished, with the advantage of non-obstruction to the vision ; (2) great saving of time
in operating ; (3) the almost entire absence of pain or fear to
the patient ; (4) the satisfactory course pursued in healing.

PALMER.

Fry, M. D., Royce D.—Bloodless Enucleation of the Tonsils under Local Anæsthesia.—*Cleveland Jour. of Med.*, February, 1900.

" The faucial tonsils are masses of lymphoid tissue imbedded
in diffuse adenoid and fibrous tissue."

" The two forms of hypertrophy are simple and hyperplastic."
In simple " the individual elements are increased in size," while
in the hyperplastic there is an " overgrowth of connective tissue."

Some thorough. chemical and physiological experiments were
made by Dr. B. G. Hannum at The Hannum Laboratory, Cleve-
land, which are enumerated in article from which the following
deduction is drawn. " An extract of the tonsillar substance
proper, *i. e.*, the lymphoid nodules and mucous glands, stripped
of their capsule and all adherent adenoid tissue, when subjected
to all known tests for all known ferments, proves conclusively
that it is devoid of any ferment product, digestive or otherwise."

The tonsil of the ruminant contains considerable mucilaginous
mucus ; that of man very little, if any ; the approximate weight
of tonsil in a ruminant is 1 to 15,000, while in man it is 1 to
115,000, from which he deduces that the tonsil in man is a
retrograde structure without function. Also deduces that
enlarged tonsils elevate the pitch of voice, while their removal
both restores it and gives the voice more flexibility and resonance ; (2) instead of the tonsils protecting against any disease,

the diseased or hypertrophied tonsils are prolific incubators in which morbific germs may be hatched, and they serve as distributing points of infection to the general system ; (3) diseased tonsils lower the general health and retard the development of the sexual organs ; (4) they do not aid digestion, (5) nor deglutition ; (6) they do not absorb saliva, as some authors claim. Cocaine is used as anæsthetic, and supra-renal extract to reduce hemorrhage.

The tonsil is exposed by the patient depressing his tongue, and is caught by the curved forceps, in its upper portion, and slightly pulled inward and forward ; the mucous membrane is incised around circumference of tonsil, then tonsil enucleated with the enucleator, with the exception of the blood vessels, which are severed with the snare.   PALMER.

Note on a Case of Acute Glaucoma the Result of an Operation for Secondary Cataract.—Charles Bell Taylor, M. D., F. R. C. S. Edin.—*The Lancet*, September 8, 1900.

The patient came under my care in his eighty-sixth year, suffering from asthma, chronic bronchitis, and constant cough. He had been blind for some years from senile cataract in the right eye and latterly the left eye had become similarly affected. Operation had not been recommended by an ophthalmic surgeon who had been previously consulted, on account of the patient's numerous infirmities, and there seemed to be little chance of ameliorating his condition. Nevertheless, as the patient was very anxious to see, and as he could not well be worse off than he was, I determined to extract the cataract on the right eye.

The operation was performed under cocaine without misadventure and without iridectomy, and although the eyeball collapsed completely on extraction of the lens—assuming the form of a tiny bird's nest—the patient made a good recovery and there was no subsequent prolapse of the iris. Twelve days later, as the pupil of the operated eye was central and freely dilatable, I ventured to divide a piece of the capsule with the needle-knife, and he returned to his home in a northern county with every prospect of good vision. I was disappointed, however, when on a visit in his neighborhood four months later, to find that he could see very little and that the slit in the capsule had closed. I was consequently compelled to remove the peccant membrane *en masse,* which I did with iris forceps through a small incision in the corneosclerotic junction. All went well for three days, but on the night of the fourth I was sent for, as he was suffering from intense pain, which had not been mitigated by the instillation of atropine. The eyeball was as hard as stone and I therefore incised the sclerotic and, punctured the hyaloid fossa, letting out a few drops of vitreous. Agony was at once changed to perfect ease. There was no further trouble, and although he has suffered severely from repeated bronchitic attacks, he now has a good-looking eye with a central pupil and excellent sight.

It has seemed to me desirable to record this case, not only on account of the success of simple extraction under most trying conditions, not only on account of the failure of discission of the capsule and the advent of acute glaucoma when that membrane was removed in its entirety, but also because of the instant arrest of the glaucomatous process by an operation which did not involve excision of the iris.

The occurrence of glaucoma, both in its simple and acute forms, though rare after operation for secondary cataract, is a contingency that has to be reckoned with, and it is noteworthy that, although its progress may be at once arrested by excision of the iris or puncture of the hyaloid fossa, it is not inhibited or prevented by iridectomy, either as a preliminary or when performed as a part of the operation of extraction for cataract. One would think that, if it were possible to cut open the eyeball and to remove so important a portion of its contents as the lens itself without misadventure or serious consequences, that any subsequent dealing with a mere shred of capsule would be almost, if not quite, danger-free. It is not so, however. Many surgeons consider that a second operation is as serious or even more serious than an extraction. Professor Nuel of Liège says that "a simple discission of capsule is quite as dangerous as an extraction for cataract"; Professor Gayet of Lyons says, "There is no operation I dread more"; Professor Kalt of Paris says, "Secondary cataracts always give me great anxiety"; and Dr. Valude (editor of the *Annales d'Oculistique*) says, "C'est la vraiment le gros avator de l'operation de la cataract, la vrai complication plus redoutable que les prolapsus iriens qui guerissent bien et que la panopthalmie si rare." Trousseau, Eperon,

Bribosa, and Critchett warn us against the disastrous consequences that occasionally follow operations for secondary
cataract and, although my experience of some thousands of cases
of extraction of cataract has on the whole been favorable, I have
still seen quite enough to warrant me in insisting that we cannot
be too careful when dealing with secondary membranous
formations.

The late Alexander Pagenstecher and, more recently, Delgardo
of Madrid, have sought to solve the problem by scooping out the
lens capsule and all at the time of extraction, but this operation
does not always attain the end in view and involves loss of
vitreous, deep anæsthesia, and conspicuous deformity of the
pupil. The late Professor Hansen used habitually to puncture
the hyaloid fossa at the time of extraction in order to secure
a clear pupil, a practice which I see has been recently revived
by Mr. Work Dodd. Other surgeons, by cross-hatching the
capsule (Swanzy), or by removing as large a portion as possible
with forceps at the time of extraction, have sought to avoid the
necessity for subsequent interference. These operations, however, are neither quite so safe nor so feasible as they seem to be,
and are apt to be followed by wrinkling of the capsule, cell proliferation, or more or less obscuration of the pupil. Besides, the
breaking up of the capsule sets free particles of lenticular cortex
which are not easily seen at the time of extraction and which,
although comparatively harmless when retained within the capsule,
become a formidable source of irritation if set free in the anterior
chamber, or when brought into contact with recently cut surfaces.
It is best, therefore, I think, as a rule, to follow Professor Knapp's
advice and to incise the capsule in its periphery, only on a level
with the upper border of the lens, to get rid of as much cortex as
possible, and to take the chance of a second operation, should
that become necessary. If it does become necessary, then we
must above all be careful to avoid any manipulation that will
involve drag on the ciliary processes. The late Sir W. Bowman
endeavored to avoid this risk by breaking up the capsule with
two needles, one in either hand. With these he penetrated the
cornea at an angle of 60° or thereabouts, pierced the capsule,
and then, by revolving the points of the needles round each
other and separating the handles, tore the opaque film asunder
without any drag on the tissues with which the capsule is con-

nected. The needles, however, are apt to dig into the vitreous humor, manipulation of the doubly impaled eyeball is difficult, and the operation is not always successful ; hence Professor Noyes of New York has suggested that we should transfix the eyeball with a Graefe's knife, and then, with two blunt hooks passed through each of the external wounds and pulling one hook against the other, establish a sufficient aperture without drag on the ciliary region. The hooks, however, can only be withdrawn with their concavities upward, and the double manipulation of the eyeball, on the stretch and with a contracted pupil, complicates matters sometimes to an embarrassing degree. I have, therefore, substituted sharp hooks so curved that they may be entered and withdrawn in any position. These operations, however, do not always attain the end in view, and we are at present practically limited to a choice of three methods when operating for secondary cataract : (1) simple discission through the cornea, as practiced by Professor Knapp and myself within a fortnight of extraction ; (2) simple discission behind the iris and through the sclera, three millimeters from the limbus, as advocated by Gama Pinto and at present practiced by Harry D. Noyes of New York ; and (3) avulsion of the membrane, as adopted in the case which I have here recorded—an operation which is habitually practiced by Professor Panas of Paris, and which may be rendered comparatively safe by first separating the circumferential attachments of the capsule.   DEADY.

Hopkins, M. D., Frederick K.—Secondary Hemorrhage Following Use of Suprarenal Extract.—*N. Y. Med. Jour.*, August 25, 1900.

The author, although very loath to believe that any deleterious effects could come from an agent fraught with such exceedingly good and helpful qualities, after several quite severe secondary hemorrhages occurring after operations in which cocaine and suprarenal solutions were combined, finally concluded that such hemorrhage is solely " due to the relaxation following the strong stimulation of the suprarenal extract." He " observed that in some persons there was an idiosyncrasy against its use, violent coryzas following its application to the nasal mucous membrane." To ascertain if others had had the same experience he communicated with several colleagues. From which replies he concludes :

"There is a general consensus of opinion that secondary hemorrhage occurs, or, anticipating its possibility, some whom we know as careful, prudent men, take no chances, but pack the fossa before allowing the patient to leave the office, thus forestalling any accident. Others continue the effect of the extract by giving the patient a solution which is to be applied to the wound at intervals for a period following the operation. Among the replies there is but one, coming from a man who had used the extract extensively, which states positively that no cases of secondary hemorrhage have been seen, and the writer does not think they occur. The unanimity of so many other observers leads me to think that this one should be classed among those prudent operators who pack carefully before dismissing the patient—though he did not state that this was his custom."

PALMER.

Fasano, Prof. A. (Naples).—**The Treatment of Laryngeal Tuberculosis.**—*The Therapist,* July 16, 1900.

(Translated from the *Klin. thera. Wochenschr.,* No. 23, 1900.)

The author merely mentions pyoktannin, menthol, soda sulphoracinic, Durante's fluid thymol, and Heryng's method of curettage and painting with lactic acid.

He considers best of all Thiocol. = potass. guaiacol sulphate.

℞ Thiocol..	1½ to 2½ grs.
Cocaine hydroch	6 grs.
Ac. boraci...	15 grs.

Used as an insufflation, while at the same time small doses of Thiocol are given internally. (Size of dose not given.)

He finishes by saying : "I think I can conclude, from my results, that Thiocol is the best antiseptic which the laboratory has produced for tuberculosis. The bacteriological experiments prove its destructive action upon the tubercle bacillus ; the clinical experiments show that Thiocol, by specifically combating the tuberculous progress, revives the biological vitality of the tissues and the trophic conditions. I am convinced that Thiocol has a future, not only in pulmonary tuberculosis, but also in laryngeal tuberculosis, when employed alone or combined with scraping out. The local application of Thiocol must here be assisted by the internal administration, as this combats the abnormal fermentation in the intestinal tract, improves appetite and nutrition, thereby rendering the system more resistive to the tuberculous process." PALMER.

Stickler, M. D., D. A.—Local Anæsthetics in the Eye, Ear, and Throat.—*Denver Critique*, August 15, 1900.

The first place is accorded to our old friend cocaine hydro-chlorate.

2. Hydrochlorate of eucaine, " A."

3. Hydrochlorate of eucaine, " B."

4. Schleich's mixture.

℞ Eucaine.. 0.2
  Sodium chloride............................... .... 0.6
  Aqua dest.

5. Holocaine.

6. Orthoform.

7. ℞ Acid. carbolici ⎫
     Menthol   ⎬ aa.. .... 1 gram.
     Cocaine hydrochlorate ⎭

or

℞ Acid. carbolici...................................... 1 gram.
  Menthol   ⎫ aa.......................... 50 gram.
  Cocaine hydrochlorate ⎭

8. Suprarenal capsule.

Schleich's mixture is used by injection for anæsthesia of deeper tissues.

℞ Orthoform........... .... 4 pts.
  Petrolatum... 30 pts.
   Sig.

One gr. placed in conjunctival sac and bandage applied. Useful in painful, relapsing ulcers of eye. Also in cancer and tuberculosis of throat.

The prescriptions No. 7 were introduced by Bonain of Bordeaux, who "has used the mixture as a local anæsthetic upon the drumhead. In the nasal fossa for exploratory punctures of the antrum through the inferior meatus, and for galvano-cautery in inflamed tissue when the ordinary solutions of cocaine are not efficacious. In the larynx, especially in the dysphagia of tuberculosis and in ulceration of the pharynx. In some of these cases the relief is marked for as much as four days from one application. In using the caustic solution for tubercular ulceration the surface should be first brushed over with cocaine solution to prevent the burning sensation. " Bonain, in summing up his experience, comes to the conclusion that the three qualities— the anæsthetic, slightly caustic and strongly antiseptic—made this application one of great usefulness."

Chloretom is advocated by Parke, Davis & Co., but little is known of it. PALMER.

Theobald, M. D., Sam'l.—A Case of Transient Spastic Convergent Strabismus.—*Johns Hopkins Hospital Bulletin*, July–August, 1900.

Spastic convergent strabismus, or strabismus from tonic spasm of the internal recti muscles, a condition to be sharply differentiated from ordinary concomitant convergent squint and from squint due to paralysis of the abducens, is one of the well-recognized ocular manifestations of hysteria ; but, apart from this, it would seem, deserves to be regarded as a rare anomaly, to which, as a rule, the text-books upon diseases of the eye devote but scant attention.

De Schweinitz, in the paragraph of less than five lines which he devotes to "spastic strabismus," ("Diseases of the Eye," third edition, p. 554), says that it "occurs only under rare circumstances in hysteria and brain disease (meningitis). It is difficult of diagnosis, periodical concomitant squint in hypermetropia being sometimes inaccurately described as due to spasm of the internal rectus (Mauthner)." Jackson, in a paragraph of equal brevity, says "deviations of the eyes due to spasms of the ocular muscles attend hysterical seizures and some forms of brain-disease. They may assist in the general diagnosis, but have little localizing value, and require no treatment apart from that of their cause" (" Diseases of the Eye," p. 234).

Fuchs, though he states that "tonic spasms of the ocular muscles are extremely rare," adds that "many cases of intermittent strabismus belong under this head," and he mentions two cases of this character which he had observed in hysterical women ("Text-Book of Ophthalmology," p. 576). Roosa says children in whom optic neuritis is found to be present are often brought to ophthalmic clinics with strabismus in its early stages which is non-paralytic. "Every careful observer," he adds, "will take great pains to determine in a given case of suddenly occurring strabismus, that there is not some cerebral lesion.   During dentition, certain children are apt to squint." This, he thinks, "may fairly be ascribed to cerebral irritation " (" Diseases of the Eye," p. 553).   Duane, in his chapter upon "movements of the eyeballs and their anomalies," in De Schweinitz and Randall's " American Text-Book of Diseases of the Eye, Ear, Throat, and Nose " (p. 511), treating of paretic and spastic squint, says " spasm, which is much less frequent than paralysis, is due to irritative lesions (meningitis, etc.), chorea, epilepsy, and hysteria ; rarely is idiopathic." Noyes, Norris and Oliver, Fick, Nettleship and Swanzy, so far as revealed by a glance through their respective treatises upon diseases of the eye, make no mention of the subject of spastic strabismus.

In Norris and Oliver's " System of Diseases of the Eye," Parinaud, treating of the ocular manifestations of hysteria, considers at some length the " anomalies of convergence " occurring in this condition.   If we would understand the anomalies of the movements of the eyes in hysteria, we must, he says, "consider that neither muscles nor nerves, but nerve centers, and, indeed, the higher centers, are affected—those whereby the movements themselves are brought into unison with psychic action "; and, he adds, " another fact connected with a study of hysterical disorders of the ocular apparatus is that they are almost always of the nature of contractures, even when they present the objective characteristics of paralysis " (vol. iv. p. 754).   In the same volume (pp. 708 and 710), Santos-Fernandez, writing of the " ocular manifestations in influenza," mentions cases of paralysis of the third and sixth nerves and of " convergent strabismus " as having been observed in this affection, while Culver, in the chapter upon " Anomalies of the Motor Apparatus of the Eye," says, " Changes in the centers of innervation as *primary* causes of strabismus are admissible only in certain definite cases," and, again, " Convergent strabismus may be due also to a *spasm of convergence*, independently of accommodation and refraction.   We have observed cases of this kind of hysteria.   It is perfectly admissible that the same phenomenon is produced in consequence of other irritations of the center of convergence " (*op. cit.*, p. 100).

Briefly described, the case which I wish to report is as follows: A little girl, seven years of age, convalescing from a pronounced attack of influenza, a marked feature of which had been persistent and severe headache, and during the course of which an otitis media had developed in the right ear, complained of diplopia, and on the following day exhibited an evident squint. At the request of the attending physician, Dr. W. D. Booker, I saw the case on the second or third day after the squint manifested itself.

There was present at this time, in both distant and near vision, a very decided convergent squint of the left eye. There were no signs of paresis of either rectus externus—each eye could be rotated outward farther than is commonly possible, and neither the extent of the squint nor the diplopia was influenced by the direction in which the head or the eyes were turned. The pupils were of normal size and there were no signs of either paralysis or spasm of the ciliary muscles. The ophthalmoscope revealed a hypermetropia of rather more than 2 D., and, as I had previously performed a tenotomy upon the little patient's mother for a pronounced esophoria, I concluded that the influenza had been the straw which had broken the camel's back, and developed a concomitant squint in a child who had, probably, inherited insufficiency of the external recti muscles and who was decidedly hypermetropic. That the trouble would be overcome without glasses or an operation seemed to me highly improbable. Dr. Booker had already prescribed iron and quinine and a nourishing diet, and the general condition of the patient was improving from day to day.

At my second visit, four days later, although the mother reported that the eyes had been straight at times during this interval (?), I found the squint unchanged except that it showed, perhaps, a greater tendency to alternate. Thinking that suppression of the accommodation might favorably influence the squint, I directed a 2-grain solution of atropia to be dropped into the eyes twice a day. Two days subsequently, the eyes being thoroughly under the influence of the atropia, the squint seemed somewhat less marked. My next visit was five days after this, and, to my gratification, I then found no trace of the squint remaining. Not only so, but even with the cover test it showed no disposition to recur, and an esophoria for distance of only 4° was shown by the Maddox rod. A decided change for the better in the general condition of the patient was also evident.

After another interval of four days, the eyes meantime having remained quite straight, the atropia was discontinued, although, I confess, I still had serious misgivings as to what would occur when the ciliary muscles began to regain their activity. However, my apprehensions proved to be groundless, for a week elapsed without any recurrence of the squint, by which time she had recovered her power of accommodation sufficiently to be able to read ordinary print. The Maddox rod now showed an esophoria for distance of only 3°, while, more noteworthy still, the vertical diplopia test showed at 12″ a so-called exophoria of 4°—a practically normal muscle balance. Since then the eyes have given no further trouble.

A few days since (April 26), nearly two months having elapsed since the disappearance of the squint, the muscle balance was tested with the following result :

$$\left. \begin{array}{l} \text{Esophoria } 20' = 1° \\ \text{No hyperphoria } 20' \end{array} \right\} \text{ Rod test.}$$

Exophoria 12″ = 1° (Vertical diplopia test).

That the squint in this case was a purely spastic one, due, doubtless, to an irritation (of influenzal origin) of the innervation center which controls the associated action of the internal recti muscles, is, in my judgment, not open to question. Had it been a concomitant squint, precipitated by the attack of influenza, as I at first supposed, it might, indeed, have disappeared under the influence of the atropia and with the improvement in the patient's general condition ; but, under such circumstances, a normal muscle balance would certainly not have been re-established in the space of a few days, as actually happened. On the contrary, a marked, and probably persistent, esophoria would certainly have been encountered.

As to abductor paresis, I have already said there were no signs whatever pointing in this direction ; but, apart from this fact, the rapid return of the lateral muscles to a condition of practical orthophoria, is as little consistent with this view of the case as it is with the view that the squint was a concomitant one.

An incomplete search through the literature of the subject has revealed only one case which bears a close resemblance to my own. In the *Archives of Pediatrics*, vol. i. p. 634, Dr. Samuel S. Adams of Washington reports an interesting case of convergent strabismus as a sequela of diphtheria, in which paresis of the external recti muscles was excluded, and which he attributed to "a spasm or over-action of the internal rectus" due to an irritation of the center of ocular adduction. The squint disappeared completely within a few days of its onset.   DEADY.

Alexander, M. D., C. M., A. Speirs (London).— Laryngeal Phthisis and its Homeopathic Treatment.—*The Jour. of the British Hom. Soc.*, July, 1900.

The doctor, following the teaching of the Organon, believes that, as this is a constitutional dyscrasia and not from local irritation, it should be treated by internal medication almost exclusively.

He reasons that, as it is estimated that every phthisical patient exhales 7,000,000,000 bacilli every twenty-four hours, those in the vicinity of a consumptive must be in such an atmosphere of bacilli that if it were transmitted by local contact probably all would be inoculated.

"Though the bacillus may be the exciting, yet it is by no means the sole cause of phthisis. For its true origin, one must go deeper, and look for a *causa causans*, inherent in, or inherited by the sufferer, a peculiar soil providing a suitable *nidus*, where the bacillus may thrive and develop, but without which it must prove as harmless as the Klebs-Loeffler bacillus often does, when found in the fauces of perfectly healthy people who have never had diphtheria at all. . .

"The soundest principle then is to treat the patient himself, and not merely the larynx, and endeavor so to alter his dyscrasia that he may no longer prove a suitable host for the bacillus, which may then quietly disappear, along with all local appearances."

A clinical report of an undoubted case of phthisis laryngea follows,—the co-existing objective and subjective symptoms are unmistakable. Cure was effected with ars. iod. and caust., and, after decided improvement set in, a change to a salubrious climate.

In discussion following Mr. Dudley Wright advocated both internal and local treatment in pure phthisis laryngea. To wit: currettage followed by rubbing in of a 10 to 40 gr. to an ounce lactic acid solution. Internally, kreos. 1x dil. gave best results.

Cases of phthisis engrafted on a syphilitic cónstitution were more amenable to treatment than those in untainted individuals.

Dr. Robinson Day reported case of woman, æt. fifty years, having quite extensive phthisical ulceration of the larynx accompanied with fibroid phthisis of the lungs, whose ulcerations healed and who is living nine years after first seen, and appears outwardly as well as at the beginning. " The patient constantly required and had to take kali bich." PALMER.

Douglass, M. D., H. Beaman.—Atrophic Rhinitis.— *The Post-Graduate,* June, 1900.

The author has discarded microbic theory of origin of this disease so ably advanced by Frankel, but considers it due rather to a lowered state of vitality or diminished physical resistance consequent upon " anæmia, struma, or syphilitic taint," poor food, unhygienic surroundings, etc. Also the wearing out of the nasal mucosa from local overtaxation of the membrane in heating, filtering, and moistening a too great a volume of air, as is sometimes noticed in persons of peculiarly wide nares or in the concave side of a deflected septum.

Treatment.—Thorough cleansing by the physician himself should be done every second day. The following preparations are mentioned :

Hydrogen dioxide (Oakland Chem. Co.), 1 to 10 or 1 to 20 ; mercury bichloride and zinc chloride, each 1 to 10,000 equal parts; this mixture is improved by addition of salt. Trichloracetic acid, one per cent. solution, as also citric acid, two to six per cent. solution, as a deodorant and astringent. Ichthyol, as a ten to twenty per cent. aqueous solution, pure, or as a salve as follows, is very highly recommended.

```
℞ Ichthyol ........  .......  ......  .......  ............  .... 4 grs.
   Menthol ......  ..........................................  5 grs.
   Vaseline ........  ....................................  ·  1 ℥
```

Ortho-chlor-phenol, ten per cent. solution in glycerine, is a powerful deodorant, in twenty-five per cent. solution a cauterizant ; only to be used in severe cases and with caution, as, if used too strong or too often, it will result in overirritation.

"The best climate for these cases is a dry, high air, the temperature making little difference. These cases do best in the mountains and especially when climbing mountains."

The galvanic current, exhibited on hot moist sponges, one half milliampere for a period of five to fifteen minutes, is held in favor by some American and German authorities.   PALMER.

Semon, Felix.—Case of Tabes, with almost Complete Laryngoplegia.—*The Jour., of Lar., Rhin. and Otol.*, March, 1900.

This being such a rare case, the author only finding one other of complete bilateral recurrent paralysis on record,—we copy report of case in full.   The other similar case was detailed by Gerhardt in Nothnagel's Spez. Pathologie und Therapie, Bd. XIII., 1896.

"A. S., a carman, aged forty years, was admitted under the care of Dr. Hughlings Jackson into the National Hospital on December 11, 1899. He had syphilis five years ago with secondary symptoms, and was treated only a few weeks. His present symptoms began fourteen months before admission with loss of control over the bladder. This was followed by numbness and shooting pains in the legs, trunk, and hands, ataxy and gastric crises. For nine months his voice had been altering, and he had had shortness of breath, but apparently no laryngeal crises.

"*Summary of Symptoms.* — Extreme general emaciation. Arteries thickened and tortuous. Double ptosis. Reflex iridoplegia. Slight weakness of the right side of the face. Extreme inco-ordination ; marked hypotonia ; can only walk when supported. Entire loss of sense of passive movement in lower extremities. Analgesia (partial) over face, over arms and upper part of chest, and over lower extremities. Severe shooting pains and gastric crises. Complete incontinence of sphincters, no anal reflex. All deep reflexes absent ; plantar reflexes show a typical tabetic response. No difficulty in swallowing ; no return of fluids through the nose.

"*Voice.*—Speaks in a loud hoarse whisper. When talking he quickly runs short of breath, and between his utterances a sort of subdued inspiratory stridor is sometimes audible. He cannot cough in the usual way, but, on attempting it, a long, noisy expiration results.

"*Palate.*—On attempted phonation the palate itself remains perfectly motionless, but the posterior arches make some rapid and feeble inward movements. The tactile sensibility is perfectly normal, but the reflex excitability is much diminished, though not completely abolished.

"*Larynx.*—During quiet respiration both vocal cords stand perfectly motionless in about the minimum width of the cadaveric position (about 3 millimeters) apart, but their posterior ends are a little nearer one another than is usual under such circumstances, and their free borders are not excavated, but perfectly straight. Neither on attempted deep inspiration nor on phonation is the slightest movement of the cords visible.

"On touching the epiglottis with a probe, no reflex movement whatever is noticeable. On touching the interarytenoid fold, regular closure of the glottis takes place immediately, without cough being produced.

"On touching the right ventricular band, reflex closure ensues. The same, more strongly and combined with feeble cough, ensues when the left ventricular band is touched. A remarkable circumstance is the comparative loudness of the voice.

" Finally, the manner in which a few fibers of the accessory and vagus have escaped (as shown by the fibrillary contraction of the palatine muscles, by the possibility of closing the glottis on peripheral stimulation, by the maintained possibility of producing tension of the vocal cords through the crico-thyroids, and by the diminished, yet not quite abolished, reflex irritation of the palate and larynx) is very remarkable." PALMER.

Webster and Thomson.—A Case of Acute Glaucoma, with Subhyaloid Hemorrhage Supervening upon Uniocular Retinitis Albuminurica.—*N. Y. Med. Jour.*, September 1, 1900.

Philip B., fifty-six years old, a cigar-packer, married, found on the morning of January 15, 1900, that he could not see to read the newspaper as usual. He consulted a physician, who told him he had a cold in his left eye and gave him a lotion. Later he consulted another physician, who said he had "fundus trouble" and that he would never see again with his left eye. This physician gave him some internal treatment, however. The attending surgeon of a dispensary which he visited examined his urine and told him his kidneys were sound, but advised him not to eat meat, potatoes, or eggs, and not to drink coffee or tea.

On the 15th of March his left eye "began to swell," and he consulted a skilled ophthalmologist, Dr. Tansley, of this city. Dr. Tansley found all the symptoms of acute glaucoma of the left eye. He attacked the disease vigorously with meiotics, which failed to give relief. As the patient was "almost crazy" with pain and as the tension of the eyeball threatened permanent loss of sight, Dr. Tansley advised an immediate operation, and, as he did not like to operate at the patient's home, on account of the unsanitary condition of the surroundings, he kindly referred him to me (Dr. Webster) and asked me to do the operation for him at the Manhattan Eye and Ear Hospital.

When I saw him, on March 19, the eyeball was red, the tension was increased, and the anterior chamber was shallow, but, owing to the meiotics that had been applied, the pupil of that eye was smaller than that of the other. The vision was reduced to perception of light. Ophthalmoscopic examination of the right eye showed what appeared to be a glaucomatous cupping of the disk (-3 D.), but the eye retained vision $= \frac{20}{20}$, had a good visual field, and was hypermetropic half a diopter. The fundus of the left eye could not be seen, on account of the opacity of the media.

I performed an iridectomy upward, under cocaine anæsthesia and with the use of suprarenal capsule extract, on the same day. Immediately after the excision of the iris the whole pupillary area was obscured by blood, which also spread itself over the anterior surface of the iris. He remained in the hospital until April 6, a period of eighteen days, during which he had treatment with a view to getting rid of the blood in the anterior chamber, but without effect. The hemorrhages were renewed as fast as the blood was absorbed, and always the anterior chamber was from a quarter to half full of blood. His urine was examined and found to be loaded with albumin and with casts of various kinds. His diet was regulated accordingly, and he was treated locally and internally, but still unsuccessfully. On the eighteenth day he was discharged from the hospital and referred back to Dr. Tansley for further treatment.

Dr. Tansley kept him under observation and treatment for a little over two weeks, and then, all perception of light being lost and the eye remaining painful and inflamed, was forced to the conclusion that enucleation should be performed. I concurred in Dr. Tansley's opinion, and on April 25 he was readmitted to the hospital and I removed the eye under anæsthesia with ether. A copious hemorrhage occurred a few hours after the operation. For this a pressure bandage was applied and the patient was kept sitting up. Two days after the enucleation, on April 27, the bandage was removed and the orbital cavity cleansed. There was a slight recurrence of the bleeding and the pressure bandage was reapplied.

On May 3 the patient was discharged with his orbital cavity in good condition and the fellow eye unaffected. DEADY.

Stein, M. D., Otto J.—Symmetrical Osteoma of the Nose, with a Report of a Case.—*The Lar.*, July, 1900.

Quite a thorough consideration of the ætiology, symptomatology, and mention of reports of recently occurring cases are included.

Clinical History.—Male, æt. twenty-eight years, the surviving member of a family of six, all of whom died of phthisis. Twelve years ago had contusion of larynx, since when has been aphonic; eleven years ago, in a fight, was struck upon the nose, which was followed by a gradual enlargement over the lateral region of the nasal. bones, continually growing, with pain or discomfort, until about four years ago. Three years before examination the ravages of consumption appeared and are progressing rapidly.

"Objectively the patient presents a classical 'frog face.' A symmetrically placed swelling, half the size of a large bird's egg, on either side of the nose between the lower and inner margin of the orbital cavities and the upper half of the dorsum of the nose, and the hanging lower jaw of the mouth-breather, combine to make up the froglike appearance of the face. External palpation of the growth defines a tumor of bony firmness, sharp in outlines, with the overlying skin normal and freely movable. The right side is slightly larger than the left. The orbital cavities are but slightly encroached upon from below. The right nasal duct is obstructed by the growth, the left one encroached upon. On anterior rhinoscopy we find the right nostril totally occluded, the left one almost so, by the protrusion of their outer walls into the cavities. This protruding, occluding mass, which

is firm and hard on palpation and offers resistance to the passage of a sharp instrument, occupies the position of the nasal
wall of the antrum.   On both sides it has grown up to and
presses against the septum, so that the finest wire cannot be
passed between the two ; at the same time the pressure has not
caused any ulceration or absorption of the septum.   On the left
side there is a depression seen on the surface of the growth, corresponding to the situation of the middle nasal fossa.   Above
and around the growth on this side, about opposite the situation
of the middle turbinal, there is a small opening, admitting a fine
probe, and through which the patient can respire and even blow
mucus.   The mucous membrane covering these tumors is pale
in color and thin, but not eroded or ulcerated, and not secreting
any noxious material.   On posterior rhinoscopy the vault of the
pharynx, as well as the posterior nares, is free from any obstruction to the passage of the light rays."

The palate is highly arched and the mucous membrane of the
pharynx the seat of a chronic catarrhal inflammation, the result
of his mouth-breathing.   Vision normal ; inability to rotate left
eye inward, divergence outward two lines, pupil dilated not responding to light.   PALMER.

Douglass, M. D., H. Beaman.—The Treatment of Hay Fever by Suprarenal Gland.—*N. Y. Med Jour.*, May 12, 1900.

After giving extracts of the few articles in which this drug has
been mentioned as applicable to this condition, he considers it
more beneficial than any other one drug, yet should not be used
to the exclusion of others.

A few doses of extract internally demonstrate distinct local
effects upon the nasal tissue. " It has no dangerous sequelæ and
no toxic action, and yet, when full doses have been given, the
effect can be easily recognized by the patients, who experience a
certain degree of vertigo, some nervous excitement, and always an
increase in frequency of the heart's action.

" In those cases in which the nasal symptoms are prominent,
particularly where there are nasal lesions, and where the development of hay fever is accompanied by much congestion, the benefit is most marked.   In nasal cases not accompanied by much
congestion the benefit is lessened, and those with perennial nasal

attacks are less relieved by the action of the drug than the simple congested cases.

"It seems that cases dependent upon a gouty or rheumatic diathesis are helped by the use of suprarenal gland, while, on the other hand, patients are not helped at all where there is a loss of blood-vessel elasticity, due to an atheromatous condition, or in those conditions of blood vessels resulting from interstitial nephritis. Cases exhibiting some degeneration of the cardiac muscle are also hopeless of any benefit from suprarenal gland.

"In hay-fever subjects having neuroses coupled with nasal lesions, and in neurasthenic subjects having general vasomotor disturbances, the best results have been observed."

Administration.—(1) local, (2) internal. (1) Nares sprayed or swabbed with twelve per cent. solution every two hours, or at longer intervals. (2) A 5-grain tablet may be taken every two hours until symptoms relieved, then lengthen intervals gradually until only two are taken in a day. PALMER.

Vallar, M.—Median Osteotomy of the Hyoid Bone as a Means of Entering the Deep Pharynx and the Base of the Tongue.—*Rev. du Chirurgie*, March, 1900.

(Translated by Dr. T. H. Manly for the *Kansas City Record.*)

Although operation in this region is fraught with much danger, on account of the proximity of important tissues—twelve cases were treated in this manner without mortality.

" OPERATIVE MANUAL.

" First, make a vertical incision through the skin and connective tissues from posterior border of symphysis to the superior border of the hyoid cartilage. In this cut, we divide no important vessels except, sometimes, a transverse branch of a vein, from one jugular to the other.

"Now we expose the body of the hyoid, the superficial aponeurosis being incised on a director, thus separating the two borders of the mylo-hyoid muscles. The hyoid now is visible at the base of the wound. This is divided in the center. The fibers of the mylo-hyoid are now separated for four centimeters —one inch and a quarter. At this stage we open the thyrohyoid membrane which invests the anterior wall of the pharynx. This is now done in such direction as special cases require.

"It is not necessary to place an osseous suture through the

divided hyoid. The membrane will be closed by suture and the divided edges of hyoid brought into contact. Osseous or fibrous union always follows with unimpaired function resulting. A preliminary tracheotomy is rarely necessary. Have employed this procedure with perfect satisfaction in several cases." PALMER.

Glascow, M. D., Wm. C.—Laryngitis a Provoking Cause of the Asthmatic Paroxysm.—*N. Y. Med. Jour.*, August 25, 1900.

The pith of the paper is in the following paragraph, to which clinical reports of four cases are added.

" It is now generally admitted that asthma is a vasomotor neurosis and that the paroxysm is provoked by some peripheral irritation of the sympathetic nerve. Experience has shown that in the greater number of cases this irritation lies in the upper portion of the respiratory tract. The posterior surface of the turbinateds, the interarytenoidal commissure, the posterior surface of the trachea, and the membrane at the bifurcation of the trachea have been demonstrated to be the most sensitive areas in the respiratory tract. It is unquestionably an irritation of one or more of these areas which produces the symptoms of reflex cough, and I think it is a similar irritation which produces the symptoms of asthma. Among these areas, according to my experience, the interarytenoidal has seemed to be the most frequent site of irritation. This is due generally to a primary laryngitis, entirely independent of any pathological condition of the nose."

Local application upon cotton applicator of carbolized-iodine solution to the interarytenoid space gives relief, partly through its anæsthetic effect, and also through the local stimulation.

PALMER.

McKernon, M. D., Jas. F.—A Contribution to the Technique of Modern Uranoplasty.—*N. Y. Med. Jour.*, June 16, 1900.

Any hypertrophy of tonsils, adenoids, or turbinateds should be removed and thoroughly healed before operating.

Chloroform anæsthesia is preferable. Preliminary tracheotomy is first performed. Smith's gag, on account of containing tongue-depressor, is best. The entrance of larynx and esophagus is covered by a large, flat, thick piece of plain sterilized gauze, with string attached, in order to keep blood, etc., from entering lungs or stomach. Parts are first cleansed with warm normal salt solution, then mopped with full-strength borolyptol.

Incisions made as usually directed. Suturing commenced at anterior extremity of incision instead of posterior.

"After the oral cavity has been cleansed with a warm normal salt solution, and the pad removed and replaced by a fresh one, a thin strip of sterilized gauze, about an inch and a half wide, is passed between the under surface of the repaired palate and the posterior pharyngeal wall. Plain sterilized gauze is used to pack the lateral incisions, and here the packing should be quite firm. Sterilized gauze is also used over the whole of the operative field, the cavity of the mouth is filled completely to the front teeth, and the gauze is pressed rather firmly against the under surface of the new palate." If dressing becomes soiled in any manner, replace immediately by fresh one. If not soiled first dressing should remain forty-eight hours, subsequently redress every day, at which time cleanse mouth with normal salt solution or formaline. Sutures should be removed gradually, only one or two each day. Do not remove before seventh or eighth day.

Nourishment to be carried on entirely *per rectum.*

The age at which to operate is from two to four years.

Reports of four successful cases are appended. PALMER.

Rose, M. D., Jno. R.—A Case of Diphtheritic Sore of the Lower Lip, with Secondary Infection of the Throat.—*Georgia Jour. of Med.,* February, 1900.

Mrs. B., the postmaster's wife and assistant, had for twenty-four hours suffered with dysphagia, throat sore and glands swollen, lower lip swollen one inch beyond the upper, with sore eighth inch in diameter. Two weeks previously lip was chapped. The next day sore increased to three-quarters of inch in diameter, and another on upper lip, both covered with a closely adherent thick whitish membrane ; pulse weak and thready, patient complained of being-weak. Membrane subsequently developed on lower part of tonsils and in larynx, with obstruction of breathing and very weak heart's action. Sundry local applications and tonics were administered, with no improvement till antitoxin was injected. Six hours after injection paralytic symptoms were relieved, and in twenty hours the patient was very comfortable and the pseudo-membrane had exfoliated. The usual gradual convalescence followed. PALMER.

BOOK REVIEWS.

ANNUAL AND ANALYTICAL CYCLOPÆDIA OF PRACTICAL MEDI-
CINE. By CHARLES E. DE M. SAJOUS, M. D.; and One Hundred Associate Editors, assisted by Corresponding Editors,
Collaborators, and Correspondents. Illustrated with Chromo-
lithographs, Engravings, and Maps. Volume V. Philadelphia, New York, Chicago: The F. A. Davis Co., Publishers,
1900. Pp. 662.

The volume under consideration should be unusually interesting to readers of the JOURNAL, covering as it does a number of
the very important diseases and conditions which are included
in our specialties.

The first article of any length in the book takes up Diseases
of the Middle Ear, giving concise and interesting accounts of
their symptoms, diagnosis, and treatment, including the newest
of the latter, both instrumental and medicinal. Directions are
given for ossiculectomy.

A short, but excellent résumé of mastoiditis is given, with the
methods of its treatment.

Diseases of the Mouth and Lips are briefly considered, occupying some ten pages of space.

The article on Myopia includes some of the latest observations
on the operative treatment of progressive myopia by the removal
of the lens.

Diseases of the Nasal Cavities receive sufficient and up-to-date
treatment, and are followed by an excellent article on adenoid
growths of the naso-pharynx.

In the article on Diseases of the Optic Nerve and Retina, by
Edward Jackson, the principal facts are well brought out in an
essay wherein scarcely a word is wasted.

Although very brief for the subject covered, most of the
important facts are brought out in very succinct language. This
article is followed by a short résumé of Diseases of the Orbit.

Under Plastic Surgery we find deformities and growths of the lips, cleft palate and rhinoplasty.

Of the articles which appeal more particularly to the general physician, one of the best is that entitled Nursery and Artificial Feeding, which covers some twenty-three pages and considers the subject from all sides. It includes directions for sterilization and Pasteurization of milk, the consideration of bacteria, the methods of examining breast milk, the conditions affecting its composition, etc. The subject is very fully covered and the matter up to date.

Other notable headings are Disorders of Pregnancy, by Dr. Currier; Abnormal Parturition, by Drs. Grandin and Marx; Pleurisy, by Dr. Alex. McPhedran; Catarrhal Pneumonia, by Dr. Solis-Cohen; Lobar Pneumonia, by Dr. Thos. G. Ashton, and Morphinomania and the Opium Habit, by the late Dr. Norman Kerr.

Like all its predecessors the present volume is well printed on good paper, and handsomely bound.

DISEASES OF THE EYE. By EDWARD NETTLESHIP, F. R. C. S., Ophthalmic Surgeon at St. Thomas' Hospital, London; Surgeon to the Royal London Ophthalmic Hospital, etc. New (6th) American from the sixth English edition, thoroughly revised by WILLIAM CAMPBELL POSEY, M. D. With a Supplement on the Detection of Color Blindness, by WILLIAM THOMSON, M. D., Professor of Ophthalmology in the Jefferson Medical College, Philadelphia. Just ready. In one 12mo volume of 562 pages, with 192 illustrations. Selections from Snellen's test-types and formulæ, and 5 colored plates. Cloth, $2.25, net. Lea Brothers & Co., Philadelphia and New York.

The present edition of this exceedingly popular work has been revised by an American editor, with a view to adapting it more especially to the wants of the American practitioner.

For this purpose special attention has been given to the methods of examination usually followed in this country, and a number of therapeutic measures have been added which have recently been largely employed by American Ophthalmologists. While the text bearing upon the different diseases of the eye has been altered as little as possible, the editor has introduced into the section on diseases of the conjunctiva the latest views regarding the bacteriological origin of several varieties of conjunctivitis, and has given descriptions of several new forms of ocular diseases. Over thirty new illustrations have been inserted, and an appendix has been added containing the laws governing the visual tests for admission into the public services of the United States. These have been obtained from the authorities at Washington and are presented for the first time in a collected form.

The appendix also contains the methods employed in examining the eyes of school children in certain American cities.

The edition contains thirty-two more pages than the preceding, is handsomely printed and bound, and needs no recommendation to ophthalmologists.

EYE, EAR, NOSE, AND THROAT : A MANUAL FOR STUDENTS AND PRACTITIONERS. By WILLIAM LINCOLN BALLENGER, M. D., Assistant Professor of Otology, Rhinology and Laryngology, in the College of Medicine of the University of Illinois, etc., and A. G. WIPPERN, M. D., Professor of Ophthalmology and Otology, Chicago Eye, Ear, and Throat College. Illustrated with 150 engravings and 6 colored plates. Lea Brothers & Co., Philadelphia and New York.

This is one of Lea's series of pocket text-books, the section on the eye being written by Dr. Wippern and the sections on ear, nose, and throat, by Dr. Ballenger. In a work of this kind brevity is a necessity, but it is only just to say that the present volume contains as much information as could well be crowded in the space between the covers ; furthermore, lack of space has not prevented sufficient treatment of important matters. Thus, in examination of the ear, we have ample descriptions of examination by means of instillations, by means of vapors and air, by transillumination ; the tests of hearing by the voice, the watch, the acoumeter, the Galton whistle, Koenig's rods, tuning forks, the range of hearing, the Weber experiment and the Rinne experiment, all briefly, but well described.

Heterophoria in all its varieties is included under anomalies of the muscles.

Suppurative diseases of the middle ear and mastoid are described fully, and the mastoid operation, as stated in the preface, is dwelt upon with marked detail; each step being given in the order usually employed by the author. It certainly is an excellent description of the operation.

Ear diseases affecting longevity are freely discussed. The

physiology and physics of obstructed nasal respiration as an ætiological factor in many nasal and naso-pharyngeal diseases are fully considered. The rationale of the symptoms of sinusitis of the accessory nasal sinuses as dependent on their peculiar topical anatomy and relation to the turbinate bodies, is explained. Under postnasal adenoids there is an explanation of the symptoms, which the author believes has not been given before.

It is altogether an admirable little book, and is well worthy of perusal by the student and general practitioner.

A MANUAL OF PERSONAL HYGIENE. Edited by WALTER L. PYLE, A. M., M. D., Assistant Surgeon to Wills Eye Hospital, Philadelphia : Fellow of the American Academy of Medicine ; former Editor of the *International Medical Magazine,* etc. Contributors: ʃ. W. Courtney, M. D. ; Walter L. Pyle, M. D.; Geo. Howard Fox, M. D. ; B. Alexander Randall, M. D. ; E. Fletcher Ingalls, M. D. ; G. N. Stewart, M. D. (Edin.) ; Charles G. Stockton, M. D. Illustrated. Philadelphia: W. B. Saunders & Co., 1900. Pp. 344. Price $1.50 net.

The preface states that "the object of this Manual is to set forth plainly the best means of developing and maintaining physical and mental vigor . . . Purely technical phraseology has been avoided as far as possible," etc.

The book covers the subject well and furnishes valuable information as to the best methods of attaining and preserving the normal standard of the various functions of the body and mind.

Under " Hygiene of the Digestive Apparatus " we find Physiology of Digestion, Hygiene of the Teeth, and Hygiene of the Gastro-intestinal Tract ; including regulation of meals and diet, proper cooking, effects of various foods, beverages, and stimulants, etc.

" Hygiene of the Skin and its Appendages " covers the various kinds of baths and their effects, clothing, and the care of the hair and nails.

" Hygiene of the Vocal and Respiratory Apparatus " inculates proper methods of breathing, the care of the nose and naso-pharynx, the care of the voice and results of improper use, and the methods of development of the chest. There are chapters on " Hygiene of the Ear and of the Eye " ; the latter including a dissertation on ametropia and eyestrain, visual tests, school hygiene, effects of various forms of artificial light, and the use of spectacles and eyeglasses in their modifications.

"Hygiene of the Brain and Nervous System" treats of prenatal influences, care of children, puberty and attendant dangers, neurasthenia, abuse of alcohol, coffee, tea, and tobacco, overwork, insomnia, etc.

The final chapter takes up the muscular system, the effects of muscular exercise, physical training—in childhood, youth, and adult life ; gymnastics, Swedish movements, amount of exercise required, and results of abuse.

We have been at some length in reciting the contents of the book, as it seems to us that it is a most excellent thing to have in every family, treating the subject in an easy, familiar manner, while presenting the scientific reasons for what it advocates, and contributing to a popular self-knowledge, by the brief, but sufficient outline of physiology of the various organs, to be found at the beginning of the respective chapters. The work should fill a want in every family.

Injuries to the Eye in their Medico-Legal Aspect. By S. Baudry, M. D., Professor in the Faculty of Medicine, University of Lille, France, etc. Translated from the original by Alfred James Ostheimer, Jr., M. D., of Philadelphia, Pa. Revised and edited by Charles A. Oliver, A. M., M. D., Attending Surgeon to the Wills Eye Hospital ; Ophthalmic Surgeon to the Philadelphia Hospital ; Member of the American and French Ophthalmological Societies, etc. With an adaptation of the Medico-Legal Chapter to the Courts of the United States of America, by Charles Sinkler, Esq., Member of the Philadelphia Bar. 5⅝ x 7¾ inches. Pages, x+161. Extra Cloth, $1.00, net. The F. A. Davis Co., publishers, 1914–16 Cherry St., Philadelphia, Pa.

This is a translation of a French work which has obtained recognition in its original form ; the English translation having been adapted to the practice of our courts by a member of the American Bar.

The various diseases and conditions of the eye resulting from traumatism are considered seriatim, with special reference to probable consequences from given causes and to the final prognosis.

There is also a chapter on "Simulated Affections of the Eye," which is valuable as containing a collection of the various methods of detection as practiced by many of the best authorities in all countries. The last chapter presents the medico-legal aspect of ocular injuries, and the rules of expert testimony as they obtain in our own courts.

It is a useful little book for the ophthalmologist, as the information is condensed and easily assimilated.

A SYSTEMATIC, ALPHABETIC REPERTORY OF HOMEOPATHIC REMEDIES. By DR. C. VON BÖNINGHAUSEN, Imperial Prussian Counselor, General Land Commissioner, Director of the Botanical Gardens, and Active or Corresponding Member of Numerous Societies. Part First. Embracing the Antipsoric, Antisyphilitic, and Antisycotic Remedies. Translated from the second German edition by C. M. BOGER, M. D.; member of I. H. A. Price, in half morocco, $3.00 ; by mail, $3.13. Philadelphia, Boericke & Tafel, 1900.

This is a repertory of fifty-two of the oldest, most needed, severest tested, and most reliable drugs applicable in treatment of chronic diseases.

The division, as in all of our materia medicas, is according to the anatomical parts, which, supplemented with a thorough index, including some of the principal symptoms, *e. g.*, nausea, vertigo, cough, etc., make reference quite easy. Each division, after a regular alphabetic list of symptoms, contains subdivisons ; namely, (*a*) Time of occurrence, (*b*) aggravation, (*c*) amelioration, and (*d*) concomitants. Under the heading of Cough there are other subdivisions ; to wit, Expectoration and Excitants.

The divisions on Coryza, Cough, Ears, Eyes, Larynx, Nose, Palate, Pharynx, and Trachea make the book especially valuable to us as specialists.

With the reputation that this author and the publisher of this work have for homeopathic productions it seems almost presumptuous for me to endeavor to give a personal recommendation, therefore I attempt none.

THE CURE FOR CONSUMPTION BY ITS OWN VIRUS. Illustrated by Numerous Cases. By J. COMPTON BURNETT, M. D. Fourth edition. Price, $1.00. By mail, $1.05. Philadelphia : Bœricke & Tafel, 1900.

An exceedingly interesting and instructive book is this to every homeopathic prescriber, which, when read, will undoubtedly impress the reader with the efficacy of high potencies of tuberculinum.

From perusal should judge that it is the same as the third edition, as it is divided into three parts. The first is Five Years' Experience in the New Cure of Consumption, to which are two additions, which together form half the text. Part III. contains the experience of other physicians.

First part consists of fifty-four full histories of tuberculous disease, including that of the lungs, cerebral meninges, lymphatics, and joints which were treated mainly by bacillinum, with occasionally other remedies to meet acute manifestations, and the great majority of which were relieved, if we may not consider them cured.

Judging from the style, the author is not one of the homeopathic extremists who usually advocate this class of drug and the very high potencies, and generally consider any departure from the strict following of the Organon heresy ; therefore, the weight of argument in this book should be considered the more.

The volume is a valuable addition to any homeopathic physician's library.

ENLARGED TONSILS CURED BY MEDICINES. By J. COMPTON BURNETT, M. D., London, England. Philadelphia : Boericke & Tafel, 1901. Price, cloth, 60 cents ; by mail, 65 cents.

This is an interesting booklet of ninety-five pages, couched in an easy, readable style, setting forth the author's idea that enlarged or diseased tonsils are only the latter and outward signs or developments of a deeper constitutional condition.

The clinical records of a number of cases are given to exemplify the action of the remedies ; of the latter, the principal ones employed are thuja, bacillinum, luet. The remedies frequently prescribed by us Americans are conspicuous by their absence, except, calc. fl. and baryta. c., which were each spoken of once.

BOOKS RECEIVED FOR REVIEW.

Rhinology, Laryngology and Otology, and their Significance in General Medicine, by E. P. Friedrich, M. D. Published by W. B. Saunders & Co.

Practical Homeopathic Therapeutics, by W. A Dewey, M. D. Published by Boericke & Tafel.

GENERAL INDEX TO VOL. XII.

CPSIA information can be obtained
at www.ICGtesting.com
Printed in the USA
BVHW08*1515041018
529297BV00008B/416/P